Ischaemic Stroke in the Young

Edited by

Turgut Tatlisumak
Department of Clinical Neuroscience
Institute of Neuroscience and Physiology
Sahlgrenska Academy at the University of Gothenburg
Department of Neurology
Sahlgrenska University Hospital
Gothenburg, Sweden

Lars Thomassen
University of Bergen
Centre for Neurovascular Diseases
Department of Neurology
Haukeland University Hospital
Bergen, Norway

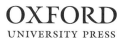

OXFORD
UNIVERSITY PRESS

OXFORD
UNIVERSITY PRESS

Great Clarendon Street, Oxford, OX2 6DP,
United Kingdom

Oxford University Press is a department of the University of Oxford.
It furthers the University's objective of excellence in research, scholarship,
and education by publishing worldwide. Oxford is a registered trade mark of
Oxford University Press in the UK and in certain other countries

© Oxford University Press 2018

The moral rights of the authors have been asserted

First Edition published in 2018

Impression: 1

Published in the United States of America by Oxford University Press
198 Madison Avenue, New York, NY 10016, United States of America

British Library Cataloguing in Publication Data

Data available

Library of Congress Control Number: 2017952354

ISBN 978–0–19–872236–6

Printed and bound by
CPI Group (UK) Ltd, Croydon, CR0 4YY

Ischaemic Stroke in the Young

Foreword

The burden of stroke on public health has been increasingly recognized with better availability of epidemiological data on stroke in different parts of the world. Stroke is now the second most common cause of death and disability worldwide. Stroke has traditionally been viewed as a disease predominantly affecting the elderly. However, among about 14 million strokes that occur in the world every year, about 2 million are ischaemic strokes that occur in persons younger than 50 years. Although the risk of stroke shows declining trends in many high-income countries, there are many studies published in the last few years showing that stroke in the young is not decreasing, but actually increasing in many geographical areas.

The consequences of stroke in the young are substantial from several perspectives. Young strokes strike at a period in life which is fragile should a serious disease occur. It often profoundly influences family life, including the children of the stroke victim. It may also influence family projects concerning future pregnancies, or possibility to obtain life insurances. Working ability may be reduced, which may carry negative socio-economical effects for the individual, the family, and society. Persons with young stroke represent a considerable part of the total disability burden of stroke, because of the accumulative effects of stroke residua and loss of function lasting a long time, and even life-long.

Ischaemic stroke in the young has long been regarded as a disease caused by a large number of rare disorders and requires large diagnostic efforts to identify. Advances in diagnostic imaging and molecular genetics have improved the identification of the rare aetiologies, and has helped to further delineate more precisely the contribution of different rare causes. Such studies have also helped to delineate the clinical syndromes and phenotypes associated with stroke, e.g., different genetic and metabolic disorders.

It remains true that a list of possible causes of young ischaemic stroke is indeed long, but recent studies have shown that traditional risk factors are also important in younger age groups. Unwanted trends in life style risk factors and their consequences may actually account for much of the apparent increase in stroke in the young as recently seen.

Another feature of ischaemic stroke of the young is the high proportion of cases where a clear cause of the stroke cannot be identified, leaving many patients without a proper diagnosis even after extensive diagnostic work-up: the cryptogenic strokes.

Our colleagues Turgut Tatlisumak and Lars Thomassen, well recognized experts in the stroke neurology field, have brought together a distinguished body of clinicians and researchers that have produced the first comprehensive textbook specifically addressing ischaemic stroke in the young. The book covers virtually all aspects of stroke in the young, from an epidemiological and risk factor perspective, to pathophysiologies, diagnostics, and therapies. Diagnostic algorithms are presented which will be very useful for clinical practice. The book also covers areas that should be prioritized for further research, as many aspects of ischaemic stroke in the young are still enigmatic.

We warmly welcome this important addition to the existing literature on stroke. The field of ischaemic stroke in the young has received its first book on the topic, and a long-recognized publication hiatus has now been filled.

October 2017

Bo Norrving, MD, PhD,
Department of Clinical Sciences,
Lund University, Sweden

Didier Leys, MD, PhD,
University of Lille,
Inserm U1171, CHU Lille, Lille, France

Contents

Contributors

Karoliina Aarnio
Clinical Neurosciences, Neurology,
University of Helsinki and
Department of Neurology, Helsinki
University Hospital, Finland

David Calvet
Neurology Department, Sainte-Anne
Hospital, Paris, France;
Paris Descartes University, Sorbonne
Paris Cité, Paris, France;
INSERM U894, Paris, France

Frank-Erik de Leeuw
Radboud University Medical
Centre, Donders Institute for Brain,
Cognition and Behaviour, Center
for Neuroscience, Department
of Neurology, Nijmegen, The
Netherlands

Merel Sanne Ekker
Radboud University Medical
Centre, Donders Institute for Brain,
Cognition and Behaviour, Center
for Neuroscience, Department
of Neurology, Nijmegen, The
Netherlands

Christian Enzinger
Department of Neurology, Medical
University of Graz, Austria; Division
of Neuroradiology, Vascular
and Interventional Radiology,
Department of Radiology, Medical
University of Graz, Austria

Franz Fazekas
Department of Neurology, Medical
University of Graz, Austria

José M. Ferro
Department of Neurosciences and
Mental Health, Neurology Service,
North Lisbon Hospital Centre and
Institute of Molecular Medicine,
University of Lisbon, Portugal

Ana Catarina Fonseca
Department of Neurosciences and
Mental Health, Neurology Service,
North Lisbon Hospital Centre and
Institute of Molecular Medicine,
University of Lisbon, Portugal

Annette Fromm
Bergen Stroke Research Group,
Department of Neurology, Centre for
Neurovascular Diseases, Haukeland
University Hospital, University of
Bergen, Norway

Thomas Gattringer
Department of Neurology, Medical
University of Graz, Austria

Eva Gerdts
Department of Heart Disease,
Haukeland University Hospital,
Bergen, Norway; Department of
Clinical Science, University of
Bergen, Norway

Bettina Henzi
Division of Paediatric Neurology,
Development and Rehabilitation,
University Children's Hospital,
Inselspital, University of Bern,
Switzerland

Katarina Jood
Institute of Neuroscience and
Physiology, Department of Clinical
Neuroscience, Sahlgrenska Academy
at University of Gothenburg, Sweden

Manfred Kaps
Department of Neurology, Justus
Liebig University, Giessen, Germany

Nicola Logallo
Center for Neurovascular Diseases,
Haukeland University Hospital,
Bergen, Norway; Department of
Clinical Medicine, University of
Bergen, Norway

Svetlana Lorenzano
Department of Neurology and
Psychiatry, Policlinico Umberto
I Hospital, Sapienza University of
Rome, Rome, Italy

Nicolas Martinez-Majander
Clinical Neurosciences, Department
of Neurology, University of Helsinki
and Department of Neurology,
Helsinki University Hospital,
Helsinki, Finland

Jean-Louis Mas
Neurology Department, Sainte-Anne
Hospital, Paris, France;
Paris Descartes University, Sorbonne
Paris Cité, Paris, France;
INSERM U894, Paris, France

Halvor Naess
Centre for Neurovascular Diseases,
Department of Neurology,
Haukeland University Hospital,
Bergen, Norway; Institute of Clinical
Medicine, University of Bergen,
Norway

Alessandro Pezzini
Department of Clinical and
Experimental Sciences, Neurology
Clinic, University of Brescia, Italy

Jukka Putaala
Clinical Neurosciences, Department
of Neurology, University of Helsinki
and Department of Neurology,
Helsinki University Hospital, Finland

Kirsi Rantanen
Clinical Neurosciences, Neurology,
University of Helsinki and
Department of Neurology, Helsinki
University Hospital, Finland

Stefan Ropele
Department of Neurology, Medical
University of Graz, Austria

Sahrai Saeed
Department of Heart Disease,
Haukeland University Hospital,
Bergen, Norway

Maja Steinlin
Division of Paediatric Neurology,
Development and Rehabilitation,
University Children's Hospital,
Inselspital, University of Bern,
Switzerland

Christian Tanislav
Department of Neurology, Justus
Liebig University, Giessen, Germany

Turgut Tatlisumak
Department of Clinical
Neuroscience, Institute of
Neuroscience and Physiology,
Sahlgrenska Academy at the
University of Gothenburg,
Department of Neurology,
Sahlgrenska University Hospital,
Gothenburg, Sweden

Lars Thomassen
University of Bergen, Centre for
Neurovascular Diseases, Department
of Neurology, Haukeland University
Hospital, Bergen, Norway

Danilo Toni
Department of Neurology and
Psychiatry, Policlinico Umberto
I Hospital, Sapienza University of
Rome, Italy

Guillaume Turc
Neurology Department, Sainte-Anne
Hospital, Paris, France;
Paris Descartes University, Sorbonne
Paris Cité, Paris, France;
INSERM U894, Paris, France

Ulrike Waje-Andreassen
Centre for Neurovascular Diseases,
Haukeland University Hospital,
Bergen, Norway; Department of
Biological and Medical Psychology,
University of Bergen, Norway

Chapter 1

Epidemiology

Merel Sanne Ekker and Frank-Erik de Leeuw

Introduction

This first chapter considers the epidemiology of stroke in young adults, in this context those who suffer from ischaemic stroke between 18 and 49 years of age. Although epidemiology can cover aetiology, diagnosis, treatment, and prognosis of disease, this chapter specifically addresses occurrence (incidence and prevalence) of disease.

We apply epidemiology as a magnifying glass to look for differences in occurrence between the sexes, seasons, and by time to find leads for potential causes of stroke in young adults. These will then be further examined in later chapters. In addition, we discuss mortality and time trends in mortality after stroke in young adults.

Incidence and prevalence

Each year, about 2 million individuals worldwide suffer a stroke between the ages of 18–49, a so-called stroke in young adults or young stroke. At a population level, the overall stroke incidence has been decreasing in high-income countries since 1980, but is rapidly increasing in the low- to middle-income countries, probably due to better awareness, detection, and stroke care (1). However, a closer look at this overall decrease of stroke incidence in high-income countries reveals that it is not present across all age categories. For example, from 1987 to 2010, Sweden experienced a decrease of 3.7% in the incidence of ischaemic stroke in people above the age of 65 years, a smaller decrease of 0.4% in people aged 45–64 years, but an increase in the incidence of ischaemic stroke of 1.3–1.6% among the younger population aged 18–44 years during this 23-year window of time (2, 3). Similar observations come from Denmark with an increasing incidence for ischaemic stroke among younger people under the age of 45 over the time period 1997–2009 (4). A prospective cohort study in Norway found a similar increase in incidence of ischaemic stroke among women aged 30–49 years and a trend for increasing incidence in men of the same age range

(5). A similar increase was also seen in France and in the Netherlands for the age group of 35–64 years (5–7). In addition, the decline in stroke incidence was not observed for patients younger than 65 years in a multicentre cohort of black and white adults in the United States, from 1987 to 2011 (8).

There are several explanations for the opposing trends over time in the incidence of stroke between 'young' and 'older' people. One explanation is that better awareness and referral to hospitals or stroke centres leads to better identification and thus to a higher incidence. With the advancements and availability of neuroimaging, for example diffusion-weighted imaging, stroke detection has improved dramatically. Patients who might have been diagnosed with other conditions, such as migraine with aura or seizures, in the 1980s or 1990s now may turn out to have magnetic resonance imaging abnormalities compatible with an ischaemic stroke. Besides better detection and diagnosis over time, the increased incidence of young stroke patients may also be due to an increase of traditional vascular risk factors, already present at a younger age. Later chapters will cover these risk factors. In this chapter, we will first use age-specific incidence to provide clues for the aetiology in young stroke patients. To provide further leads for (novel) risk factors, we will examine seasonal and sex variation in ischaemic stroke.

Aetiology

The Trial of ORG 10172 in Acute Stroke Treatment (TOAST) classification is commonly used to define the cause of ischaemic stroke. The definite cause of the stroke remains uncertain ('5b. Undetermined after extensive evaluation') in many more young stroke patients than in elderly stroke patients. The percentage of this so-called cryptogenic stroke in young adults ranges between 25% and 35%, which is much higher than that in older stroke patients (9). Cardioembolic stroke (20%) and dissections of cervical or cerebral arteries (15%) are common causes of stroke that are more often seen in young adults (9, 10). Chapters 3–6 will address the aetiology in young stroke patients in more detail.

Seasonal variation

When taking a closer look at incidence data of stroke, it seems that there is variation in the occurrence of ischaemic stroke incidence by month or season. Observations about weather and season are best studied in countries without large variations in climate between regions within seasons. While some studies did not observe differences in stroke incidence between seasons (11, 12), others showed a peak incidence in winter and summer (13, 14). This may provide leads for potential new causes of stroke. A possible explanation is that with higher temperatures, the levels of coagulation factors increase due to dehydration (13, 15). Seasonal variation of stroke occurrence could not be explained by monthly or seasonal variation in the prevalence of risk factors (13). Spontaneous dissections of the cervical arteries show mild seasonal variation, with a higher prevalence during winter. The 'winter' peak might be associated with infectious disease. Traumatic dissections (e.g. due to even minor trauma caused by cycling accidents, playing golf, or other outdoor activities) may have a higher incidence in summer (16, 17).

Overall, data about seasonal variation of stroke are inconclusive. Study design, climate per country, and other meteorological variables (e.g. drought, humidity, and air pollution) may differ and people's behaviour may change due to weather conditions, all influencing the risk of stroke (18). None of these variations are investigated specifically for young adults, which could be interesting, especially in patients with cryptogenic stroke.

Sex differences

When the incidence of ischaemic stroke is stratified by age, the incidence is higher for men in most age categories. However, there is excess risk in women aged 20–29 years in Finland (9). In a similar study in the Netherlands, this excess risk was observed for women aged 25–49 years (Fig. 1.1).

This excess risk in young women may be explained by risk factors specific for this age. Pregnancy and the subsequent puerperium are typical episodes in a young women's life at reproductive age that are associated with an increased

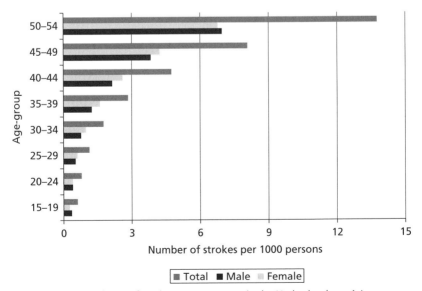

Fig. 1.1 Point prevalence of strokes per age group in the Netherlands on 1 January 2011, showing a higher incidence for women in the age group from 25 to 49 years.
Source: data from LINH, LMR and CBS-Mortality statistics; data modified by RIVM, the Netherlands.

risk for ischaemic stroke due to changes in coagulation and pregnancy-related complications (preeclampsia, gestational hypertension and diabetes, and haemolysis, elevated liver enzymes and low platelets (HELLP) syndrome) (19, 20). Another typical risk factor that is associated with a higher risk in young women is oral contraceptive use (21). Migraine is also more frequent in young patients, especially in women (female:male ratio 3:1), and migraine with aura is associated with a higher risk of ischaemic stroke (9). Women having migraine with aura have a relative risk ratio of 2 for ischaemic stroke, with an even higher risk in patients with a higher migraine attack frequency. This relative risk ratio increases even more to 9–10 in women with migraine who also smoke and use oral contraceptives (22–24). Finally, there is some overrepresentation of a few other, rare diseases with a high thromboembolic risk including the antiphospholipid syndrome, systemic lupus erythematosus, and Sneddon syndrome (25, 26). Chapter 12 will cover the specific risk factors and specific aetiology of young stroke in women more extensively.

In almost all age groups above 30 years in the Finnish study and above 45–49 years in the Dutch study mentioned earlier, incidence of ischaemic stroke is higher in men, most likely due to the higher prevalence of traditional risk factors. The traditional risk factors are present in virtually every man over the age of 44 years, and are even present in the majority of the very young patients (18–25 years) (9). The prevalence of hypertension and diabetes, two major risk factors for ischaemic stroke, have dramatically increased over the last decade and are already present in young adults (6, 10, 27). Smoking has not decreased in young men and women, in contrast with the older population. The prevalence of obesity is stable among young women, but has increased in men over the last years (27). Another non-traditional risk factor more specific for younger stroke patients, both men and women, can be illicit drug use, which is considered to be much higher now than it was 10 years ago (6, 7, 9, 27, 28). More discussion on risk factors can be found in Chapter 2.

Prognosis

Apart from sex differences in incidence and presence of risk factors, there is also a discrepancy in prognosis after stroke between women and men. While a poorer prognosis after stroke in elderly women (>70 years of age) has been recognized, only a few studies have addressed this in young female stroke patients (29, 30). The Dutch FUTURE study showed that young women have a two- to threefold higher risk of a poor outcome and worse functional performance compared to young men, independent of stroke severity or pre-stroke functioning (31). A smaller Spanish study reported similar results (32). No conclusive explanation for this difference has been proposed. More details about treatment and prognosis in women are given in Chapter 12.

Mortality and morbidity

Mortality

Stroke is an important cause of death in young adults under 45 years of age. In the United States, more than 2800 deaths per year are attributed to stroke and a quarter of these are attributable to ischaemic stroke (8, 33). In the Netherlands, the 20-year mortality after acute stroke in adults aged 18–50 years was high compared with the expected mortality in this age category (26.8% (95% confidence interval 21.9–31.8%) versus 7.6%) (34). Cardiovascular co-morbidity is still the most important predictor for long-term mortality.

Time trends

When we look in more detail at the time course of mortality across age groups, there is a consistent decline in the elderly patients. The Framingham study showed a significant decrease in case fatality after ischaemic stroke between 1950 and 2004, but only for men, not in women (35). Numbers for young adults were different here, too. Young male stroke patients were at higher risk for mortality after ischaemic stroke, compared with women (33). There is not only an excess risk of dying immediately after the stroke, but this risk remains elevated during the decades after the stroke (34, 36).

Post-stroke epilepsy

A contributing factor to the higher risk of death, even years after a stroke, might be the occurrence of post-stroke epilepsy. This important and very disabling consequence of stroke is, with an incidence of approximately 10%, common in young stroke patients (37, 38). Future studies investigating if it is desirable to give prophylactic treatment with antiepileptics and who would benefit from it, might positively influence the incidence of post-stroke epilepsy and consequently the mortality rates. Development and research into other neuroprotective agents can contribute too.

Conclusion

When stroke strikes young, we have to take a closer look, not only to find aetiologies and risk factors but also to inform patients about their prognosis. Epidemiology has revealed differences between stroke in the elderly and among the young. This is illustrated by increasing incidence and mortality, a higher proportion of unspecified aetiologies, a higher frequency of rare and specific risk factors, and more pronounced sex differences of stroke at a younger age. Under the age of 35 years, stroke predominantly occurs in women; above 35 years, more men suffer a stroke, possibly due to differences in specific and traditional risk factors between these age groups. In terms of aetiology, the proportion of those with a cryptogenic stroke is higher in young adults, leaving many patients without a proper diagnosis even after extensive diagnostic work-up. Few studies have addressed geographical and seasonal influences in young adults. However, by using epidemiology as a magnifying glass, for example, by assessing sex- and age-specific incidence in great detail, new aetiologies and trigger factors might be discovered. Finally, young stroke patients appear to have a rather poor prognosis and high risk of mortality, both immediately and years after their stroke.

Young stroke is an acute disease with life-long consequences. Due to the low absolute number of cases, future research should unquestionably be carried out in a collaborative way.

References

1. **Feigin VL, Lawes CM, Bennett DA, Barker-Collo SL, Parag V.** Worldwide stroke incidence and early case fatality reported in 56 population-based studies: a systematic review. Lancet Neurol. 2009;8(4):355–69.

2. **Rosengren A, Giang KW, Lappas G, Jern C, Toren K, Bjorck L.** Twenty-four-year trends in the incidence of ischemic stroke in Sweden from 1987 to 2010. Stroke. 2013;44(9):2388–93.

3. **Medin J, Nordlund A, Ekberg K.** Increasing stroke incidence in Sweden between 1989 and 2000 among persons aged 30 to 65 years: evidence from the Swedish Hospital Discharge Register. Stroke. 2004;35(5):1047–51.

4. **Demant MN, Andersson C, Ahlehoff O, Charlot M, Olesen JB, Gjesing A**, et al. Temporal trends in stroke admissions in Denmark 1997-2009. BMC Neurol. 2013;13:156.

5. **Vangen-Lonne AM, Wilsgaard T, Johnsen SH, Carlsson M, Mathiesen EB.** Time trends in incidence and case fatality of ischemic stroke: the Tromsø study 1977–2010. Stroke. 2015;46(5):1173–79.

6. **Vaartjes I, O'Flaherty M, Capewell S, Kappelle J, Bots M.** Remarkable decline in ischemic stroke mortality is not matched by changes in incidence. Stroke. 2013;44(3):591–97.

7. **Bejot Y, Daubail B, Jacquin A, Durier J, Osseby GV, Rouaud O**, et al. Trends in the incidence of ischaemic stroke in young adults between 1985 and 2011: the Dijon Stroke Registry. J Neurol Neurosurg Psychiatry. 2014;85(5):509–13.

8. **Koton S, Schneider AL, Rosamond WD, Shahar E, Sang Y, Gottesman RF**, et al. Stroke incidence and mortality trends in US communities, 1987 to 2011. JAMA. 2014;312(3):259–68.

9. **Putaala J, Metso AJ, Metso TM, Konkola N, Kraemer Y, Haapaniemi E**, et al. Analysis of 1008 consecutive patients aged 15 to 49 with first-ever ischemic stroke: the Helsinki young stroke registry. Stroke. 2009;**40**(4):1195–203.

10. **Ferro JM, Massaro AR, Mas JL.** Aetiological diagnosis of ischaemic stroke in young adults. Lancet Neurol. 2010;**9**(11):1085–96.

11. **Raj K, Bhatia R, Prasad K, Srivastava MV, Vishnubhatla S, Singh MB.** Seasonal differences and circadian variation in stroke occurrence and stroke subtypes. J Stroke Cerebrovasc Dis. 2015;**24**(1):10–16.

12. **Rothwell PM, Wroe SJ, Slattery J, Warlow CP.** Is stroke incidence related to season or temperature? The Oxfordshire Community Stroke Project. Lancet. 1996;**347**(9006):934–36.

13. **Han MH, Yi HJ, Kim YS, Kim YS.** Effect of seasonal and monthly variation in weather and air pollution factors on stroke incidence in Seoul, Korea. Stroke. 2015;**46**(4):927–35.

14. **Khan FA, Engstrom G, Jerntorp I, Pessah-Rasmussen H, Janzon L.** Seasonal patterns of incidence and case fatality of stroke in Malmo, Sweden: the STROMA study. Neuroepidemiology. 2005;**24**(1–2):26–31.

15. **Berginer VM, Goldsmith J, Batz U, Vardi H, Shapiro Y.** Clustering of strokes in association with meteorologic factors in the Negev Desert of Israel: 1981–1983. Stroke. 1989;**20**(1):65–69.

16. **Yamada SM, Goto Y, Murakami M, Hoya K, Matsuno A.** Vertebral artery dissection caused by swinging a golf club: case report and literature review. Clin J Sport Med. 2014;**24**(2):155–57.

17. **Maroon JC, Gardner P, Abla AA, El-Kadi H, Bost J.** "Golfer's stroke": golf-induced stroke from vertebral artery dissection. Surg Neurol. 2007;**67**(2):163–68.

18. **McArthur K, Dawson J, Walters M.** What is it with the weather and stroke? Expert Rev Neurother. 2010;**10**(2):243–49.

19. **O'Neal MA, Feske SK.** Stroke in pregnancy: a case-oriented review. Pract Neurol. 2016;**16**(1):23–34.

20. **Miller BR, Strbian D, Sundararajan S.** Stroke in the young: patent foramen ovale and pregnancy. Stroke. 2015;**46**(8):e181–83.

21. **Roach RE, Helmerhorst FM, Lijfering WM, Stijnen T, Algra A, Dekkers OM.** Combined oral contraceptives: the risk of myocardial infarction and ischemic stroke. Cochrane Database Syst Rev. 2015;**8**:CD011054.

22. **Kurth T, Chabriat H, Bousser MG.** Migraine and stroke: a complex association with clinical implications. Lancet Neurol. 2012;**11**(1):92–100.

23. **Kurth T, Slomke MA, Kase CS, Cook NR, Lee IM, Gaziano JM**, et al. Migraine, headache, and the risk of stroke in women: a prospective study. Neurology. 2005;**64**(6):1020–26.

24. **Schurks M, Rist PM, Bigal ME, Buring JE, Lipton RB, Kurth T.** Migraine and cardiovascular disease: systematic review and meta-analysis. BMJ. 2009;**339**:b3914.

25. **Brey RL, Stallworth CL, McGlasson DL, Wozniak MA, Wityk RJ, Stern BJ**, et al. Antiphospholipid antibodies and stroke in young women. Stroke. 2002;**33**(10):2396–400.

26. **Urbanus RT, Siegerink B, Roest M, Rosendaal FR, de Groot PG, Algra A.** Antiphospholipid antibodies and risk of myocardial infarction and ischaemic

stroke in young women in the RATIO study: a case-control study. Lancet Neurol. 2009;**8**(11):998–1005.

27. **Wieberdink RG, Ikram MA, Hofman A, Koudstaal PJ, Breteler MM.** Trends in stroke incidence rates and stroke risk factors in Rotterdam, the Netherlands from 1990 to 2008. Eur J Epidemiol. 2012;**27**(4):287–95.

28. **George MG, Tong X, Kuklina EV, Labarthe DR.** Trends in stroke hospitalizations and associated risk factors among children and young adults, 1995–2008. Ann Neurol. 2011;**70**(5):713–21.

29. **Appelros P, Stegmayr B, Terent A.** Sex differences in stroke epidemiology: a systematic review. Stroke. 2009;**40**(4):1082–90.

30. **Appelros P, Stegmayr B, Terent A.** A review on sex differences in stroke treatment and outcome. Acta Neurol Scand. 2010;**121**(6):359–69.

31. **Synhaeve NE, Arntz RM, van Alebeek ME, van Pamelen J, Maaijwee NA, Rutten-Jacobs LC,** et al. Women have a poorer very long-term functional outcome after stroke among adults aged 18–50 years: the FUTURE study. J Neurol. 2016;**263**(6):1099–105.

32. **Martinez-Sanchez P, Fuentes B, Fernandez-Dominguez J, de Los Ortega-Casarrubios M, Aguilar-Amar MJ, Abenza-Abildua MJ,** et al. Young women have poorer outcomes than men after stroke. Cerebrovasc Dis. 2011;**31**(5):455–63.

33. **Poisson SN, Glidden D, Johnston SC, Fullerton HJ.** Deaths from stroke in US young adults, 1989–2009. Neurology. 2014;**83**(23):2110–15.

34. **Rutten-Jacobs LC, Arntz RM, Maaijwee NA, Schoonderwaldt HC, Dorresteijn LD, van Dijk EJ,** et al. Long-term mortality after stroke among adults aged 18 to 50 years. JAMA. 2013;**309**(11):1136–44.

35. **Carandang R, Seshadri S, Beiser A, Kelly-Hayes M, Kase CS, Kannel WB,** et al. Trends in incidence, lifetime risk, severity, and 30-day mortality of stroke over the past 50 years. JAMA. 2006;**296**(24):2939–46.

36. **Rutten-Jacobs LC, Arntz RM, Maaijwee NA, Schoonderwaldt HC, Dorresteijn LD, van Dijk EJ,** et al. Cardiovascular disease is the main cause of long-term excess mortality after ischemic stroke in young adults. Hypertension. 2015;**65**(3):670–75.

37. **Arntz RM, Rutten-Jacobs LC, Maaijwee NA, Schoonderwaldt HC, Dorresteijn LD, van Dijk EJ,** et al. Poststroke epilepsy is associated with a high mortality after a stroke at young age: follow-up of Transient Ischemic Attack and Stroke Patients and Unelucidated Risk Factor Evaluation Study. Stroke. 2015;**46**(8):2309–11.

38. **Arntz R, Rutten-Jacobs L, Maaijwee N, Schoonderwaldt H, Dorresteijn L, van Dijk E,** et al. Post-stroke epilepsy in young adults: a long-term follow-up study. PloS One. 2013;**8**(2):e55498.

Chapter 2

Risk factors

Jukka Putaala and
Nicolas Martinez-Majander

Introduction

Ischaemic stroke is a multifactorial disease with a wide range of modifiable and non-modifiable risk factors, all acting somewhere in the causal chain between exposure and disease. In addition to well-documented vascular risk factors that influence the risk over the years or decades with fairly well understood mechanisms of association, a multitude of temporal, that is, dynamic risk factors (sometimes called 'triggers' if immediately preceding the stroke) have been identified. Such factors, including acute infections, pregnancy and postpartum stage, binge drinking, and recent illicit drug use, may not constantly increase the individual's risk of stroke but act or are measurable in some periods of time while absent during most of the time. A patent foramen ovale (PFO)—although present since birth—could also be considered as a dynamic risk factor as shunt through a PFO from the venous to arterial side of circulation may occur only after a physical strain causing a Valsalva manoeuvre.

Many of the unconventional risk factors associated with young-onset stroke can also predispose to stroke at older ages, but there are rationales to regard them as young-age specific: (a) the factor exists only at young age (e.g. oestrogen-containing contraception, pregnancy, puerperium); (b) the factor exists at all ages, but a statistically stronger association has been demonstrated for younger ages (e.g. PFO, migraine); or (c) the factor is related to risk behaviour in the population that is more common at younger ages (e.g. illicit drug use, heavy drinking, binge drinking, smoking). Common to all of these is that mechanisms of associations are incompletely understood.

In young patients, unconventional risk factors, genetic factors, and temporal triggers may play a greater role than in elderly stroke patients. However, recent large studies have shown a high prevalence of traditional risk factors also in young stroke patients and the risk factor profile today resembles more that of old stroke patients than it seemed a few decades ago.

In the first part of this chapter, we review the burden of traditional vascular risk factors in young stroke patients as well as their strength of association. In the second part, we focus mainly on exogenous risk factors that can be considered specific to young adults and discuss their evidence base. Certain risk factors, for example, reproductive health-related conditions, cardiac interatrial abnormalities, and genetic thrombophilia, are discussed thoroughly elsewhere in this book, and only briefly mentioned here from the risk factor viewpoint. Rare monogenetic diseases with early-onset stroke as a manifestation of the condition are not discussed in this chapter.

Traditional risk factors

Prevalence

Fig. 2.1 illustrates the high prevalence of traditional vascular risk factors in the largest recent multicentre cohorts to date on ischaemic stroke in young adults. The five most prevalent risk factors in these studies were abdominal obesity defined as high waist circumference (64.1%), current smoking (37.0–55.5%), physical inactivity (48.2%), hypertension (22.4–46.6%), and dyslipidaemia (24.4–45.8%) (1–3). These studies represent European hospital-based data with variable enrolment periods and at least some patient selection. Upper age cut-off also varied from 45 to 55 years and the Stroke in Young Fabry Patients (sifap1) study included both transient ischaemic attack and ischaemic stroke. These data, nevertheless, confirm that traditional vascular risk factors are among the main players in cerebrovascular ischaemic events at a young age.

Diabetes mellitus was relatively rare in these studies (3.6–10.3%) without subtypes of diabetes being reported. In the single-centre Helsinki Young Stroke Registry (4), among patients aged 15–49 years, the frequency of type 1 (T1D) and type 2 (T2D) diabetes mellitus was 4.4% and 6.0%, respectively, reflecting one of the world's highest prevalence of T1D in Finland (5). Atrial fibrillation, a highly prevalent and undetected risk factor among elderly stroke patients, is rare in the young (6).

The 15 Cities Young Stroke Study and sifap1 study provide the most compelling data on age- and sex-specific differences in the prevalence of traditional risk factors in young stroke patients. In the former study, men had their first-ever ischaemic stroke at an older age than women. Men also more frequently harboured dyslipidaemia or coronary heart disease, or smoked, than did women (1). In both sexes, the prevalence of a family history of stroke, dyslipidaemia, smoking, hypertension, diabetes mellitus, coronary heart disease, peripheral arterial disease, and atrial fibrillation increased with age. After

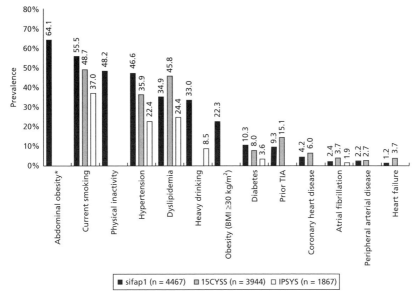

Fig. 2.1 Prevalence of well-documented risk factors in the three largest to date multicentre cohorts of young ischaemic stroke patients: sifap1 (Stroke in Young Fabry Patients) had an age limit of 18–55 years, 15CYSS (15 Cities Young Stroke Study) had an age limit of 15–49 years, and IPSYS (Italian Project on Stroke in Young Adults) had an age limit of 18–45 years. * High waist circumference; BMI, body mass index; TIA, transient ischaemic attack.

adjusting for age and gender, this study observed no differences in the risk factor prevalence between southern, central, and northern European patient populations.

The sifap1 study demonstrated a striking clustering of vascular risk factors with increasing age (Fig. 2.2), especially with physical inactivity, arterial hypertension, dyslipidaemia, obesity, and diabetes mellitus (2). Regarding sex-specific differences, dyslipidaemia, smoking, hypertension, cardiovascular disease, diabetes mellitus, and high-risk alcohol consumption clustered in men. Dyslipidaemia and cardiovascular disease showed the strongest gender disparity (favouring women) particularly in age groups of 35 years or greater. Women were, in turn, more often physically inactive or were obese also at younger ages (<35 years).

Strength of associations

The magnitude of the effect of traditional vascular risk factors for young-onset ischaemic stroke has been assessed in relatively few studies. Albeit with highly

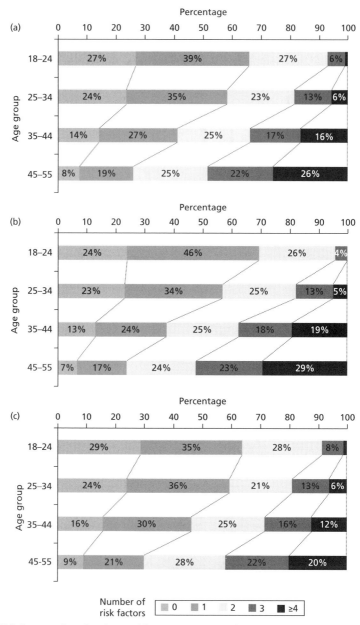

Fig. 2.2 Frequencies of patients with none, 1, 2, 3, and 4 or more well-documented risk factors in the Stroke in Young Fabry Patients Study in (a) all patients, (b) men, and (c) females.

Reproduced from Stroke, 44(1), von Sarnowski B, Putaala J, Grittner U, Gaertner B, Schminke U, Curtze S, Huber R, Tanislav C, Lichy C, Demarin V, Basic-Kes V, Ringelstein EB, Neumann-Haefelin T, Enzinger C, Fazekas F, Rothwell PM, Dichgans M, Jungehulsing GJ, Heuschmann PU, Kaps M, Norrving B, Rolfs A, Kessler C, Tatlisumak T, Lifestyle risk factors for ischemic stroke and transient ischemic attack in young adults in the Stroke in Young Fabry Patients study, pp. 119–125, Copyright (2013), with permission from Wolters Kluwer Health, Inc.

variable point estimates, the associations of hypertension (odds ratio (OR) range 1.9–18.7) (7–13) and smoking (OR range 1.4–7.8) (7–11, 13, 14) with stroke have been fairly well demonstrated for young-onset stroke in multi-ethnic populations. For smoking, a cumulative dose–response effect has also been shown (14, 15).

The association of diabetes and young-onset ischaemic stroke has not been as consistent as for hypertension and smoking, with several studies finding an association (7, 8, 13), others finding no association (9, 11, 14), and some finding association only in men (10). In the studies showing an association, the OR for diabetes or elevated fasting blood glucose varied from 3.3 to 22.9, with variation depending on sex and ethnicity (7, 8, 10, 13). Data are limited regarding the risk differences regarding diabetes subtypes, although T1D seemingly is associated with greater risk of young-onset stroke than T2D (16). Only a few studies investigated manifested cardiac disease or separately atrial fibrillation in young adults. Smaller studies reported ORs ranging from 2.7 to 3.3 (9, 10, 13) for different combinations of cardiac disease, with no data available separately for atrial fibrillation.

It is plausible that the link between dyslipidaemia and ischaemic stroke is more complex than in the elderly, since atherosclerotic conditions underlying young strokes are much less frequent. The association between low high-density lipoprotein (HDL) cholesterol and young-onset ischaemic stroke has been suggested by several case–control studies, with a size of 83% lower odds per 1 standard deviation increment (8, 11). Of the other lipid particles that have been subject to more intense research, apolipoproteins A-I (ApoA-I) and B (ApoB) have many advantages over conventional lipid measurements and provide a more precise estimation of cardiovascular risk, including ischaemic stroke (17). One small study observed an association between ApoB, an inverse association between ApoA-I, and a strong independent association between ApoB/ApoA-I ratio and ischaemic stroke in the young (OR 4.0; 95% confidence interval (CI), 1.6–10.0) (18). No association was found for the conventional lipid particles in that study when adjusted for age, sex, lifestyle factors, and high-sensitive C-reactive protein. Atherogeneity of lipid particles may thus not play a major role in young-onset ischaemic stroke while other functions of the lipid particles may be more relevant. In particular, HDL cholesterol, besides its reverse cholesterol transport action, may act as a modulator of platelet and coagulation responses and vascular endothelium (19). These beneficial effects of HDL cholesterol might explain the observed inverse association of HDL and young-onset ischaemic stroke. Furthermore, a meta-analysis suggested that lipoprotein(a) has a stronger association for the risk of ischaemic stroke at young age compared with older ages independent of other risk factors (20).

In addition to proatherosclerotic functions, lipoprotein(a) may be involved in prothrombotic and antifibrinolytic functions (21).

A body mass index (BMI) of >30 kg/m^2 was associated with early-onset ischaemic stroke in a recent population-based case–control study of 1201 cases and 1154 controls (age 15–49 years) with an OR of 1.6 (95% CI, 1.3–1.9) when adjusted for demographic factors. Yet, this association diminished after further adjustment for smoking, hypertension, and diabetes mellitus suggesting that the effect of obesity may be mediated by these risk factors (22). An association between metabolic syndrome and young-onset ischaemic stroke has been shown by one study (8). We found no studies assessing unhealthy diet as a risk factor for young stroke.

Psychosocial distress and depression can be considered as well-documented risk factors for stroke in general (17). Also at young age, psychosocial distress (23), and both unipolar and bipolar depression, but also anxiety disorders (24, 25), showed a positive association with ischaemic stroke in a few studies, with a roughly two to five times greater risk compared to age- and sex-matched individuals without these disorders after adjustment for confounders.

The role of sleep disorders has not been extensively investigated in younger patients, but interestingly, a large longitudinal study of patients with obstructive sleep apnoea suggested a higher stroke risk for women aged 35 years or less compared to older age groups and a relatively higher risk for women compared to men (26).

How much do traditional risk factors explain ischaemic strokes at a young age?

Population attributable risk (PAR) characterizes the independent contribution of a risk factor to the burden of the disease, indicating a proportion of cases that would not occur in a population if the factor was eliminated. Although PAR is a practical epidemiologic measure, limited data exist on the PARs for young-onset stroke. Rohr and colleagues suggested PAR-% ranging from 13.2% to 22.1% for diabetes mellitus, 17.2% to 40.5% for current smoking, and 21.3% to 53.5% for hypertension, depending on sex and ethnicity. PAR for hypertension was highest for African Americans (7). Except for the high PAR range for diabetes, these PARs are roughly in accordance for those demonstrated for general ischaemic stroke patients in the INTERSTROKE study (17).

Some traditional risk factors manifesting exceptionally early in life may contribute relatively more to the young-onset stroke than the usual-onset forms of the same risk factor. An illustrative example supporting this hypothesis comes from a longitudinal study comparing patients with early-onset form and usual-onset form of T2D with diabetes-free controls (27). Patients with the early-onset form of T2D had a ten times higher risk of ischaemic stroke compared to those with usual-onset T2D during a mean follow-up of 3.9 years despite a similar delay from diagnosis to starting of insulin treatment. This finding suggests that patients with the early-onset form of T2D are literally 'losing their relative protection of youth'.

Risk factors considered specific to young adults

The risk factors discussed in the previous section represent conditions with a well-established strength of association in general. Importantly, there is a range of unconventional risk factors, of which many can be considered specific to young adults. However, the association of such risk factors is frequently inconsistently demonstrated between studies, or may have been found in a single study or suggested by case-reports only. Dose-dependency and time-dependency are often incompletely shown, something that would be needed to increase the probability of a causal role of the particular risk factor. Furthermore, most of the unconventional risk factors are found fairly frequently in the population and concomitant conditions may be needed to elevate the risk of thrombosis over the critical threshold.

Cardiac interatrial abnormalities, oral contraceptive use, pregnancy, and puerperium as risk factors are thoroughly discussed elsewhere in this book (see Chapters 5 and 12), but shall be mentioned here due to their associations with other risk factors discussed in this chapter. Briefly, case–control studies suggest an association with PFO and ischaemic stroke particularly at younger ages (30), although such an association remains to be proved in population-based studies (31). An increased risk of ischaemic stroke has also been shown for combined oral contraceptives (COCs) with high dose of oestrogen (28) and puerperium (29).

Migraine

A number of hospital-based or population-based case–control and cohort studies mostly including young patients have addressed the role of migraine as a risk factor for ischaemic stroke, especially in young adults. Three meta-analyses of these observational studies produced different results (32–34).

Etminan et al. showed in their meta-analysis (2005) that the pooled relative risk for ischaemic stroke in any type of migraine was 2.2 (95% CI, 1.9–2.5), for migraine with aura (MA) 2.3 (95% CI, 1.6–3.2), and for migraine without aura (MO) 1.8 (95% CI, 1.1–3.2) (32). In contrast, Schurks et al. and Spector et al. found no association for MO (relative risk 1.2; 95% CI, 0.9–1.7 and 1.2; 95% CI, 0.9–1.8, respectively) in the two most recent meta-analyses (33–34).

The latest meta-analysis by Spector et al. included 13 case–control studies and 8 cohort studies with 622,381 patients and was able to address several confounding factors, such as hypertension, smoking, COCs, cholesterol, cardiac disease, and family history of migraine or stroke. In that study, the pooled adjusted OR for ischaemic stroke in patients with any type of migraine was 2.0 (95% CI, 1.7–2.4) and for MA, 2.3 (95% CI, 1.5–3.3) (34). Most notably, MA can thus be considered a risk factor for ischaemic stroke, while evidence for MO as a stroke risk factor remains inconsistent.

Smoking and COCs modulate the risk of ischaemic stroke in young women with migraine: smoking increases the risk up to 10-fold, COCs by 13.9–16.9-fold, and the triple combination of these factors further increases the risk with an OR of 34–35 (35). According to some studies, increased stroke risk may also be related to a recent onset of migraine and a high frequency of attacks (36–38).

Case–control studies also show that PFO is twice as common in patients with ischaemic stroke with MA than in those without (39, 40), leading to a hypothesis that paradoxical embolism might be one of the possible pathways linking MA and ischaemic stroke. Another hypothesis underlying the migraine–stroke link is that stroke could be caused by adverse effects of specific migraine medications. This hypothesis seems to hold true only for overuse of ergotamines, but not for therapeutic doses of them nor any doses of triptans (41). Finally, migraine and ischaemic stroke might share common genetic pathways, although the genetic overlap appears stronger for MO than MA (42), contradicting the epidemiologic evidence on MA especially as a stroke risk factor. Further research is needed to improve our understanding of the role of migraine as a risk factor for ischaemic stroke.

Alcohol abuse

The associations of both long-term (13, 24, 43) and recent heavy drinking (10) with young-onset ischaemic stroke have been fairly well established, with at least some dose–response effect demonstrated. Over 8-fold increases in women (43) and 15-fold increases regardless of sex (13) in risk have been found with long-term heavy drinking. Consuming high amounts of alcohol during one drinking session or binge drinking characterizes many young patients' drinking habits (44). Alcohol thus acts both as a chronic risk factor and as a transient trigger for ischaemic stroke in young adults. The specific mechanisms of how alcohol may contribute to an increased risk of ischaemic stroke include vulnerability to cardiac arrhythmias and effects on haemostasis, fibrinolysis, and blood clotting. Heavy drinkers are also more likely to suffer from head and neck trauma predisposing to cervical artery dissection (45).

Illicit drug use

Illicit drug use appears to be an important cause of stroke in geographic regions where their use is frequent. In a large multicentre study conducted in the Baltimore–Washington area, recent use of illicit drugs was detected in 12.1% and illicit drug use appeared as a probable cause in 4.7% of their ischaemic stroke patients aged 15–44 (46). According to Kaku et al., stroke risk is approximately 6.5-fold higher (95% CI, 3.1–13.6) among young drug abusers compared to non-users (47).

Amphetamine and related substances

Amphetamine-like substances, including methamphetamine, phenylpropanolamine, and methylphenidate, are used as central nervous system stimulants and appetite suppressors. Possible mechanisms causing stroke include acute hypertensive crisis, vasospasm, accelerated atherosclerosis, or platelet activation and aggregation with thrombus formation. A large population-based study from Texas, USA, showed a fivefold increased risk of haemorrhagic stroke associated with amphetamine abuse. However, no increased risk of ischaemic strokes was observed (48). Another study from Petitti et al showed an OR of 7.0 (95% CI, 2.8–17.9) for cocaine or amphetamine use, or both, for all strokes in young women after adjustment for confounders (49). A more recent study utilizing US inpatient registry data suggested a lower risk of ischaemic stroke for amphetamine users aged 15–54 (OR 2.21, 95% CI, 2.12–2.30) (50).

Cocaine

Cocaine is the second most commonly used illicit drug after marijuana and the most common illicit drug associated with stroke. Cocaine can be taken orally, intranasally, or intravenously whereas crack cocaine is smoked. A recent population-based case–control study showed that acute cocaine use within 24 hours was strongly associated with increased risk of ischaemic stroke compared to never-users (OR 6.4; 95% CI, 2.2–18.6), especially with the crack cocaine (OR 7.9; 95% CI, 1.8–35.0) (51). Infrequent use was not associated with increased risk, but frequent use (more than once a week) increased the risk twofold also after excluding acute users. A pure registry-based study again suggested a lower risk for cocaine use (OR 1.32; 95% CI, 1.30–1.34) (50). The possible mechanisms causing stroke are similar to those of amphetamine-like substances. Furthermore, infections induced by cocaine use can lead to endocarditis and secondary vasculitis (52).

Opiates

With heroin, derived from opium, most strokes are ischaemic and thought to be caused by hypoventilation or hypotension, or both, as well as by infective endocarditis, cardioembolism, and vasculitis. Heroin can be snorted, smoked, or injected either intravenously or subcutaneously. Apart from case series (53), virtually no systematic data are available on the strength of association of heroin use with ischaemic stroke. As with cocaine, most likely there are differences in the risk depending on the route and timing of administration.

Cannabis

The most important cannabinoid, delta-9-tetrahydrocannabinol, is also the most widely used illicit drug worldwide. When smoked, its rapid absorption leads to euphoria, relaxation, and self-confidence. Case reports of cannabis-associated strokes are infrequent, but support a causal link (54). After adjusting for confounders, marijuana had an independent but weak association (OR 1.17; 95% CI, 1.15–1.20) with ischaemic stroke at the age of 15–54 years based on US inpatient data, with the highest incidence for the age group of 25–34 years (50). Frequent use of cannabis may be needed to increase the risk substantially (55). However, it still remains inconclusive whether cannabis stands as an independent risk factor for ischaemic stroke in the young or merely reflects the 'cannabis lifestyle', with several concomitant stroke risk factors, such as cigarette smoking (56).

Chronic and acute infections

Both chronic and acute infections increase the risk of acute ischaemic stroke (57). In particular, chronic dental infections, human immunodeficiency virus, and chronic and active *Chlamydia pneumoniae* infection and its elevated antibodies were associated with ischaemic stroke in the young (58–63), while other pathogens have not been systemically studied in young patients. Chronic infections can affect the risk of stroke by damaging vascular endothelium, influencing or interfering with other risk factors (e.g. altering serum lipids towards a more atherogenic profile), triggering platelet activation, and creating a procoagulant state (57).

Meanwhile, acute infections are associated with an increased risk of ischaemic stroke when occurring within the preceding weeks prior to the index stroke—respiratory tract infections being the most common type of these infections (64–66). Some case–control studies indicate an association between acute infection and cervical artery dissection, the most common cause of ischaemic stroke in the young (67). Systematic studies evaluating the association specifically in young adults are scarce, however (65, 68). In a retrospective analysis of 681 ischaemic stroke patients under the age of 50, up to 10.7% had preceding infections within 4 weeks prior to stroke, the most common being upper respiratory tract infections (54%), followed by gastrointestinal (13%), chest (11%), and skin or mucous membrane (11%) infections (69).

Acute infections may lead to alterations in immunohaematological mecha-nisms and several systemic manifestations of inflammation, including increased concentrations of C-reactive protein, elevated anticardiolipin antibody levels, and reduced concentrations of circulating antithrombotic proteins. As a result, modulation of anticoagulant pathways, initiation of extrinsic coagulation path-ways, and increased platelet reactivity, as well as endothelial dysfunction were reported (70).

Antiphospholipid antibodies

Antiphospholipid syndrome (APS)—more prevalent in young women than in the general population—is a significant risk factor for arterial, venous, and small vessel thrombosis and can lead to pregnancy-related complications such as pre-eclampsia or miscarriages (71). APS diagnosis requires two positive blood tests at least 12 weeks apart showing the presence of antiphospholipid antibodies (aPL) reacting against proteins that bind to phospholipids on plasma membranes: lupus anticoagulant, anticardiolipin antibodies of immunoglobu-lin G or M isotype, or both, in medium or high titre, or anti-β_2-glycoprotein-I antibodies (72). In addition, antibodies to prothrombin are commonly tested.

Presence of aPL alone may independently contribute to the risk of ischaemic stroke. Earlier case–control studies, albeit with rather small sample sizes, have fairly well established the role of aPL as a risk factor for first ischaemic stroke at young age in patients mostly free from systemic lupus erythematosus (73–78). Recently, Urbanus and co-workers showed in their analysis of 175 women aged under 50 years with first-ever ischaemic stroke and 628 healthy controls that risk for ischaemic stroke was considerable in patients with lupus anticoagulant (OR 43.1; 95% CI, 12–152.0) and those with anti-β_2-glycoprotein-I antibod-ies (OR 2.3 for a cut-off 90th percentile of control subjects; 95% CI, 1.2–3.7) (79). Possibly due to the small number of cases with anticardiolipin or antipro-thrombin antibodies, these were not related to higher risk for ischaemic stroke. Moreover, Urbanus et al. found a significant synergy of additional risk factors in women with lupus anticoagulant compared with healthy controls: the OR for ischaemic stroke was 201.0 (95% CI, 22.1–1828.0) in oral contraceptive users and 87.0 in smokers (95% CI, 14.5–523.0). In contrast, in women without lupus anticoagulant, the OR for ischaemic stroke was only 2.9 (95% CI, 1.8–4.6) and 2.2 (1.5–3.4), respectively (79).

Inherited haematological conditions

Sickle cell disease

Sickle cell disease (SCD) is more frequent among people with ancestors from tropical and sub-Saharan regions; approximately 7–8% of people of African ancestry carry the sickle cell trait among the US population (80). SCD can affect any organ or tissue in the body, but stroke—both ischaemic (75%) and haemorrhagic (25%)—is one of the most severe and frequent complication of SCD. Stroke incidence in children is approximately 1% per year (81), with cumulative risks of 11% by the age of 20, 15% by the age of 30, and 25% by the age of 45 years (82). As more children with SCD survive, the disease also more frequently affects young adults, in whom haemorrhagic subtype is the primary presentation. Most of the well-known risk factors for stroke in SCD were identified from paediatric studies, while limited data exist for young adults. The stroke risk factors include genotype (highest risk for HbSS), hypertension, increasing age, and low baseline haemoglobin (81, 83).

Genetic thrombophilia

A recent systematic review including two case–control, seven case-only, and two cohort studies concluded that genetic contribution is significant especially to young-onset ischaemic stroke (84). Several genetic variants have been investigated as risk factors for ischaemic stroke in the young, of which the most prevalent and commonly screened are factor V Leiden G1691A and prothrombin G20210A mutations. Studies have also assessed candidate genes encoding fibrinogen (*FGA* and *FGB*) or platelet glycoproteins (*ITGB3* and *ITGA2*), genes involved in homocysteine metabolism (*MTHFR* C677T), lipid metabolism (*APOE*), and inflammation. The associations have remained largely inconclusive for young adults— also regarding well-known rare inherited thrombophilias, protein C, protein S, and antithrombin III deficiencies. Yet, most of these single-gene variants have shown a substantially strong association with paediatric stroke (85).

Regarding factor V Leiden G1691A, the most recent case–control study of Hamedani et al. did not support an association with young-onset ischaemic stroke (86), but for the prothrombin G20210A mutation, the same group found a significant association. However, the association appeared only for patients aged 15–42 years (OR 2.5; 95% CI, 1.2–28.1), not for those aged 42–49 years (87). This association was confirmed in their meta-analysis for adults aged 55 years or younger, although with attenuated strength (OR 1.5; 95% CI, 1.1–2.0).

Conclusion

In contrast to past belief, recent studies have shown that traditional, modifiable vascular risk factors are highly prevalent in young adults with ischaemic stroke. Surprisingly little is known about the strength of association and PAR of these well-documented risk factors. Studies are also warranted to characterize the stroke risk associated with the early-onset forms of traditional risk factors.

Another challenge will be to decipher the mechanisms of association of unconventional risk factors—those typically considered young-age specific—and investigate potential novel young-age-specific risk factors, such as air pollution (88) and work- and stress-related precipitants (89).

Acknowledgements

The authors were supported by grants from the Helsinki University Central Hospital Research Funds (JP; NMM) and Doctoral School of Health Sciences, University of Helsinki (NMM).

References

1. **Putaala J, Yesilot N, Waje-Andreassen U, Pitkaniemi J, Vassilopoulou S, Nardi K**, et al. Demographic and geographic vascular risk factor differences in European young adults with ischemic stroke: the 15 cities young stroke study. Stroke. 2012;**43**:2624–30.

2. **von Sarnowski B, Putaala J, Grittner U, Gaertner B, Schminke U, Curtze S**, et al. Lifestyle risk factors for ischemic stroke and transient ischemic attack in young adults in the Stroke in Young Fabry Patients study. Stroke. 2013;**44**:119–25.

3. **Pezzini A, Grassi M, Lodigiani C, Patella R, Gandolfo C, Zini A**, et al. Predictors of long-term recurrent vascular events after ischemic stroke at young age: the Italian Project on Stroke in Young Adults. Circulation. 2014;**129**:1668–76.

4. **Putaala J, Metso AJ, Metso TM, Konkola N, Kraemer Y, Haapaniemi E**, et al. Analysis of 1008 consecutive patients aged 15 to 49 with first-ever ischemic stroke: the Helsinki Young Stroke Registry. Stroke. 2009;**40**:1195–203.

5. **Harjutsalo V, Sjoberg L, Tuomilehto J.** Time trends in the incidence of type 1 diabetes in Finnish children: a cohort study. Lancet. 2008;**371**:1777–82.

6. **Prefasi D, Martinez-Sanchez P, Rodriguez-Sanz A, Fuentes B, Filgueiras-Rama D, Ruiz-Ares G**, et al. Atrial fibrillation in young stroke patients: do we underestimate its prevalence? Eur J Neurol. 2013;**20**:1367–74.

7. **Rohr J, Kittner S, Feeser B, Hebel JR, Whyte MG, Weinstein A**, et al. Traditional risk factors and ischemic stroke in young adults: the Baltimore-Washington Cooperative Young Stroke Study. Arch Neurol. 1996;**53**:603–607.

8. **Lipska K, Sylaja PN, Sarma PS, Thankappan KR, Kutty VR, Vasan RS**, et al. Risk factors for acute ischaemic stroke in young adults in South India. J Neurol Neurosurg Psychiatry. 2007;**78**:959–63.

9. **Naess H, Nyland HI, Thomassen L, Aarseth J, Myhr KM.** Etiology of and risk factors for cerebral infarction in young adults in western Norway: a population-based case-control study. Eur J Neurol. 2004;**11**:25–30.

10. **Haapaniemi H, Hillbom M, Juvela S.** Lifestyle-associated risk factors for acute brain infarction among persons of working age. Stroke. 1997;**28**:26–30.

11. **Albucher JF, Ferrieres J, Ruidavets JB, Guiraud-Chaumeil B, Perret BP, Chollet F.** Serum lipids in young patients with ischaemic stroke: a case-control study. J Neurol Neurosurg Psychiatry. 2000;**69**:29–33.

12. **Bandasak R, Narksawat K, Tangkanakul C, Chinvarun Y, Siri S.** Association between hypertension and stroke among young Thai adults in Bangkok, Thailand. Southeast Asian J Trop Med Public Health. 2011;**42**:1241–48.

13. **You RX, McNeil JJ, O'Malley HM, Davis SM, Thrift AG, Donnan GA.** Risk factors for stroke due to cerebral infarction in young adults. Stroke. 1997;**28**:1913–18.

14. **Love BB, Biller J, Jones MP, Adams HP, Jr, Bruno A.** Cigarette smoking. A risk factor for cerebral infarction in young adults. Arch Neurol. 1990;**47**:693–98.

15. **Bhat VM, Cole JW, Sorkin JD, Wozniak MA, Malarcher AM, Giles WH,** et al. Dose-response relationship between cigarette smoking and risk of ischemic stroke in young women. Stroke. 2008;**39**:2439–43.

16. **Hagg S, Thorn LM, Putaala J, Liebkind R, Harjutsalo V, Forsblom CM,** et al. Incidence of stroke according to presence of diabetic nephropathy and severe diabetic retinopathy in patients with type 1 diabetes. Diabetes Care. 2013;**36**:4140–46.

17. **O'Donnell MJ, Xavier D, Liu L, Zhang H, Chin SL, Rao-Melacini P,** et al. Risk factors for ischaemic and intracerebral haemorrhagic stroke in 22 countries (the INTERSTROKE study): a case-control study. Lancet. 2010;**376**:112–23.

18. **Sabino AP, De Oliveira Sousa M, Moreira Lima L, Dias Ribeiro D, Sant'Ana Dusse LM, Das Gracas Carvalho M,** et al. ApoB/ApoA-I ratio in young patients with ischemic cerebral stroke or peripheral arterial disease. Transl Res. 2008;**152**:113–18.

19. **van der Stoep M, Korporaal SJ, Van Eck M.** High-density lipoprotein as a modulator of platelet and coagulation responses. Cardiovasc Res. 2014;**103**:362–71.

20. **Nave AH, Lange KS, Leonards CO, Siegerink B, Doehner W, Landmesser U,** et al. Lipoprotein (a) as a risk factor for ischemic stroke: a meta-analysis. Atherosclerosis. 2015;**242**:496–503.

21. **Boffa MB, Koschinsky ML.** Lipoprotein (a): truly a direct prothrombotic factor in cardiovascular disease? J Lipid Res. 2016;**57**:745–57.

22. **Mitchell AB, Cole JW, McArdle PF, Cheng YC, Ryan KA, Sparks MJ,** et al. Obesity increases risk of ischemic stroke in young adults. Stroke. 2015;**46**:1690–92.

23. **Wang L, Wang KS.** Age differences in the associations of behavioral and psychosocial factors with stroke. Neuroepidemiology. 2013;**41**:94–100.

24. **Chiu YC, Bai YM, Su TP, Chen TJ, Chen MH.** Ischemic stroke in young adults and preexisting psychiatric disorders: a nationwide case-control study. Medicine (Baltimore). 2015;**94**:e1520.

25. **Lee HC, Lin HC, Tsai SY.** Severely depressed young patients have over five times increased risk for stroke: a 5-year follow-up study. Biol Psychiatry. 2008;**64**:912–15.

26. **Chang CC, Chuang HC, Lin CL, Sung FC, Chang YJ, Hsu CY,** et al. High incidence of stroke in young women with sleep apnea syndrome. Sleep Med. 2014;**15**:410–14.

27. **Hillier TA, Pedula KL.** Complications in young adults with early-onset type 2 diabetes: losing the relative protection of youth. Diabetes Care. 2003;**26**:2999–3005.

28. **Roach RE, Helmerhorst FM, Lijfering WM, Stijnen T, Algra A, Dekkers OM.** Combined oral contraceptives: the risk of myocardial infarction and ischemic stroke. Cochrane Database Syst Rev. 2015;**8**:CD011054.

29. **Kittner SJ, Stern BJ, Feeser BR, Hebel R, Nagey DA, Buchholz DW,** et al. Pregnancy and the risk of stroke. N Engl J Med. 1996;**335**:768–74.

30. **Alsheikh-Ali AA, Thaler DE, Kent DM.** Patent foramen ovale in cryptogenic stroke: incidental or pathogenic? Stroke. 2009;**40**:2349–55.

31. **Davis D, Gregson J, Willeit P, Stephan B, Al-Shahi Salman R, Brayne C.** Patent foramen ovale, ischemic stroke and migraine: systematic review and stratified meta-analysis of association studies. Neuroepidemiology. 2013;**40**:56–67.

32. **Etminan M, Takkouche B, Isorna FC, Samii A.** Risk of ischaemic stroke in people with migraine: systematic review and meta-analysis of observational studies. BMJ. 2005;**330**:63.

33. **Schurks M, Rist PM, Bigal ME, Buring JE, Lipton RB, Kurth T.** Migraine and cardiovascular disease: systematic review and meta-analysis. BMJ. 2009;**339**:b3914.

34. **Spector JT, Kahn SR, Jones MR, Jayakumar M, Dalal D, Nazarian S.** Migraine headache and ischemic stroke risk: an updated meta-analysis. Am J Med. 2010;**123**:612–24.

35. **Bousser MG.** Estrogens, migraine, and stroke. Stroke. 2004;**35**:2652–56.

36. **Kurth T, Schurks M, Logroscino G, Buring JE.** Migraine frequency and risk of cardiovascular disease in women. Neurology. 2009;**73**:581–88.

37. **Donaghy M, Chang CL, Poulter N, European Collaborators of The World Health Organisation Collaborative Study of Cardiovascular Disease and Steroid Hormone Contraception.** Duration, frequency, recency, and type of migraine and the risk of ischaemic stroke in women of childbearing age. J Neurol Neurosurg Psychiatry. 2002;**73**:747–50.

38. **MacClellan LR, Giles W, Cole J, Wozniak M, Stern B, Mitchell BD,** et al. Probable migraine with visual aura and risk of ischemic stroke: the stroke prevention in young women study. Stroke. 2007;**38**:2438–45.

39. **Lamy C, Giannesini C, Zuber M, Arquizan C, Meder JF, Trystram D,** et al. Clinical and imaging findings in cryptogenic stroke patients with and without patent foramen ovale: the PFO-ASA Study. Atrial Septal Aneurysm. Stroke. 2002;**33**:706–11.

40. **Sztajzel R, Genoud D, Roth S, Mermillod B, Le Floch-Rohr J.** Patent foramen ovale, a possible cause of symptomatic migraine: a study of 74 patients with acute ischemic stroke. Cerebrovasc Dis. 2002;**13**:102–106.

41. **Wammes-van der Heijden EA, Rahimtoola H, Leufkens HG, Tijssen CC, Egberts AC.** Risk of ischemic complications related to the intensity of triptan and ergotamine use. Neurology. 2006;**67**:1128–34.

42. **Malik R, Freilinger T, Winsvold BS, Anttila V, Vander Heiden J, Traylor M,** et al. Shared genetic basis for migraine and ischemic stroke: a genome-wide analysis of common variants. Neurology. 2015;**84**:2132–45.

43. **Nightingale AL, Farmer RD.** Ischemic stroke in young women: a nested case-control study using the UK General Practice Research Database. Stroke. 2004;**35**:1574–78.

44. **Taylor JR, Combs-Orme T.** Alcohol and strokes in young adults. Am J Psychiatry. 1985;**142**:116–18.

45. **Hillbom M, Numminen H.** Alcohol and stroke: pathophysiologic mechanisms. Neuroepidemiology. 1998;**17**:281–87.

46. **Sloan MA, Kittner SJ, Feeser BR, Gardner J, Epstein A, Wozniak MA,** et al. Illicit drug-associated ischemic stroke in the Baltimore-Washington Young Stroke Study. Neurology. 1998;**50**:1688–93.

47. **Kaku DA, Lowenstein DH.** Emergence of recreational drug abuse as a major risk factor for stroke in young adults. Ann Intern Med. 1990;**113**:821–27.

48 Westover AN, McBride S, Haley RW. Stroke in young adults who abuse amphetamines or cocaine: a population-based study of hospitalized patients. Arch Gen Psychiatry. 2007;**64**:495–502.

49. Petitti DB, Sidney S, Quesenberry C, Bernstein A. Stroke and cocaine or amphetamine use. Epidemiology. 1998;**9**:596–600.

50. Rumalla K, Reddy AY, Mittal MK. Recreational marijuana use and acute ischemic stroke: a population-based analysis of hospitalized patients in the United States. J Neurol Sci. 2016;**364**:191–96.

51. Cheng YC, Ryan KA, Qadwai SA, Shah J, Sparks MJ, Wozniak MA, et al. Cocaine use and risk of ischemic stroke in young adults. Stroke. 2016;**47**:918–22.

52. Neiman J, Haapaniemi HM, Hillbom M. Neurological complications of drug abuse: pathophysiological mechanisms. Eur J Neurol. 2000;**7**:595–606.

53. Brust JC, Richter RW. Stroke associated with addiction to heroin. J Neurol Neurosurg Psychiatry. 1976;**39**:194–99.

54. Hackam DG. Cannabis and stroke: systematic appraisal of case reports. Stroke. 2015;**46**:852–56.

55. Hemachandra D, McKetin R, Cherbuin N, Anstey KJ. Heavy cannabis users at elevated risk of stroke: evidence from a general population survey. Aust N Z J Public Health. 2016;**40**:226–30.

56. Barber PA, Pridmore HM, Krishnamurthy V, Roberts S, Spriggs DA, Carter KN, et al. Cannabis, ischemic stroke, and transient ischemic attack: a case-control study. Stroke. 2013;**44**:2327–29.

57. Grau AJ, Urbanek C, Palm F. Common infections and the risk of stroke. Nat Rev Neurol. 2010;**6**:681–94.

58. Syrjanen J, Peltola J, Valtonen V, Iivanainen M, Kaste M, Huttunen JK. Dental infections in association with cerebral infarction in young and middle-aged men. J Intern Med. 1989;**225**:179–84.

59. Grau AJ, Becher H, Ziegler CM, Lichy C, Buggle F, Kaiser C, et al. Periodontal disease as a risk factor for ischemic stroke. Stroke. 2004;**35**:496–501.

60. Benjamin LA, Bryer A, Emsley HC, Khoo S, Solomon T, Connor MD. HIV infection and stroke: current perspectives and future directions. Lancet Neurol. 2012;**11**:878–90.

61. Anzini A, Cassone A, Rasura M, Ciervo A, Beccia M, Di Lisi F, et al. Chlamydia pneumoniae infection in young stroke patients: a case--control study. Eur J Neurol. 2004;**11**:321–27.

62. Bandaru VC, Boddu DB, Laxmi V, Neeraja M, Kaul S. Seroprevalence of Chlamydia pneumoniae antibodies in stroke in young. Can J Neurol Sci. 2009;**36**:725–30.

63. Piechowski-Jozwiak B, Mickielewicz A, Gaciong Z, Berent H, Kwiecinski H. Elevated levels of anti-Chlamydia pneumoniae IgA and IgG antibodies in young adults with ischemic stroke. Acta Neurol Scand. 2007;**116**:144–49.

64. Grau AJ, Buggle F, Heindl S, Steichen-Wiehn C, Banerjee T, Maiwald M, et al. Recent infection as a risk factor for cerebrovascular ischemia. Stroke. 1995;**26**:373–79.

65. Syrjanen J, Valtonen VV, Iivanainen M, Kaste M, Huttunen JK. Preceding infection as an important risk factor for ischaemic brain infarction in young and middle aged patients. Br Med J (Clin Res Ed). 1988;**296**:1156–60.

66. **Zurru MC, Alonzo C, Brescacin L, Romano M, Camera LA, Waisman G,** et al. Recent respiratory infection predicts atherothrombotic stroke: case-control study in a Buenos Aires healthcare system. Stroke. 2009;**40**:1986–90.

67. **Guillon B, Berthet K, Benslamia L, Bertrand M, Bousser MG, Tzourio C.** Infection and the risk of spontaneous cervical artery dissection: a case-control study. Stroke. 2003;**34**:e79–81.

68. **Nagaraja D, Christopher R, Tripathi M, Kumar MV, Valli ER, Patil SA.** Preceding infection as a risk factor of stroke in the young. J Assoc Physicians India. 1999;**47**:673–75.

69. **Heikinheimo T, Broman J, Haapaniemi E, Kaste M, Tatlisumak T, Putaala J.** Preceding and poststroke infections in young adults with first-ever ischemic stroke: effect on short-term and long-term outcomes. Stroke. 2013;**44**:3331–37.

70. **Emsley HC, Hopkins SJ.** Acute ischaemic stroke and infection: recent and emerging concepts. Lancet Neurol. 2008;**7**:341–53.

71. **Cervera R, Asherson RA.** Clinical and epidemiological aspects in the antiphospholipid syndrome. Immunobiology. 2003;**207**:5–11.

72. **Miyakis S, Lockshin MD, Atsumi T, Branch DW, Brey RL, Cervera R,** et al. International consensus statement on an update of the classification criteria for definite antiphospholipid syndrome (APS). J Thromb Haemost. 2006;**4**:295–306.

73. **Brey RL, Hart RG, Sherman DG, Tegeler CH.** Antiphospholipid antibodies and cerebral ischemia in young people. Neurology. 1990;**40**:1190–96.

74. **Brey RL, Stallworth CL, McGlasson DL, Wozniak MA, Wityk RJ, Stern BJ,** et al. Antiphospholipid antibodies and stroke in young women. Stroke. 2002;**33**:2396–400.

75. **Nencini P, Baruffi MC, Abbate R, Massai G, Amaducci L, Inzitari D.** Lupus anticoagulant and anticardiolipin antibodies in young adults with cerebral ischemia. Stroke. 1992;**23**:189–93.

76. **Toschi V, Motta A, Castelli C, Paracchini ML, Zerbi D, Gibelli A.** High prevalence of antiphosphatidylinositol antibodies in young patients with cerebral ischemia of undetermined cause. Stroke. 1998;**29**:1759–64.

77. **Blohorn A, Guegan-Massardier E, Triquenot A, Onnient Y, Tron F, Borg JY,** et al. Antiphospholipid antibodies in the acute phase of cerebral ischaemia in young adults: a descriptive study of 139 patients. Cerebrovasc Dis. 2002;**13**:156–62.

78. **Singh K, Gaiha M, Shome DK, Gupta VK, Anuradha S.** The association of antiphospholipid antibodies with ischaemic stroke and myocardial infarction in young and their correlation: a preliminary study. J Assoc Physicians India. 2001;**49**:527–29.

79. **Urbanus RT, Siegerink B, Roest M, Rosendaal FR, de Groot PG, Algra A.** Antiphospholipid antibodies and risk of myocardial infarction and ischaemic stroke in young women in the RATIO study: a case-control study. Lancet Neurol. 2009;**8**:998–1005.

80. **Hassell KL.** Population estimates of sickle cell disease in the U.S. Am J Prev Med. 2010;**38**:S512–21.

81. **Ohene-Frempong K, Weiner SJ, Sleeper LA, Miller ST, Embury S, Moohr JW,** et al. Cerebrovascular accidents in sickle cell disease: rates and risk factors. Blood. 1998;**91**:288–94.

82. **Moser FG, Miller ST, Bello JA, Pegelow CH, Zimmerman RA, Wang WC**, et al. The spectrum of brain MR abnormalities in sickle-cell disease: a report from the Cooperative Study of Sickle Cell Disease. AJNR Am J Neuroradiol. 1996;**17**:965–72.

83. **Strouse JJ, Lanzkron S, Urrutia V.** The epidemiology, evaluation and treatment of stroke in adults with sickle cell disease. Expert Rev Hematol. 2011;**4**:597–606.

84. **Cheng YC, Cole JW, Kittner SJ, Mitchell BD.** Genetics of ischemic stroke in young adults. Circ Cardiovasc Genet. 2014;**7**:383–92.

85. **Kenet G, Lutkhoff LK, Albisetti M, Bernard T, Bonduel M, Brandao L**, et al. Impact of thrombophilia on risk of arterial ischemic stroke or cerebral sinovenous thrombosis in neonates and children: a systematic review and meta-analysis of observational studies. Circulation. 2010;**121**:1838–47.

86. **Hamedani AG, Cole JW, Cheng Y, Sparks MJ, O'Connell JR, Stine OC**, et al. Factor V leiden and ischemic stroke risk: the Genetics of Early Onset Stroke (GEOS) study. J Stroke Cerebrovasc Dis. 2013;**22**:419–23.

87. **Jiang B, Ryan KA, Hamedani A, Cheng Y, Sparks MJ, Koontz D**, et al. Prothrombin G20210A mutation is associated with young-onset stroke: the genetics of early-onset stroke study and meta-analysis. Stroke. 2014;**45**:961–67.

88. **Yitshak Sade M, Novack V, Ifergane G, Horev A, Kloog I.** Air pollution and ischemic stroke among young adults. Stroke. 2015;**46**:3348–53.

89. **Kivimaki M, Jokela M, Nyberg ST, Singh-Manoux A, Fransson EI, Alfredsson L**, et al. Long working hours and risk of coronary heart disease and stroke: a systematic review and meta-analysis of published and unpublished data for 603,838 individuals. Lancet. 2015;**386**:1739–46.

Chapter 3

Classification

Christian Tanislav and Manfred Kaps

Introduction

Classifying ischaemic strokes according to the underlying aetiology is complex, as stroke is a heterogeneous disorder with numerous potential mechanisms. However, with advances in research and methodology, many causes for stroke have been identified (1–5). The attribution of stroke aetiology is therefore an essential part of individual patient care as well as stroke research.

In adult stroke patients below the age of 55 years, more than 70% of the subjects suffer from brain infarction, and 20% of the patients present with a transient ischaemic attack (TIA) (6). A TIA occurs mostly without visible acute ischaemic lesions (6); nevertheless, similar mechanisms for the temporary brain ischaemia are presumed. Therefore the expansion of classifications for strokes will encompass all acute cerebral ischaemic events. For clinical practice, a classification should have a direct link to the mechanism, examining all information obtained in the workup and other related case history and aggregating them to a specific pathophysiology.

Requirements should be identified for developing a stroke classification system. The classification should be reliable with high inter-rater agreement, and the performance should not result in additional time effort or other consumption of resources. The widely used TOAST (Trial of Org 10172 in Acute Stroke Treatment) classification for ischaemic stroke differentiates five aetiological classes (7). Many studies demonstrated that outcomes such as recurrence rates or mortality differ for the different stroke subtypes, making the classification also a prognostic one (8–11). Moreover, in recent clinical trials intended to prove the effectiveness of different treatments, the TOAST classification served as a reliable tool for selecting suitable patients (12–14). In spite of the advantages of accurate stroke subtyping, procedural difficulties need to be challenged. The final decision regarding the assigned classification is guided by the clinician's interpretation. There are promising new developments that have evolved from the TOAST study to substantiate the taken decision. The revised TOAST criteria, as applied in the STOPStroke study, aimed to rate the assigned stroke subtypes according to the sustaining evidence (15). This algorithm was improved by standardizing its application, even by providing a web-based option, thereby obtaining an excellent intra- and inter-operator reliability (16, 17). A further approach for simplifying the use of TOAST was the development of the ASCO (A: atherosclerosis; S: small-vessel disease; C: cardiac pathology; O: other causes) and ASCOD classifications (18, 19). Comparable to the algorithm computed by Ay and co-workers in the STOPStroke study, ASCO recodes the TOAST subtypes and attributes to each category an evidence level (18, 19). The ASCOD addresses dissections in a particular way, coding it as 'D', thus as a separate subgroup (18, 19).

The keys points of criticism for TOAST are its inaccuracy in subtyping undetermined aetiologies in young stroke patients (20) especially as in those patients, not being able to explain mechanisms is more often experienced than in elderly patients (4, 21–23). New techniques such as brain magnetic resonance imaging (MRI) provide additional information allowing the discernment between infarcts of embolic pattern and those caused by small artery occlusion. This may be particularly of interest in those patients with no obvious aetiology. The recently published scheme for the embolic stroke of undetermined source (ESUS) would be especially beneficial to further characterize the high proportion of young stroke patients with an inconclusive stroke workup (24).

Due to its widespread use in clinical practice as well as in research, the TOAST stroke classification provides a solid basis for new developments. However, for young stroke patients, unique features of this group need to be considered to identify additional classifications. For comparability, the TOAST framework should remain as the fundamental core.

Is TOAST the right approach for classifying young patients with an ischaemic cerebrovascular event?

The TOAST classification was developed for classifying different stroke aetiologies within a clinical trial, the Trial of Org 10172 in Acute Stroke Treatment (7). This trial investigated in a blinded, placebo controlled, and randomized design the effect of a low-molecular-weight heparinoid in acute stroke patients (7). The investigators aimed to develop a simple system for classifying stroke subtypes according to the underlying mechanism. Based on clinical features and on data collected in the stroke workup (MRI/computed tomography (CT) studies, cardiac imaging (echocardiography, electrocardiogram, etc.), and imaging of the brain arteries including ultrasound and laboratory assessments for prothrombotic states) different raters assign the categories for patients included in the study. Five categories were defined: (a) large-artery atherosclerosis (LAA), (b) cardioembolism (CE), (c) small artery disease (SAD), (d) stroke of other determined aetiology (OD), and (e) stroke of undetermined aetiology (7). Within this trial the TOAST classification provided reliable results with good inter-observer agreements. Subsequently, the classification was applied in many studies and became the most common classification system for stroke subtyping. Currently the TOAST classification is widely used in clinical trials as well as in usual clinical routine (11, 17, 25).

The first three classes of stroke subtypes in TOAST (LAA, CE, and SAD) are closely related to vascular disease and vascular risk factors including hypertension, diabetes, hyperlipidaemia, and smoking. In general, many of the patients present these aetiologies (20); in long-term evaluations, the proportion of these stroke subtypes remains consistent. It underscores that the methodology is robust to withstand influences from new developments in the field (Fig. 3.1) (26). Nonetheless, it is also obvious that the proportion of undetermined aetiologies is high (Fig. 3.1). While aetiologies related to vascular risk factors (LAA, CE, and SAD) represent 55–62% of the stroke patients, the proportion

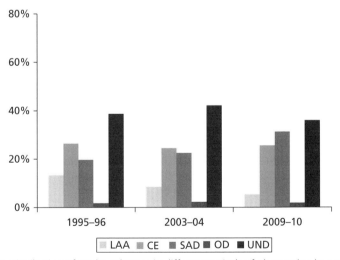

Fig. 3.1 Distribution of stroke subtypes in different periods of observation in a general stroke population without age restrictions. LAA, large artery atherosclerosis; CE, cardioembolism; SAD, small artery disease; OD, other determined aetiology; and UND, undetermined aetiology. Values on the vertical scale indicate percentages.
Source: data from Neuroepidemiology, 44(1), Kolominsky-Rabas PL, Wiedmann S, Weingartner M, Liman TG, Endres M, Schwab S, et al, Time trends in incidence of pathological and etiological stroke subtypes during 16 years: the Erlangen Stroke Project, pp. 24–9, Copyright (2015), Karger Publishers.

of patients of undetermined aetiology remains a remarkable subgroup with 36–42% of the patients (26).

Addressing young stroke patients and the distribution of TOAST stroke subtypes, the definition of 'young' matters. To establish a cut-off for being young is challenging, however several studies in young stroke populations used different cut-offs for defining young adults including subjects younger than 45–55 years (5, 21, 22). The definition is important, as the vascular disease might be an age-dependent pathology, even in a young stroke population. With increasing age, vascular risk factors increase proportionately; as a result, stroke subtypes related to vascular burden become more common (Fig. 3.2, Table 3.1).

The Stroke in Young Fabry Patients (sifap1) study demonstrated an age-dependent increase in the number of patients with TOAST subtypes of LAA, CE, and SAD. Comparable findings were observed in different studies even applying different age limits for the definition of young (Table 3.1). Recent studies resulted in comparable proportions of stroke subtypes due to similar age brackets (3–5, 22, 23, 27–31)—two studies published in 2013 comprised more than 3000 patients each and provide the most reliable results (4, 5).

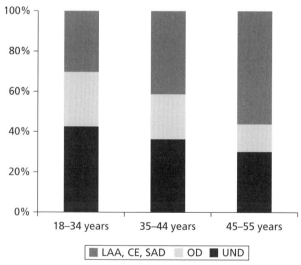

Fig. 3.2 Distribution of stroke subtypes in different age groups in the Stroke in Young Fabry Patients study population (18–55 years). LAA, large artery atherosclerosis; CE, cardioembolism; SAD, small artery disease; OD, other determined aetiology; and UND, undetermined aetiology.

Adapted from Stroke, 44(2), Rolfs A, Fazekas F, Grittner U, Dichgans M, Martus P, Holzhausen M, et al, Acute cerebrovascular disease in the young: the Stroke in Young Fabry Patients study, pp. 340–9, Copyright (2013), with permission from Wolters Kluwer Health, Inc.

Table 3.1 Distribution of aetiologies according to the TOAST classification in selected studies with young stroke populations

Reference	Country/year	Age range (years)	N	LAA	CE	SAD	OD	UND
Cerato et al. (22)	Italy/2004	16–49	273	16	24	17	19	24
Rasura et al. (23)	Italy/2006	14–47	394	12	33	3	28	24
Varona et al. (30)	Spain/2007	15–45	272	21	17	0	26	36
Jovanovic et al. (31)	Serbia/2008	15–45	865	14	20	14	20	32
Putaala et al. (3)	Finland/2009	15–49	1008	8	20	14	25	33
Pezzini et al. (27)	Italy/2011	<45	1017	11	30	5	36	18
Tancredi et al. (29)	Italy/2013	16–44	324	9	19	16	29	27
Yesilot Barlas et al. (4)	Europe/2013	15–49	3301	9	17	12	22	40
Rolfs et al. (5)	Europe/2013	18–55	5032	19	17	13	18	33

Indicated values are percentages.

CE, cardioembolism, LAA, large artery atherosclerosis, OD, other determined aetiology; SAD, small artery disease, UND, undetermined aetiology.

Yesilot Barlas and colleagues investigated younger patients which resulted in a slightly lower proportion of strokes attributed to LAA and the higher percentages of undetermined aetiologies (4). In line with these findings and further larger-scale studies, the same trend in the allocation of stroke subtypes could be noted (3–5, 25). In a comparison of baseline data between patients included in the sifap1 study (5025 participants) and a corresponding stroke population ($N = 15,997$; <56 years; patients with an ischaemic stroke or TIA derived from a large-scale registry of the Institute of Quality Assurance Hesse of the Federal State of Hesse, GQH, Germany), no pertinent differences in proportions of stroke subtypes were detected (25). The correlation between higher age and stroke aetiologies related to a vascular burden (LAA, CE, and SAD) was also supported in this analysis; in comparison to the Hesse registry, the age distribution in the sifap1 study was skewed to the younger age categories (Fig. 3.3), so in comparing subgroups in the registry, a slightly higher proportion of patients with stroke aetiologies LAA, CE, and SAD were observed (Fig. 3.3) (25).

In summary, the bulk of clinical studies demonstrate strong support for the reliability of subtyping young strokes to LAA, CE, and SAD according to the definition of TOAST. LAA, CE, and SAD are stroke aetiologies associated with the presence of vascular risk factors. In conclusion, for classifying young strokes to these categories, the TOAST scheme can be recommended as it can

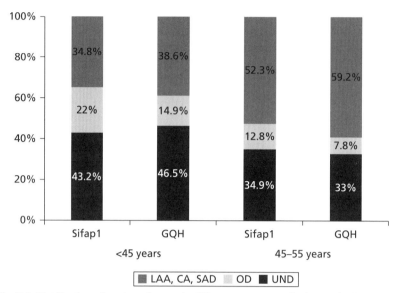

Fig. 3.3 Distribution of stroke subtypes in different age groups in the Stroke in Young Fabry Patients (Sifap1) study versus the stroke registry from the Institute of Quality Assurance Hesse of the Federal State of Hesse (GQH), Germany. LAA, large artery atherosclerosis; CE, cardioembolism; SAD, small artery disease; OD, other determined aetiology; and UND, undetermined aetiology.

Adapted from BMC Neurol, 14(45), Tanislav C, Grittner U, Misselwitz B, Jungehuelsing GJ, Enzinger C, von SB, et al, Lessons from everyday stroke care for clinical research and vice versa: comparison of a comprehensive and a research population of young stroke patients, Copyright (2014), BioMed Central Ltd, reproduced under the Creative Commons License 2.0.

address 30–60% of the young stroke victims who are affected by vascular risk factors.

How to deal with the high number of patients of undetermined aetiology

A weak point of the TOAST classification is the poor differentiation when subtyping the undetermined aetiology. Despite the systematic diagnostic approaches, the increasing knowledge about uncommon causes for stroke and the more accurate diagnostic procedures including vascular imaging, coagulopathy testing, and genetic screening, in a substantial proportion of young patients the aetiology remains unclear (Table 3.1). This group includes patients with no obvious cause for stroke despite intensive diagnostic workup, as well as those individuals with incomplete cases, due to insufficient scope and timing of diagnostic workups. Furthermore, patients with two concurrent aetiologies might also be allocated to this group, as the TOAST classification does not specifically address them (7). These inaccuracies result in an overestimation in this group.

Therefore, approaches to reduce the high number of patients with unexplained strokes would target a shifting from the subtype of undetermined aetiology to either those aetiologies related to vascular risk factors (LAA, CE, and SAD), or to the category of other determined aetiologies. The latter appears more appropriate in the context of young patients, as in this specific stroke population uncommon causes for stroke is more frequently expected than in older patients (5).

New approaches for more accurate stroke subtyping might have an influence in reducing high proportions of undetermined aetiology and would allow a more differentiated view on the heterogeneity within this class. In this context, the ASCO classification for stroke might represent a promising alternative (19). With a simple new labelling of the TOAST classes LAA, CE, SAD, and other determined aetiologies into A for LAA, S for SAD, C for CE, and O for other determined aetiologies and with additional grading for each category regarding the plausibility (five levels: 1 for definitely potential cause, 2 for uncertain causality, 3 for unlikely causality, 0 for disease completely absent, and 9 for insufficient workup) and the evidence level which sustain the diagnosis (three levels: A for direct evidence, B for indirect evidence, and C for weak evidence), the ASCO classification enables a more differentiated categorization of stroke subtypes (19). Taking into account all possibilities according to combinatory rules, a concise and simple application in the clinical routine as well as subjected in medical education programmes, the ASCO classification would not contribute to a better handling with the issue. However, in clinical trials, with need of precisely selecting patients for proving different circumstances, the ASCO classification might be promising in particular cases. For investigating the distribution of patent foramen ovale (PFO) within the sifap1 study, the ASCO classification was applied for identifying pure cryptogenic patients. In patients with ASCO class 1–3 (with findings indicating a potential aetiology), the PFO frequency was lower than in those patients classified with ASCO 0 (no evidence for any potential stroke causes); within ASCO 0 the frequency of PFO increased dramatically when dichotomizing according to the presence of vascular risk factors (Fig. 3.4) (unpublished data).

Other determined aetiologies, the uncommon causes?

Stroke of other determined aetiology summarizes 10–30% of the young stroke cases (Table 3.1)—the younger the ischaemic patients are, the likelier the case is

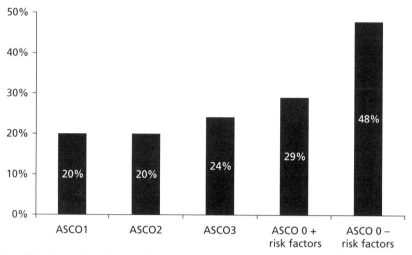

Fig. 3.4 Distribution of PFO using the ASCO classification; the frequency of PFO is the highest in the ASCO 0 class without vascular risk factors.

Reproduced from Stroke, 48(1), Huber R, Grittner U, Weidemann F, Thijs V, Tanislav C, Enzinger C, Fazekas F, Wolf M, Hennerici MG, McCabe DJ, Putaala J, Tatlisumak T, Kessler C, von Sarnowski B, Martus P, Kolodny E, Norrving B, Rolfs A, Patent Foramen Ovale and Cryptogenic Strokes in the Stroke in Young Fabry Patients Study, pp. 30–35, Copyright (2017), with permission from Wolters Kluwer Health, Inc.

'other determined aetiology' (Fig. 3.3). Table 3.2 presents a selection of uncommon causes of stroke in young adults. In this chapter the different uncommon causes will be briefly described—details on pathogenesis and further information will be provided in more detail in the following chapters of this book.

Arterial dissection is one of the most important pathologies in the TOAST subtype of other determined aetiology. Proportions provided in the literature encompass 2–15% of all strokes among young patients (3–5, 22, 30). The relatively high percentage of dissection in young stroke in the latest studies may be a result of the increasing availability of MRI, which became widely used over time as a standard procedure for many stroke patients. With imaging of the vascular status by MRI, dissections are more likely to be deciphered. In contrast, the pathology of moyamoya vasculopathy remains unaffected by this development (5). In Asian patients, the moyamoya vasculopathy represents one of the most common and significant non-atherosclerotic vasculopathies, but it also occurs worldwide (32–34). However, in the Western hemisphere, moyamoya pathology is significantly less common (32–34). The relationship between migraines and strokes has been described in several publications (35). The risk of a stroke occurring is particularly pronounced in young women having migraines with aura, smokers, and women current taking oral contraceptives (35). Coagulopathies may play a role in the pathogenesis of stroke in young adults, but for most disorders it is difficult to establish a cause and effect

Table 3.2 Selected uncommon causes for stroke in young patients

Non-atherosclerotic angiopathies	Dissection of the brain-supplying arteries
	Moyamoya disease and syndrome
	Fibromuscular dysplasia
	Susac's syndrome, Sneddon's syndrome
	Migraine-related strokes
	Cerebral amyloid angiopathy
	Reversible cerebral vasoconstriction syndrome
	Vessel aneurysm
Genetic disorders	Fabry disease
	CADASIL
	MELAS
	Marfan syndrome
	Neurofibromatosis
	Sturge–Weber disease
Haematological conditions	Hypercoagulable states due to: deficiencies of protein S, protein C, or antithrombin; factor V Leiden mutation, prothrombin gene G20210A mutation
	Antiphospholipid syndrome
	Sickle cell disease
	Thrombotic thrombocytopenic purpura
	Hyperviscosity syndromes
	Acute disseminated intravascular coagulation
	Myeloproliferative disorders
Inflammatory disorders	Vasculitis (primary angiitis of the CNS, Sjögren syndrome, Wegener's granulomatosis)
	Takayasu arteritis
	Temporal arteritis
	Behçet syndrome
	Neurosarcoidosis
	HIV
	Varicella zoster virus
	Neurosyphilis
	Tuberculous meningitis
Iatrogenic	Peri-interventional
	Drug-induced event

relationship with certainty (36). The antiphospholipid antibody syndrome represents an exception to this observation—in one systematic review, antiphospholipid antibodies were identified as an independent factor for ischaemic strokes in young patients (36).

Primary cerebral angiitis is more frequent in young male patients than in women (37). The vasculitis related to infections is more prevalent in individuals with human immunodeficiency virus (HIV), so this pathology is more common in developing countries with a high HIV prevalence (37). Rare genetic disorders such as cerebral autosomal dominant arteriopathy with subcortical infarcts and leucoencephalopathy (CADASIL), mitochondrial encephalopathy with lactic acidosis and stroke-like episodes (MELAS), or Fabry disease, an X-linked storage disorder, are of relevance as stroke pathologies (5, 38, 39). However they represent a small proportion of patients and some of the genetic variants may lead to isolated neurological phenotypes, becoming clinically apparent with strokes. As other markers indicating the disorders in these cases are missing, clinicians are less aware considering these pathologies for diagnosis.

In summary, while pathologies such as dissections moved into the focus of interest, also influenced by the expansion of new diagnostic techniques such as MRI, rare pathologies including genetic disorders are rather neglected. As these are of great relevance for the patient as well as for other potentially affected family members, diagnosing these disorders should be shifted into the focus of educational programmes.

Due to the lack of comprehensive evidence regarding rare causes for stroke, linking a disorder to the actual cerebrovascular event remains challenging. Thus, the final verdict and the stroke subtype classification are at the physician's discretion.

Approaches for dissecting undetermined aetiologies

Patients classified by TOAST as undetermined aetiology subsume three heterogeneous categories. The first category includes those patients with an unclear aetiology despite extensive diagnostic workup; in the second category, patients with two or more possible aetiologies for stroke are represented; and a third group includes those patients with an insufficient diagnostic workup.

Undetermined aetiology despite extensive workup: the real cryptogenic stroke

It is still true that clinicians will encounter patients without a single specific finding indicating a stroke mechanism even after comprehensive examinations are performed. For avoiding misunderstandings, the term stroke of undetermined aetiology should therefore be explicitly reserved for these pure cryptogenic strokes, with no obvious aetiology despite extensive/sufficient diagnostic workup.

The development of new imaging techniques enabled the precise detection of brain infarctions. The accumulated data demonstrating an infarction pattern indicates potential stroke mechanisms (24). Even if no stroke aetiology is sustained by findings detected in the diagnostic workup, inevitably leading to subtyping a stroke of undetermined aetiology, the infarction pattern may indicate an embolic or non-embolic mechanism. In this context, the differentiation between lacunar and non-lacunar infarction patterns, as applied in the ESUS definition, seems to be the most appropriate approach (24). Similar to the discussion carried out above, for the diagnosis of ESUS a minimum standard of workup is required. Imaging criteria for a lacunar stroke as applied for ESUS addresses the location and size of lesion. All other infarction patterns, except a single lesion 1.5 cm in size (≤2.0 cm on MRI diffusion images) in the distribution of the small penetrating cerebral arteries (visualization by CT requires delayed imaging >24–48 hours after stroke onset) may be interpreted as being of embolic origin, of cardiac provenance, or as originating from a brain-supplying artery (24). Patients without evidence of an acute lesion, mainly with TIAs (symptoms lasting <24 hours) will be missed in this situation.

As discussed above, the imaging-based identification of embolic strokes without any further findings related to an embolic aetiology may be a result of either cardiac or an arterio-arterial embolization. However, in young stroke victims without vascular risk factors, an occult atrial fibrillation appears more likely. Nevertheless, clinicians should be aware of this uncertainty, especially when experiencing a stroke of undetermined aetiology with an embolic pattern in the brain imaging. This situation does not automatically link to a specific treatment regimen. Several studies investigated different treatment approaches in ESUS, mainly aiming at proving the benefit of using new oral anticoagulants (40, 41). They will provide further information regarding the best treatment strategy in ESUS.

Undetermined aetiology, when two or more evident causes are detected

Using the label of undetermined aetiology for patients with two or more possible causes for stroke is confusing. However, for these patients the TOAST classification does not provide further characterization. Many of these patients possesses a pronounced vascular burden, so in the majority of the cases two aetiologies related to vascular risk factors (LAA, CE, SAD) compete for the diagnosis. Even if approaches for determining the likelihood for each individual aetiology were developed, they may not adjust entirely the uncertainty in establishing one of them (15). Differentiating between strokes caused by SAD and cerebrovascular events due to LAA or CE, the interpretation of findings in the brain imaging would help in settling a definitive diagnosis (15). However, clinicians will probably process this information prior to this question arising, so this condition might be an exceptional situation.

However, even after extensive clinical evaluation or other supportive tools for facilitating the final decision in such controversial situations, the actual diagnosis is at the clinician's discretion. If in doubt, documenting the uncertainty would be more reasonable as compared to potentially establishing a false diagnosis. For this purpose, classifying these patients in their own category rather than subsuming them in the undetermined class would be more satisfactory.

Unclear aetiology due to insufficient workup

There is a variety of reasons for an insufficient diagnostic workup in stroke patients. In part this might be due to the patient refusing examinations, other factors such as the availability of diagnostic procedures, timing of examinations, or poor local standards could also hinder a comprehensive workup. However, the latest evidence suggests that a minimum standard of diagnostics is required to rule out aetiologies potentially causative for strokes in young adults (Table 3.3) (20, 24). In these patients, causes such as dissections, Fabry disease, hypercoagulable states, or other uncommon causes will be identified

Table 3.3 Requirements in the stroke workup in young adults, for ensuring a reliable detection of pathologies related to vascular risk factors

Workup	Required procedure	Additional procedures
Brain imaging	◆ Brain MRI/CT (MRI preferable)	
Vascular imaging	◆ Ultrasound extracranial/intracranial brain arteries (Doppler/duplex)	◆ MR-angiography ◆ CT-angiography ◆ DSA
Cardiac evaluation	◆ 24 h ECG ◆ Transthoracic echocardiography ◆ Transoesophageal echocardiography	◆ Implanted event recorder
Screening for coagulopathies	◆ Deficiencies of protein S, protein C, or antithrombin ◆ Factor V Leiden mutation ◆ Prothrombin gene G20210A mutation ◆ Antiphospholipid syndrome ◆ Other coagulopathies ◆ Pathogenicity for the stroke mechanism for all coagulopathies remains the physician's appreciation	
Diagnostics for other uncommon causes	◆ Specific procedures required, according to the physician's appreciation	

before they are assigned as differential diagnoses. Most promising would be diagnostics for unveiling aetiologies related to vascular risk factors (LAA, CE, and SAD); they would imply the performance of routine diagnostic procedures such as ultrasound studies of the brain-supplying arteries, brain imaging, or cardiac rhythm analysis including electrocardiograms. Epidemiological studies revealed a considerable vascular burden with high proportions of hypertension, diabetes, and hypercholesterolaemia in stroke patients with insufficient workup, suggesting in many of them that conventional aetiologies (including LAA, CE, or SAD) most likely caused the event (20). In this context, more educational programmes and mandatory guidelines containing minimum standards for the evaluation of stroke aetiologies might minimize the proportion of patients with poor diagnostic workup. Minimum standards in the aetiological workup should include procedures for detecting frequent causes for stroke in this age category. The extent might be determined by the availability of diagnostic procedures as well as financial limitations.

Paradoxical embolism across a PFO: an undetermined aetiology?

In stroke patients with a detected PFO with no other potential causes for their ischaemic stroke, the proposed pathomechanism is paradoxical embolism. The pathogenicity of a PFO in the scope of embolism remains uncertain, as a PFO is a common finding in many healthy individuals (42). In few cases the paradoxical embolism might be directly visualized while performing a transoesophageal echocardiography. Hence, in the majority of cases the mechanism of a paradoxical embolism is eventually a suspected pathology. Different conditions increase the likelihood for the occurrence of paradoxical embolism; therefore findings which indicate an increased venous thromboembolic activity may sustain this proposed mechanism. In this context, the evidence for deep vein thrombosis or pulmonary embolism, presenting concomitant to the cerebrovascular event, is of high relevance (43). Conditions known for triggering the occurrence of venous thromboembolic events (e.g. long-distance flights) as well as the detection of an embolic pattern in the brain imaging may also underline paradoxical embolism as potentially responsible for the cerebrovascular event.

The classification of a suspected paradoxical embolism as a cardioembolic event should be avoided. Albeit an embolic entity, the paradoxical embolism is underscored by a mechanism that differs fundamentally from the genuine embolization from a cardiac source. The latter is a result of a primary cardiac pathology with a consecutive development of thrombotic aggregates, whereas in paradoxical embolism, the heart serves only as a component of the vascular system enabling the right-to-left shunt. Although the most often detected right-to-left shunting is as a result of a PFO, shunting can occur at any level in the vascular system, enabling the passage of venous thrombotic material into the arterial system (44). The mechanism of paradoxical embolism in an aetiological classification should be addressed in a general manner and as its own class rather than being focused only on a PFO. Factors which may enforce the suspected pathophysiology of a paradoxical embolism need specific consideration when classifying cerebrovascular events related to paradoxical embolism.

Revised and adapted classification for young strokes

In this chapter, we aimed to assess the present evidence supporting stroke subtyping in young patients and reassemble all information for an adapted classification. Due to the broad variation in clinical practice as well as in research, the TOAST stroke classification system provides a solid basis for the development of new classifications (7). New approaches such as the ASCO classification are promising, but not highly suitable for vast utilization in clinical practice (19). The implementation of ASCO or other models will always compete with TOAST, a classification with many points of criticism, but in principle, a reasonably straightforward categorization of stroke mechanisms. Therefore, the right approach favours TOAST as a baseline, incorporating its strengths and trying to ameliorate uncertainties.

In the context of young stroke patients, we adapted TOAST to a new classification (Table 3.4), incorporating reliable aspects and improving the handling in uncertain situations. The discretionary utilization of TOAST for classifying aetiologies related to vascular risk factors (LAA, CE, and SAD) is suitable and it addresses a considerable proportion of young patients (3, 4). As demonstrated in several studies, the younger the patients, the higher the likelihood that aetiologies related to vascular risk factors decreases (5). However, with decreasing age the relevance of uncommon stroke causes increases (5). Despite intensive workup, in many young stroke patients the stroke mechanism remains uncertain. Therefore, the TOAST category of undetermined aetiology captures a considerable proportion of patients. In this context, we propose only those strokes which remain pure cryptogenic should be allocated to this category. Patients with insufficient stroke workup and those with two competing aetiologies should be addressed in a specific manner as their own categories. Also, patients with suspected paradoxical embolism should be addressed separately, rather than being classified as either cardioembolic or undetermined aetiology. The outline of the revised TOAST classification adapted for young strokes patients is presented in Table 3.4.

Table 3.4 Stroke subtypes according to TOAST adapted for young strokes

	Stroke subtype	Definition
Sufficient workup*	Large artery atherosclerosis (LAA)	Imaging findings of abnormality of either significant (<50%) stenosis or occlusion of a major brain artery or branch of a cortical artery, presumably due to atherosclerosis
	Small artery disease (SAD)	Clinical lacunar syndromes without evidence of cerebral cortical dysfunction. Or imaging evidence of a relevant acute infarction <20 mm within the territory of basal or brainstem-penetrating arteries in the absence of any other pathology in the parent artery at the site of the origin of the penetrating artery
	Cardioembolism (CE)	Major risk for cardioembolism: ♦ Permanent or paroxysmal atrial fibrillation ♦ Sustained atrial flutter ♦ Intracardiac thrombus ♦ Sick sinus syndrome ♦ Recent myocardial infarction ♦ Atrial myxoma or other cardiac tumours ♦ Infectious endocarditis ♦ Valvular vegetations ♦ Congestive heart failure ♦ Prosthetic cardiac valve ♦ Mitral stenosis
	Paradoxical embolism related to PFO or other venous–arterial shunting	
	Likely	Evidence for a right-to-left shunting and the concomitant evidence for either pulmonary embolism or deep vein thrombosis or thrombus detected within a patent foramen ovale or conditions known for facilitating the occurrence of venous embolic events (e.g. long-distance flights) preceding or associated with the cerebrovascular event *or* Evidence for a non-lacunar stroke (see definition below) in the brain imaging CT/MRI (preferable MRI)
	Possible	The single evidence for a right-to-left shunting without the direct evidence or factors associated with an increased venous thrombotic activity as indicated above
	Other determined causes (OD)	See Table 3.2
	Two or more possible causes	The presence of >1 evident mechanism

(continued)

Table 3.4 Continued

	Stroke subtype	Definition
	Undetermined aetiology	No obvious aetiology after sufficient workup
	Without ischaemic brain lesion in the CT/MRI (preferably MRI)	No evidence for a lesion indicating an acute brain ischaemia
	Lacunar ischaemic lesion in the brain CT/MRI (preferably MRI) (non-ESUS)	A lacunar lesion is defined as a single subcortical infarct ≤1.5 cm (≤2.0 cm on MRI diffusion images) in largest dimension and in the distribution of the small/penetrating cerebral arteries. Visualization by CT usually needs delayed imaging greater than 24–48 h after the stroke onset
	Non-lacunar ischaemic lesion/lesions in the CT/MRI (preferably MRI) (ESUS)	*Non-lacunar infarcts* are defined as any lesion involving the cortex or one or more lesions >1.5 cm (>2 cm if detected by MRI diffusion-weighted imaging) in largest diameter when detected exclusively subcortical Visualization by CT usually needs delayed imaging greater than 24–48 h after the stroke onset
Insufficient workup*	**Unclear aetiology**	Allocating aetiology is not possible due to insufficient workup

CE, cardioembolism; LAA, large artery atherosclerosis; OD, other determined aetiology; SAD, small artery disease; UND, undetermined aetiology.

* Criteria for sufficient workup are indicated in Table 3.3.

To summarize, classifying strokes is a procedure used to categorize patients into subgroups of similar/comparable aetiologies. In comparison to a general stroke population, mechanisms in young stroke patients are not characterized by a specific pathology, but the proportion of the different subgroups may be different. In this context, specific aetiologies should be addressed separately instead of summarizing them in generic classes. The proposed classification allows a more concise insight within the different stroke causes. It may be useful for educational programmes as well as for selecting the appropriate patients for clinical studies. Our classification for young stroke patients does not urge a specific therapeutic regimen within each class. Decisions regarding therapy are guided by other factors rather than simply a stroke subtype classification.

References

1. **Carolei A, Marini C, Ferranti E, Frontoni M, Prencipe M, Fieschi C.** A prospective study of cerebral ischemia in the young. Analysis of pathogenic determinants. The National Research Council Study Group. Stroke. 1993;**24**(3):362–67.

2. **Rolfs A**, **Bottcher T**, **Zschiesche M**, **Morris P**, **Winchester B**, **Bauer P**, et al. Prevalence of Fabry disease in patients with cryptogenic stroke: a prospective study. Lancet. 2005;**366**(9499):1794–96.

3. **Putaala J**, **Metso AJ**, **Metso TM**, **Konkola N**, **Kraemer Y**, **Haapaniemi E**, et al. Analysis of 1008 consecutive patients aged 15 to 49 with first-ever ischemic stroke: the Helsinki young stroke registry. Stroke. 2009;**40**(4):1195–203.

4. **Yesilot Barlas N.**, **Putaala J**, **Waje-Andreassen U**, **Vassilopoulou S**, **Nardi K**, **Odier C**, et al. Etiology of first-ever ischaemic stroke in European young adults: the 15 cities young stroke study. Eur J Neurol. 2013;**20**(11):1431–39.

5. **Rolfs A**, **Fazekas F**, **Grittner U**, **Dichgans M**, **Martus P**, **Holzhausen M**, et al. Acute cerebrovascular disease in the young: the Stroke in Young Fabry Patients study. Stroke. 2013;**44**(2):340–49.

6. **Tanislav C**, **Grittner U**, **Fazekas F**, **Thijs V**, **Tatlisumak T**, **Huber R**, et al. Frequency and predictors of acute ischaemic lesions on brain magnetic resonance imaging in young patients with a clinical diagnosis of transient ischaemic attack. Eur J Neurol. 2016;**23**(7):1174–82.

7. **Adams HP, Jr.**, **Bendixen BH**, **Kappelle LJ**, **Biller J**, **Love BB**, **Gordon DL**, et al. Classification of subtype of acute ischemic stroke. Definitions for use in a multicenter clinical trial. TOAST. Trial of Org 10172 in Acute Stroke Treatment. Stroke. 1993;**24**(1):35–41.

8. **Crichton S**, **Barratt B**, **Spiridou A**, **Hoang U**, **Liang SF**, **Kovalchuk Y**, et al. Associations between exhaust and non-exhaust particulate matter and stroke incidence by stroke subtype in South London. Sci Total Environ. 2016;**568**:278–84.

9. **Heuschmann PU.** Incidence of stroke in Europe at the beginning of the 21st century. Stroke. 2009;**40**(5):1557–63.

10. **Ois A**, **Cuadrado-Godia E**, **Rodriguez-Campello A**, **Giralt-Steinhauer E**, **Jimenez-Conde J**, **Lopez-Cuina M**, et al. Relevance of stroke subtype in vascular risk prediction. Neurology. 2013;**81**(6):575–80.

11. **Kolominsky-Rabas PL**, **Weber M**, **Gefeller O**, **Neundoerfer B**, **Heuschmann PU.** Epidemiology of ischemic stroke subtypes according to TOAST criteria: incidence, recurrence, and long-term survival in ischemic stroke subtypes: a population-based study. Stroke. 2001;**32**(12):2735–40.

12. **Connolly SJ**, **Ezekowitz MD**, **Yusuf S**, **Eikelboom J**, **Oldgren J**, **Parekh A**, et al. Dabigatran versus warfarin in patients with atrial fibrillation. N Engl J Med. 2009;**361**(12):1139–51.

13. **Hankey GJ**, **Patel MR**, **Stevens SR**, **Becker RC**, **Breithardt G**, **Carolei A**, et al. Rivaroxaban compared with warfarin in patients with atrial fibrillation and previous stroke or transient ischaemic attack: a subgroup analysis of ROCKET AF. Lancet Neurol. 2012;**11**(4):315–22.

14. **Sacco RL**, **Diener HC**, **Yusuf S**, **Cotton D**, **Ounpuu S**, **Lawton WA**, et al. Aspirin and extended-release dipyridamole versus clopidogrel for recurrent stroke. N Engl J Med. 2008;**359**(12):1238–51.

15. **Ay H**, **Furie KL**, **Singhal A**, **Smith WS**, **Sorensen AG**, **Koroshetz WJ.** An evidence-based causative classification system for acute ischemic stroke. Ann Neurol. 2005;**58**(5):688–97.

16. **Ay H**, **Benner T**, **Arsava EM**, **Furie KL**, **Singhal AB**, **Jensen MB**, et al. A computerized algorithm for etiologic classification of ischemic stroke: the Causative Classification of Stroke System. Stroke. 2007;**38**(11):2979–84.

17. McArdle PF, Kittner SJ, Ay H, Brown RD, Jr., Meschia JF, Rundek T, et al. Agreement between TOAST and CCS ischemic stroke classification: the NINDS SiGN study. Neurology. 2014;**83**(18):1653–60.

18. Amarenco P, Bogousslavsky J, Caplan LR, Donnan GA, Wolf ME, Hennerici MG. The ASCOD phenotyping of ischemic stroke (updated ASCO phenotyping). Cerebrovasc Dis. 2013;**36**(1):1–5.

19. Amarenco P, Bogousslavsky J, Caplan LR, Donnan GA, Hennerici MG. New approach to stroke subtyping: the A-S-C-O (phenotypic) classification of stroke. Cerebrovasc Dis. 2009;**27**(5):502–8.

20. Li L, Yiin GS, Geraghty OC, Schulz UG, Kuker W, Mehta Z, et al. Incidence, outcome, risk factors, and long-term prognosis of cryptogenic transient ischaemic attack and ischaemic stroke: a population-based study. Lancet Neurol. 2015;**14**(9):903–13.

21. Spengos K, Vemmos K. Risk factors, etiology, and outcome of first-ever ischemic stroke in young adults aged 15 to 45 - the Athens young stroke registry. Eur J Neurol. 2010;**17**(11):1358–64.

22. Cerrato P, Grasso M, Imperiale D, Priano L, Baima C, Giraudo M, et al. Stroke in young patients: etiopathogenesis and risk factors in different age classes. Cerebrovasc Dis. 2004;**18**(2):154–59.

23. Rasura M, Spalloni A, Ferrari M, De CS, Patella R, Lisi F, et al. A case series of young stroke in Rome. Eur J Neurol. 2006;**13**(2):146–52.

24. Hart RG, Diener HC, Coutts SB, Easton JD, Granger CB, O'Donnell MJ, et al. Embolic strokes of undetermined source: the case for a new clinical construct. Lancet Neurol. 2014;**13**(4):429–38.

25. Tanislav C, Grittner U, Misselwitz B, Jungehuelsing GJ, Enzinger C, von SB, et al. Lessons from everyday stroke care for clinical research and vice versa: comparison of a comprehensive and a research population of young stroke patients. BMC Neurol. 2014;**14**:45.

26. Kolominsky-Rabas PL, Wiedmann S, Weingartner M, Liman TG, Endres M, Schwab S, et al. Time trends in incidence of pathological and etiological stroke subtypes during 16 years: the Erlangen Stroke Project. Neuroepidemiology. 2015;**44**(1):24–29.

27. Pezzini A, Grassi M, Lodigiani C, Patella R, Gandolfo C, Casoni F, et al. Predictors of migraine subtypes in young adults with ischemic stroke: the Italian project on stroke in young adults. Stroke. 2011;**42**(1):17–21.

28. Smajlovic D, Salihovic D, Ibrahimagic OC, Sinanovic O. Characteristics of stroke in young adults in Tuzla Canton, Bosnia and Herzegovina. Coll Antropol. 2013;**37**(2):515–19.

29. Tancredi L, Martinelli BF, Braga M, Santilli I, Scaccabarozzi C, Lattuada P, et al. Stroke care in young patients. Stroke Res Treat. 2013;**2013**:715380.

30. Varona JF, Guerra JM, Bermejo F, Molina JA, Gomez de la CA. Causes of ischemic stroke in young adults, and evolution of the etiological diagnosis over the long term. Eur Neurol. 2007;**57**(4):212–18.

31. Jovanovic DR, Beslac-Bumbasirevic L, Raicevic R, Zidverc-Trajkovic J, Ercegovac MD. Etiology of ischemic stroke among young adults of Serbia. Vojnosanit Pregl. 2008;**65**(11):803–809.

32. Hallemeier CL, Rich KM, Grubb RL, Jr., Chicoine MR, Moran CJ, Cross DT, III, et al. Clinical features and outcome in North American adults with moyamoya phenomenon. Stroke. 2006;**37**(6):1490–96.

33. **Kraemer M**, **Heienbrok W**, **Berlit P.** Moyamoya disease in Europeans. Stroke. 2008;**39**(12):3193–200.

34. **Liu W**, **Xu G**, **Liu X.** Neuroimaging diagnosis and the collateral circulation in moyamoya disease. Interv Neurol. 2013;**1**(2):77–86.

35. **Bousser MG**, **Welch KM.** Relation between migraine and stroke. Lancet Neurol. 2005;**4**(9):533–42.

36. **Brey RL.** Antiphospholipid antibodies in young adults with stroke. J Thromb Thrombolysis. 2005;**20**(2):105–12.

37. **Onwuchekwa AC**, **Onwuchekwa RC**, **Asekomeh EG.** Stroke in young Nigerian adults. J Vasc Nurs. 2009;**27**(4):98–102.

38. **Tatlisumak T**, **Putaala J**, **Innila M**, **Enzinger C**, **Metso TM**, **Curtze S**, et al. Frequency of MELAS main mutation in a phenotype-targeted young ischemic stroke patient population. J Neurol. 2016;**263**(2):257–62.

39. **Tan RY**, **Markus HS.** CADASIL: migraine, encephalopathy, stroke and their inter-relationships. PLoS One. 2016;**11**(6):e0157613.

40. **Diener HC**, **Easton JD**, **Granger CB**, **Cronin L**, **Duffy C**, **Cotton D**, et al. Design of Randomized, double-blind, Evaluation in secondary Stroke Prevention comparing the EfficaCy and safety of the oral Thrombin inhibitor dabigatran etexilate vs. acetylsalicylic acid in patients with Embolic Stroke of Undetermined Source (RE-SPECT ESUS). Int J Stroke. 2015;**10**(8):1309–12.

41. **Perera KS**, **Vanassche T**, **Bosch J**, **Giruparajah M**, **Swaminathan B**, **Mattina KR**, et al. Embolic strokes of undetermined source: prevalence and patient features in the ESUS Global Registry. Int J Stroke. 2016;**11**(5):526–33.

42. **Hagen PT**, **Scholz DG**, **Edwards WD.** Incidence and size of patent foramen ovale during the first 10 decades of life: an autopsy study of 965 normal hearts. Mayo Clin Proc. 1984;**59**(1):17–20.

43. **Tanislav C**, **Puille M**, **Pabst W**, **Reichenberger F**, **Grebe M**, **Nedelmann M**, et al. High frequency of silent pulmonary embolism in patients with cryptogenic stroke and patent foramen ovale. Stroke. 2011;**42**(3):822–24.

44. **Lochner P**, **Tezzon F**, **Nardone R**, **Tanislav C.** Paradoxical brain embolism caused by an arterial-venous fistula: a diagnostic pitfall. Neurol Sci. 2010;**31**(3):341–43.

Chapter 4

Vascular aetiology

Annette Fromm

Large artery atherosclerosis

Atherosclerosis is a multifactorial, slowly progressing, chronic inflammatory disease, characterized by the development of atherosclerotic lesions (atheroma, plaques) mainly from the innermost layer of the arterial wall, the intima, but secondarily also involving the media and adventitia layers. The disease begins in infancy and progresses with individual variations in time and location through-out lifetime, dependent on cardiovascular risk factors such as hypertension, diabetes, smoking, and genetic predisposition. Its course may be excessive as demonstrated in post-endarterectomy cases and by post-interventional in-stent stenoses. Atherosclerosis affects the entire artery tree, but involves mostly systemic large- and medium-sized arteries, most commonly the aorta, carotid, coronary, and peripheral arteries (1). Atherosclerosis has further been associated with infections. Chronic inflammation leads to multifocal plaque development, mostly asymmetrical and predominantly at bifurcations, branch points, and curvatures of the arterial tree due to flow alterations, whereas straight artery segments often remain spared (2). Inflammation-mediated neovascularization and intraplaque haemorrhage, along with lipid core necrosis and fibrous cap thinning, differentiate the stable from the unstable, vulnerable plaque prone to rupture (3). Plaque rupture preferentially occurs in areas of fibrous cap thinning secondary to inflammatory processes. The presence of features of vulnerability is not necessarily related to a more advanced degree of stenosis.

Atherosclerosis in brain-supplying arteries is the origin of several mechanisms behind ischaemic cerebrovascular events. These include atheroembolism, thromboembolism from atherosclerotic plaque surface, occlusion due to plaque rupture and thrombosis, reduced perfusion distal to steno-occlusive plaques, and dissection or subintimal haematoma (4).

In stroke medicine, the term large artery atherosclerosis (LAA) commonly covers extra- and intracranial brain-supplying arteries histologically categorized as large to medium-sized arteries. Large and medium-sized arteries differ regarding their content of elastic tissue, smooth muscle cell layers, and vasa vasorum. However, a clear definition of which medium-sized arteries in particular are to be counted in the LAA category has not been established.

LAA is an increasing cause of age-related stroke above the age of 45 years (5, 6). Only 4.9% of European ischaemic stroke patients aged 44 or younger had in ultrasound examination stenosis of 50% or greater or occlusion of at least one brain-supplying cervical artery, of which two-thirds were considered symptomatic (7). Non-stenotic plaques were common, particularly in males. LAA as an overall cause of stroke has been diagnosed in 4% of the population aged 18–44 (5). However, depending on the diagnostic workup and the stroke classification system used, the identification of LAA as the cause of stroke differs significantly. There is evidence for symptomatic atherosclerotic disease with low-grade stenosis presenting features of plaque instability, which does not meet mostly rigid stroke classification criteria. Atherosclerotic disease has been suggested to be a relevant contributor to stroke of undetermined cause (8).

In intracranial arteries, the prevalence of large artery stenosis differs widely across ethnicities, being highest in Asian populations (9). In Europe, supratentorial intracranial stenosis or occlusion was identified in 10.8% of ischaemic stroke patients younger than 45 years compared to 15.5% of middle-aged patients (45–55 years), of which 8.8% and 11.2% respectively were evaluated as symptomatic (7).

Carotid artery disease

The bifurcation, sinus, and siphon are the carotid artery segments most prone to atherosclerosis (Fig. 4.1), regardless of ethnicity, gender, and age (10). Most clinical decision-making is based on the degree of stenosis. However, the correlation between the degree of stenosis and ischaemic events is not entirely consistent. Other lesion characteristics, such as molecular and cellular processes responsible for plaque composition, have therefore been suggested as potential markers of plaque vulnerability which has an impact on stroke risk.

The majority of infarcts caused by carotid artery disease are of an embolic nature arising from unstable plaque rupture, ulceration, and atheroembolism, or from atherothrombosis and thromboembolism. Embolism from cardiac or more proximal arterial sources has to be considered. Traditionally postulated haemodynamic insufficiency distally to high-grade carotid stenosis or occlusion is probably the mechanism of cerebral infarction in only a small percentage of ischaemic strokes. External watershed infarcts in border zones between the anterior and the middle cerebral artery circulation and between the middle and the posterior cerebral artery circulation may actually be caused by embolism, while internal watershed infarcts in the centrum ovale area may be predominantly true haemodynamic infarcts (11). Carotid artery disease further occurs frequently in association with underlying non-atherosclerotic conditions such as dissections or—more rarely—disorders such as fibromuscular dysplasia,

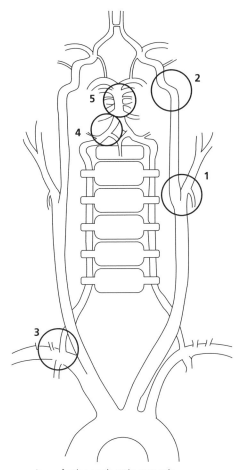

Fig. 4.1 Most common sites of atherosclerotic stenosis.
1. Carotid bifurcation and sinus
2. Carotid siphon
3. Vertebral artery origin, proximal portion and Subclavian artery
4. Intradural vertebral artery
5. Basilar artery

direct tumour infiltration, or secondary arterial disease, for example, subsequent to radiation therapy.

Stroke symptoms vary widely and depend on the size of the thromboembolic clot, the location and size of the endangered artery, and the location and size of the endangered brain area. The extent of the infarcted area depends on the anatomical location of the occlusion and on the sufficiency of existing collateral pathways. The most devastating carotid strokes are due to 'carotid-T occlusion' including the proximal middle and anterior cerebral artery (e.g. due to anterograde thrombosis), leaving brain perfusion to a retrograde collateral supply via border zone arteries over the convexity of the brain. Catastrophic strokes are further due to occlusion of the distal internal carotid proximal to an incomplete circle of Willis and distal to or involving the branching of the ophthalmic artery. The lack of collateral supply via the anterior and/or the posterior communicating artery and via the ophthalmic artery results in severe hypoperfusion.

Transient monocular blindness (amaurosis fugax) is frequently caused by small particles (cholesterol crystals, platelet complexes, calcium emboli) occluding minor retinal vessels. Concurrent hemispheric symptoms are rare due to small embolus size, and vision is usually completely restored after an attack. The 2-year risk of stroke due to high-grade carotid stenosis (>70%) was found to be threefold higher for patients with initial hemispheric transient ischaemic attack (TIA) (43.5%) compared to retinal TIA (16.6%) in the North American Symptomatic Carotid Endarterectomy Trial (NASCET). Transient monocular blindness is not to be confused with migrainous sensations, which frequently appear with colourful or flashing light events.

In the European general population, the prevalence of asymptomatic moderate (≥50%) and severe (≥70%) atherosclerotic carotid stenosis has recently been estimated to be 0.2% and 0.1% respectively in males, and 0% for both degrees of stenosis in females aged 50 years or younger. The prevalence increases with age and the number of risk factors (12). Overall, severe asymptomatic carotid artery stenosis has been associated with an annual stroke risk of 2–5% (13).

However, angiographic abnormalities are common in young ischaemic stroke patients (14, 15). A large, multinational European young stroke study based on ultrasound imaging recently reported an overall prevalence of atherosclerotic carotid artery stenosis of 50% and above and occlusion in 4.9% of patients aged 18–44 years (3.4% symptomatic), and in 11.0% of those aged 45–55 years (9.2% symptomatic) (7). Overall, extracranial carotid artery disease was detected in 9.5% of patients aged 18–44, and in 27.6% of those aged 45–55, reflecting the contributing role of premature atherosclerosis to early-onset stroke (16). Non-stenotic plaques were observed more frequently among males and middle-aged patients (7). Further, increased carotid intima–media thickness as a marker of atherosclerotic disease is common among young and middle-aged ischaemic stroke patients (17). Besides the risk of death due to stroke, patients with asymptomatic carotid stenosis have an even greater risk of vascular death due to myocardial infarction (18).

Vertebrobasilar artery disease

Vertebrobasilar disease is most commonly caused by atherosclerosis, influenced by gender and race, and associated with multiple ischaemic episodes and a high risk of early recurrent stroke (19). Vertebral artery atherosclerosis accounts for approximately 20% of all posterior circulation strokes (20). However, it is less frequent than carotid artery atherosclerosis. The subclavian artery, the origin and the most proximal portion of the extracranial vertebral artery, the intradural vertebral artery, and the basilar artery are most frequently affected (Fig. 4.1). Anterior and posterior circulation atherosclerosis do not necessarily coexist. Thrombotic processes may be—but are not only—formed at the site of pre-existing atherosclerotic lesions. Thrombus extension from the intracranial vertebral artery into the basilar artery is common. Artery-to-artery or cardiac embolism mostly leads to occlusive disease at the top of the basilar, in the posterior cerebral arteries, or in the distal vertebral arteries, superior cerebellar arteries, and posterior inferior cerebellar arteries. Occlusive vertebrobasilar disease often presents severely, particularly when intracranial arteries are involved, and is frequently characterized by clinical fluctuations. Infarction of the brainstem and the cerebellum frequently leads to fatal oedema.

In unilateral extracranial vertebral artery occlusion, a potentially broad collateral supply may derive from cervical branches, from the occipital branch of the external carotid artery, via the circle of Willis and the posterior communicating artery, or from compensation via the contralateral vertebral artery. However, the sufficiency of the collateral supply depends on gradually temporal development of a stenosis. Even in bilateral vertebral artery occlusion, intracranial locations are associated with far more severe clinical presentations than extracranial occlusions which are favoured in their collateral supply.

Subclavian steal phenomenon is caused by stenosis or occlusion of the subclavian or the innominate artery leading to impaired blood flow, blood pressure, and pulse to the affected upper limb, compensated for by various degrees of retrograde 'steal' from the posterior circulation via the ipsilateral vertebral artery. In case of insufficient collateralization, the phenomenon may present with headache, transient symptoms deriving from the originally supplied but eventually hypoperfused region of the brain, or with claudication in the affected arm. However, subclavian steal rarely becomes symptomatic and its prevalence is thus unknown.

Other vascular causes of steno-occlusive vertebrobasilar disease are aneurysms, arterial dissection, fibromuscular dysplasia, and lipohyalinosis—subintimal fat accumulation causing functional occlusion and ischaemic lacunar lesions independently from atherosclerotic disease. Mechanical factors such as compression of the extracranial vertebral artery by cervical spondylosis, trauma, or sudden rotation or manipulation of the neck may cause arterial injury.

In European young ischaemic stroke patients, the frequency of extra- and intracranial vertebrobasilar flow abnormalities was approximately similar to the prevalence of extracranial carotid artery stenosis and occlusion (10.3% vs 9.5%), and more pronounced in patients aged 45–55 years than younger patients (12.1% vs 6.9%) (7).

Intracranial occlusive disease

Intracranial LAA is a major cause of TIA and ischaemic stroke throughout the world, but shows significant ethnological and geographical differences regarding its prevalence (9). Occlusive intracranial disease most often affects medium-sized arteries and their proximal branches (Fig. 4.2): the anterior, middle, and posterior cerebral arteries; the posterior and anterior inferior cerebellar arteries; and the distal basilar artery (21). Among Caucasians, 1–7% of ischaemic strokes have been accredited to intracranial atherosclerosis in US Americans and western Europeans.

However, embolic strokes are far more frequent than stroke caused by intracranial atherosclerotic lesions. The majority of emboli affect the middle cerebral artery territory due to anatomical accessibility and high blood flow volume. Embolus size, composition, and organization determine at which level middle cerebral artery branches are occluded. One single embolus may occlude a major segment, or lead to migration to several serially arranged arteries by dissolution into minor fragments and particles. Without the use of advanced imaging techniques, it usually is not possible to distinguish whether intracranial stenosis or occlusion is caused by embolism, atherosclerosis, thrombosis, thrombosis together with atherosclerosis, dissection, or other entities. However, the documentation of partial or complete recanalization by follow-up studies may rather point to embolic sources or dissection.

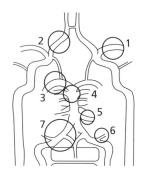

Fig. 4.2 Intracranial atherosclerosis. 1. Middle cerebral artery. 2. Anterior cerebral artery. 3. Posterior cerebral artery. 4. Distal basilar artery. 5. Anterior inferior cerebellar artery. 6. Posterior inferior cerebellar artery. 7. Intradural vertebral artery.

Occlusions in the territories of the anterior cerebral artery and the posterior cerebral artery are much less common. Nevertheless, anterior cerebral artery ischaemia secondary to vasospasm after aneurysmal subarachnoid haemorrhage is not uncommon. The posterior cerebral artery may even be bilaterally involved in a top-of-the-basilar occlusion, either by embolization or anterograde thrombosis. The common anatomical variant of a persisting 'fetal' posterior cerebral artery with its origin from the intracranial internal carotid artery may lead to posterior cerebral artery ischaemia due to embolization from the anterior circulation.

In European young ischaemic stroke patients, 24.1% of those with extracranial internal carotid artery stenosis or occlusion additionally had intracranial stenosis or occlusion (7). Stenosis or occlusion in the intracranial arteries (11.2% and 3.2%, respectively) was overall more common than in the extracranial internal carotid artery (4.2% and 5.2%, respectively). They were mostly related to the middle cerebral artery (12.2%), and were symptomatic in 10.4%. The prevalence of intracranial stenosis increased with age (7). However, to what extent atherosclerosis was the process behind the referred stenoses and occlusions remains uncertain.

Aortic atheroma

Atherosclerotic plaques of the thoracic aorta have attracted attention during the search for sources of cerebral and peripheral embolism. The question is whether aortic atherosclerosis is a risk factor for stroke, a marker of generalized atherosclerosis, or just an innocent parallel bystander. In a community-based study, 51% of randomly selected people aged 45 years or older presented with aortic atheroma, predominantly in the descending part. The presence of atheroma increased with age and vascular risk factors (22). Atheromas in the descending aorta are also more frequently found in stroke patients undergoing transoesophageal echocardiography than in unselected patients, and among stroke patients are associated with extracranial and intracranial atherosclerosis. Diastolic flow reversal and retrograde embolization from complex plaques is assumed to be a mechanism of stroke, but scientific evidence for a true cause-and-effect relationship is currently lacking, and atherosclerosis in the descending aorta so far remains a marker of generalized atherosclerosis and high vascular risk (23). However, ulcerated aortic plaques, including those localized in the ascending or the horizontal aorta, were previously convincingly associated with cerebrovascular events, especially among patients with otherwise unknown cause of stroke (24, 25).

Small vessel disease

Small vessel disease (SVD) affects vessels of the microvasculature. In stroke medicine, the term is usually used for stenosis and occlusion affecting small terminal arteries and arterioles sized less than 400 μm in diameter deriving from the carotid or vertebrobasilar circulation, including the deep penetrating lenticulostriate, thalamoperforating, and paramedian brainstem branches. The cerebral regions supplied are predominantly the deep and central subcortical regions including the caudate nucleus, globus pallidus and putamen, thalamus, internal capsule, centrum semiovale, central brainstem, and cerebellum. Typical entities of SVD are lacunar infarcts due to complete infarction of one single perforating branch, white matter hyperintensities due to incomplete infarction, microbleeds, and various degrees of brain atrophy.

Lacunar infarctions are categorized as strictly subcortical lesions with a diameter of less than 15 mm. However, diagnosis of SVD can be uncertain and may easily be confused with other aetiologies. Microatheroma and hypertension-related lipohyalinosis are probably the most common underlying conditions in the development of SVD, but diabetes mellitus, microembolization, fibrinoid necrosis, amyloid deposition, and arteritis also contribute. Haemodynamic perfusion failure subsequent to more proximal large artery disease is also possible (e.g. in the centrum semiovale). However, the true cause of lacunar-appearing infarction may only be clarified by histopathologic investigation.

Lesions vary from clinically silent infarcts to strategic infarcts affecting cortical functions by disruption of circuits between cortical and subcortical or between different cortical regions. Apart from motor-sensory syndromes, SVD frequently causes a variety of neuropsychological disturbances. Lacunar strokes are strongly predisposing for vascular dementia, and stroke recurrence, symptomatic or silent, pre-existing white matter hyperintensities, infarct volume, and cerebral atrophy, particularly of the medial temporal lobe, have been identified as determinants (26).

About 13.5% of young ischaemic stroke patients in Europe suffer stroke due to SVD (5). However, the prevalence of pre-existing deep and periventricular white matter hyperintensities are associated with age, seen in 6–7% of young stroke patients only from the age of about 45 years, but rare or even absent at younger ages. Microbleeds, assumed markers for and contributors to SVD, are probably rare at young age (27).

Dissections

A majority of ischaemic strokes among young adults arise from cervical artery dissection (CeAD). Dissections occur about twice as often in the carotid arteries compared to the vertebral arteries, and in 13–16% of cases, multiple arteries are affected. The mean patient age for CeAD is 44–46 years, slightly higher in carotid artery dissection than in vertebral artery dissection (28). Dissections typically occur at mobile, not anchored artery courses. Common sites of CeAD are the pharyngeal portion of the internal carotid artery, the movable distal part of the proximal vertebral artery (V1) close to its entrance into the intervertebral foramina at C5 or C6, and the more distal atlas loop (V3). Dissections of the atlas loop can extend into the intracranial (V4) or transforaminal segment (V2). Intracranial dissections most commonly occur in the supraclinoid portion of the internal carotid artery, the proximal middle cerebral artery (M1), and the intracranial vertebral artery segment (V4), frequently involving the basilar artery (Fig. 4.3) (29).

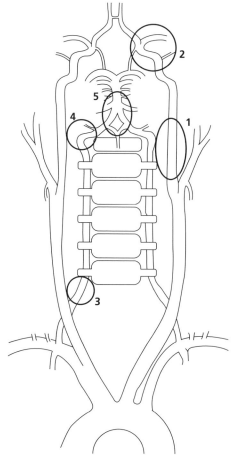

Fig. 4.3 Most common sites of dissection.
1. Pharyngeal carotid artery
2. Supraclinoid carotid artery and proximal middle cerebral artery
3. Distal extraforaminal vertebral artery
4. Atlas loop
5. Intracranial vertebral artery and proximal basilar artery

CeAD is a heterogeneous and multifactorial disease. Cervical trauma including sport activities and cervical manipulation, recent infection, and genetic factors probably play roles in pathogenesis (30). Associations with, for example, vasculopathies, connective tissue abnormalities, intracranial aneurysms, hyperhomocysteinaemia, and migraine have been discussed. The relevance of vascular risk factors is still unclear, but associations with hypertension, smoking, and inverse associations with overweight and hypercholesterolaemia have been suggested (31).

CeAD secondary to intimal tear or rupture of the vasa vasorum leads to mural haematoma in the arterial wall, causing compression or occlusion of the arterial lumen (subintimal dissection), or segmental aneurysmal dilation (subadventitial dissection). Local symptoms as headache, neck pain, Horner's syndrome, cranial nerve palsy (IX, X, XII), tinnitus, and cervical root palsy are attributable to mechanisms such as artery distension, sympathetic nerve or cranial nerve stretching, and cervical root compression. They frequently precede embolic ischaemic events from the intimal tear or haemodynamic events due to high-grade stenosis within a few minutes to several weeks. Involvement of intracranial arteries may lead to pseudoaneurysm formation, rupture, and subarachnoid haemorrhage because of their more vulnerable anatomical construction. Further, carotid artery dissection may lead to retinal ischaemia and vertebral artery dissection may cause cervical spinal cord infarcts. However, a considerable number of CeADs and intracranial dissections remain undiagnosed due to only subtle, misleading, or even asymptomatic clinical manifestation.

CeAD was recently diagnosed as causative in 10.4% of young European stroke patients, with equal frequencies of carotid artery dissection and vertebral artery dissection (32). However, CeAD is rarely known at the time of acute stroke treatment aiming at immediate recanalization. But intravenous recombinant tissue plasminogen activator thrombolysis has similar safety and efficacy in CeAD as in other causes of ischaemic stroke. Also, endovascular procedures, including intra-arterial thrombolysis, mechanical clot extraction, and stenting, may be indicated (33). There is no evidence for superiority of either anticoagulant or antiplatelet therapy in prevention of stroke or death after CeAD (34).

Recurrence rates of dissections and ischaemic events are low. Mortality rates are probably less than 5%. Yet, incidence and outcome estimations may be diffused by a lack of early diagnosis in malignant fatal infarctions, or the lack of diagnosis in the large number of patients with no, minor, or only local symptoms. Normalization and stabilization of the dissected artery should be achieved before resuming activities involving forced or sudden head movements (30).

Dolichoectasia

Dolichoectasia (DE) is common in elderly patients, but cases are also reported from the age of 3 months, and associations with disorders more typical for young populations have been suggested. DE is characterized by elongation, sometimes tortuosity and/or dilatation of at least one cerebral artery due to outward remodelling. Single segments or entire arteries may be affected, and spanning across bifurcations is possible.

Pathophysiology probably involves biological, anatomical, and haemo-dynamic features. Rarefication of elastic tissue and fragmentation of the elastic lamina in the medial layer have been described (35). Vascular risk factors, imbalance of metalloproteinases, metabolic lysosomal storage disorders (e.g. Fabry disease, Pompe disease), and alterations of elastic fibres (e.g. in Marfan syndrome and tortuosity syndrome) may influence medial layer components (36). The degree of connectivity between the anterior and the posterior circulation may be associated with flow and diameter in the latter. Thus, atherosclerosis in the anterior circulation or an insufficient circle of Willis may partly explain the coexistence with DE in the posterior circulation (37). Associations with ischaemic cardiac disease and aortic aneurysms have also been described.

DE may present with cerebral infarction, TIA or cerebral haemorrhage, cranial nerve, brainstem, or third ventricle compression, subarachnoid haemorrhage due to rupture of dolichoectatic arteries, or DE may even be asymptomatic. Mechanical traction, kinking, and occlusion of penetrating arteries may be stroke mechanisms, but also thrombosis or artery-to-artery embolization. Cerebral infarctions are rather distally distributed, for example, in the thalamus, midbrain, or occipital lobes, or present with lacunar infarcts and white matter hyperintensities (38).

The prevalence of DE has been estimated to 12% in all-age stroke populations, with the basilar artery as the most frequently reported location in 80%. Diagnostic criteria for basilar artery DE include a diameter greater than 4.5 mm, and considerations regarding the laterality of its course and the height of the bifurcation on computed tomography scan. For the anterior circulation, no validated diagnostic criteria are available to date.

Vascular comorbidity

Atherosclerosis is the main cause of *coronary heart disease* (CHD) (39). In European young ischaemic stroke and TIA patients, CHD has been found in 4.2% and established myocardial infarction in 3.1% at the time of the index event (40). A composite prevalence of CHD and myocardial infarction among young ischaemic stroke patients has been reported for 6.0% in data derived from 15 European stroke centres (41). Further, acute coronary disease is associated with recurrent arterial events and vascular death after ischaemic stroke, leading to significantly higher mortality among young stroke patients compared to matching controls over time (42).

The prevalence of *peripheral artery disease* (PAD) is dependent on age, risk factor profile, and concomitant manifestations of atherosclerotic disease at other sites. Clinical symptoms of PAD vary, and the disease is frequently under-diagnosed. PAD guidelines suggest PAD in general to be asymptomatic in 20–50%, or presenting with atypical leg pain in 30–40%, with typical claudication in 10–35%, and with critical ischaemia in 1–3% (43).

In European young ischaemic stroke patients, PAD was prevalent in 2.2% (40). Further, the presence of PAD was identified as one of the strongest predictors of 5-year mortality (44).

Cerebrovascular disease, CHD, and PAD together account for 4.35 million deaths, 49% of all deaths in Europe each year (45). All three have serious implications for morbidity (Fig. 4.4) and mortality (46). One-year event rates increase with the number of symptomatic arterial disease sites (47), suggesting thorough vascular investigation to be necessary in deciding further preventive treatment. Among patients with atrial fibrillation, atherosclerotic vascular disease (e.g. PAD, aortic atheroma, and myocardial infarction) are predictors of stroke, thromboembolism, and mortality (48).

Despite its impact, there are, to date, no sufficient prospective data available regarding generalized atherosclerotic disease in all major vascular beds in young ischaemic stroke populations.

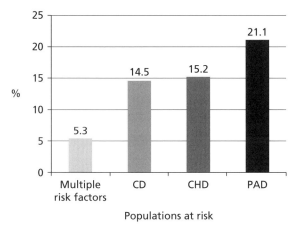

Fig. 4.4 Cardiovascular events within 1 year of diagnosis in patients with multiple risk factors, cerebrovascular disease (CD), coronary heart disease (CHD), and peripheral arterial disease (PAD).

Source: data from JAMA, 297(11), Steg PG, Bhatt DL, Wilson PW, D'Agostino R, Sr., Ohman EM, Rother J, et al. One-year cardiovascular event rates in outpatients with atherothrombosis, pp. 1197–206, Copyright (2007), American Medical Association.

References

1. **Corti R, Fuster V.** Imaging of atherosclerosis: magnetic resonance imaging. Eur Heart J. 2011;**32**(14):1709–19.

2. **Warboys CM, Amini N, de Luca A, Evans PC.** The role of blood flow in determining the sites of atherosclerotic plaques. F1000 Med Rep. 2011;**3**:5.

3. **Thim T, Hagensen MK, Bentzon JF, Falk E.** From vulnerable plaque to atherothrombosis. J Intern Med. 2008;**263**(5):506–16.

4. **Brott TG, Halperin JL, Abbara S, Bacharach JM, Barr JD, Bush RL,** et al. 2011 ASA/ ACCF/AHA/AANN/AANS/ACR/ASNR/CNS/SAIP/SCAI/SIR/SNIS/SVM/SVS guideline on the management of patients with extracranial carotid and vertebral artery disease: executive summary: a report of the American College of Cardiology Foundation/American Heart Association Task Force on Practice Guidelines, and the American Stroke Association, American Association of Neuroscience Nurses, American Association of Neurological Surgeons, American College of Radiology, American Society of Neuroradiology, Congress of Neurological Surgeons, Society of Atherosclerosis Imaging and Prevention, Society for Cardiovascular Angiography and Interventions, Society of Interventional Radiology, Society of NeuroInterventional Surgery, Society for Vascular Medicine, and Society for Vascular Surgery. Catheter Cardiovasc Interv. 2013;**81**(1):E76–123.

5. **Rolfs A, Fazekas F, Grittner U, Dichgans M, Martus P, Holzhausen M,** et al. Acute cerebrovascular disease in the young: the Stroke in Young Fabry Patients study. Stroke. 2013;**44**(2):340–49.

6. **Putaala J, Metso AJ, Metso TM, Konkola N, Kraemer Y, Haapaniemi E,** et al. Analysis of 1008 consecutive patients aged 15 to 49 with first-ever ischemic stroke: the Helsinki young stroke registry. Stroke. 2009;**40**(4):1195–203.

7. **von Sarnowski B, Schminke U, Tatlisumak T, Putaala J, Grittner U, Kaps M,** et al. Prevalence of stenoses and occlusions of brain-supplying arteries in young stroke patients. Neurology. 2013;**80**(14):1287–94.

8. **Fromm A, Haaland OA, Naess H, Thomassen L, Waje-Andreassen U.** Atherosclerosis in Trial of Org 10172 in Acute Stroke Treatment Subtypes among Young and Middle-Aged Stroke Patients: The Norwegian Stroke in the Young Study. J Stroke Cerebrovasc Dis. 2016;**25**(4):825–30.

9. **Gorelick PB, Wong KS, Bae HJ, Pandey DK.** Large artery intracranial occlusive disease: a large worldwide burden but a relatively neglected frontier. Stroke. 2008;**39**(8):2396–99.

10. **Solberg LA, Eggen DA.** Localization and sequence of development of atherosclerotic lesions in the carotid and vertebral arteries. Circulation. 1971;**43**(5):711–24.

11. **Sorgun MH, Rzayev S, Yilmaz V, Isikay CT.** Etiologic subtypes of watershed infarcts. J Stroke Cerebrovasc Dis. 2015;**24**(11):2478–83.

12. **de Weerd M, Greving JP, Hedblad B, Lorenz MW, Mathiesen EB, O'Leary DH,** et al. Prevalence of asymptomatic carotid artery stenosis in the general population: an individual participant data meta-analysis. Stroke. 2010;**41**(6):1294–97.

13. **Inzitari D, Eliasziw M, Gates P, Sharpe BL, Chan RK, Meldrum HE,** et al. The causes and risk of stroke in patients with asymptomatic internal-carotid-artery stenosis. North American Symptomatic Carotid Endarterectomy Trial Collaborators. N Engl J Med. 2000;**342**(23):1693–700.

14. **Adams HP, Jr., Kappelle LJ, Biller J, Gordon DL, Love BB, Gomez F,** et al. Ischemic stroke in young adults. Experience in 329 patients enrolled in the Iowa Registry of stroke in young adults. Arch Neurol. 1995;**52**(5):491–95.

15. **Ji R, Schwamm LH, Pervez MA, Singhal AB.** Ischemic stroke and transient ischemic attack in young adults: risk factors, diagnostic yield, neuroimaging, and thrombolysis. JAMA Neurol. 2013;**70**(1):51–57.

16. **Kittner SJ, Singhal AB.** Premature atherosclerosis: A major contributor to early-onset ischemic stroke. Neurology. 2013;**80**(14):1272–73.

17. **Fromm A, Haaland OA, Naess H, Thomassen L, Waje-Andreassen U.** Risk factors and their impact on carotid intima-media thickness in young and middle-aged ischemic stroke patients and controls: the Norwegian Stroke in the Young Study. BMC Res Notes. 2014;**7**:176.

18. **Norris JW, Zhu CZ, Bornstein NM, Chambers BR.** Vascular risks of asymptomatic carotid stenosis. Stroke. 1991;**22**(12):1485–90.

19. **Marquardt L, Kuker W, Chandratheva A, Geraghty O, Rothwell PM.** Incidence and prognosis of > or = 50% symptomatic vertebral or basilar artery stenosis: prospective population-based study. Brain. 2009;**132**(Pt 4):982–88.

20. **Wehman JC, Hanel RA, Guidot CA, Guterman LR, Hopkins LN.** Atherosclerotic occlusive extracranial vertebral artery disease: indications for intervention, endovascular techniques, short-term and long-term results. J Interv Cardiol. 2004;**17**(4):219–32.

21. **Caplan LR, Gorelick PB, Hier DB.** Race, sex and occlusive cerebrovascular disease: a review. Stroke. 1986;**17**(4):648–55.

22. **Agmon Y, Khandheria BK, Meissner I, Schwartz GL, Petterson TM, O'Fallon WM,** et al. Relation of coronary artery disease and cerebrovascular disease with atherosclerosis of the thoracic aorta in the general population. Am J Cardiol. 2002;**89**(3):262–67.

23. **Katsanos AH, Giannopoulos S, Kosmidou M, Voumvourakis K, Parissis JT, Kyritsis AP,** et al. Complex atheromatous plaques in the descending aorta and the risk of stroke: a systematic review and meta-analysis. Stroke. 2014;**45**(6):1764–70.

24. **Guidoux C, Mazighi M, Lavallée P, Labreuche J, Meseguer E, Cabrejo L,** et al. Aortic arch atheroma in transient ischemic attack patients. Atherosclerosis. 2013;**231**(1):124–28.

25. **Amarenco P, Röther J, Michel P, Davis SM, Donnan GA.** Aortic arch atheroma and the risk of stroke. Curr Atheroscler Rep. 2006;**8**(4):343–46.

26. **Pohjasvaara T, Mantyla R, Salonen O, Aronen HJ, Ylikoski R, Hietanen M,** et al. How complex interactions of ischemic brain infarcts, white matter lesions, and atrophy relate to poststroke dementia. Arch Neurol. 2000;**57**(9):1295–300.

27. **Fazekas F, Enzinger C, Schmidt R, Dichgans M, Gaertner B, Jungehulsing GJ,** et al. MRI in acute cerebral ischemia of the young: the Stroke in Young Fabry Patients (sifap1) Study. Neurology. 2013;**81**(22):1914–21.

28. **Debette S, Grond-Ginsbach C, Bodenant M, Kloss M, Engelter S, Metso T,** et al. Differential features of carotid and vertebral artery dissections: the CADISP study. Neurology. 2011;**77**(12):1174–81.

29. **Caplan LR.** Dissections of brain-supplying arteries. Nat Clin Pract Neurol. 2008;**4**(1):34–42.

30. **Debette S, Leys D.** Cervical-artery dissections: predisposing factors, diagnosis, and outcome. Lancet Neurol. 2009;**8**(7):668–78.

31. **Debette S, Metso T, Pezzini A, Abboud S, Metso A, Leys D**, et al. Association of vascular risk factors with cervical artery dissection and ischemic stroke in young adults. Circulation. 2011;**123**(14):1537–44.

32. **von Sarnowski B, Schminke U, Grittner U, Fazekas F, Tanislav C, Kaps M**, et al. Cervical artery dissection in young adults in the stroke in young Fabry patients (sifap1) study. Cerebrovasc Dis. 2015;**39**(2):110–21.

33. **Arnold M, Fischer U, Bousser MG.** Treatment issues in spontaneous cervicocephalic artery dissections. Int J Stroke. 2011;**6**(3):213–18.

34. **CADISS Trial Investigators, Markus HS, Hayter E, Levi C, Feldman A, Venables G**, et al. Antiplatelet treatment compared with anticoagulation treatment for cervical artery dissection (CADISS): a randomised trial. Lancet Neurol. 2015;**14**(4):361–67.

35. **Caplan LR.** Dilatative arteriopathy (dolichoectasia): What is known and not known. Ann Neurol. 2005;**57**(4):469–71.

36. **Pico F, Labreuche J, Amarenco P.** Pathophysiology, presentation, prognosis, and management of intracranial arterial dolichoectasia. Lancet Neurol. 2015;**14**(8):833–45.

37. **Gutierrez J, Sultan S, Bagci A, Rundek T, Alperin N, Elkind MS**, et al. Circle of Willis configuration as a determinant of intracranial dolichoectasia. Cerebrovasc Dis. 2013;**36**(5–6):446–53.

38. **Gutierrez J.** Dolichoectasia and the risk of stroke and vascular disease: a critical appraisal. Curr Cardiol Rep. 2014;**16**(9):525.

39. **Hansson GK.** Inflammation, atherosclerosis, and coronary artery disease. N Engl J Med. 2005;**352**(16):1685–95.

40. **von Sarnowski B, Putaala J, Grittner U, Gaertner B, Schminke U, Curtze S**, et al. Lifestyle risk factors for ischemic stroke and transient ischemic attack in young adults in the Stroke in Young Fabry Patients study. Stroke. 2013;**44**:119–125.

41. **Putaala J, Yesilot N, Waje-Andreassen U, Pitkaniemi J, Vassilopoulou S, Nardi K**, et al. Demographic and geographic vascular risk factor differences in European young adults with ischemic stroke: the 15 cities young stroke study. Stroke. 2012;**43**(10):2624–30.

42. **Waje-Andreassen U, Naess H, Thomassen L, Eide GE, Vedeler CA.** Long-term mortality among young ischemic stroke patients in western Norway. Acta Neurol Scand. 2007;**116**(3):150–56.

43. **Hirsch AT, Haskal ZJ, Hertzer NR, Bakal CW, Creager MA, Halperin JL**, et al. ACC/AHA 2005 Practice Guidelines for the management of patients with peripheral arterial disease (lower extremity, renal, mesenteric, and abdominal aortic): a collaborative report from the American Association for Vascular Surgery/Society for Vascular Surgery, Society for Cardiovascular Angiography and Interventions, Society for Vascular Medicine and Biology, Society of Interventional Radiology, and the ACC/AHA Task Force on Practice Guidelines (Writing Committee to Develop Guidelines for the Management of Patients With Peripheral Arterial Disease): endorsed by the American Association of Cardiovascular and Pulmonary Rehabilitation; National Heart, Lung, and Blood Institute; Society for Vascular Nursing; TransAtlantic Inter-Society Consensus; and Vascular Disease Foundation. Circulation. 2006;**113**(11):e463–654.

44. **Putaala J, Curtze S, Hiltunen S, Tolppanen H, Kaste M, Tatlisumak T.** Causes of death and predictors of 5-year mortality in young adults after first-ever ischemic stroke: the Helsinki Young Stroke Registry. Stroke. 2009;**40**(8):2698–703.

45. **Allender S, Scarborough P, Peto V, Rayner M.** European Cardiovascular Disease Statistics. Brussels: European Heart Network; 2008.

46. **Hirsch AT, Criqui MH, Treat-Jacobson D, Regensteiner JG, Creager MA, Olin JW,** et al. Peripheral arterial disease detection, awareness, and treatment in primary care. JAMA. 2001;**286**(11):1317–24.

47. **Steg PG, Bhatt DL, Wilson PW, D'Agostino R, Sr., Ohman EM, Rother J,** et al. One-year cardiovascular event rates in outpatients with atherothrombosis. JAMA. 2007;**297**(11):1197–206.

48. **Anandasundaram B, Lane DA, Apostolakis S, Lip GY.** The impact of atherosclerotic vascular disease in predicting a stroke, thromboembolism and mortality in atrial fibrillation patients: a systematic review. J Thromb Haemost. 2013;**11**(5):975–87.

Chapter 5

Cardiac aetiology

Guillaume Turc, David Calvet,
and Jean-Louis Mas

Cardioembolism is responsible for approximately 20% of ischaemic strokes in young adults, a notably smaller proportion than that of older patients (30%), in which atrial fibrillation (AF) is much more frequent (1). Compared with other aetiologies, cardioembolic strokes are associated with a more severe clinical presentation, and a higher mortality (2). A cardioembolic aetiology (Box 5.1) should be suspected when (a) a potential cardioembolic source is identified; (b) there are neurological clues suggestive of an embolic mechanism; and (c) there is a lack of evidence of other causes of stroke (3). The following clinical features are significantly more frequent in patients with a definite cardioembolic disease: a sudden onset of stroke, decreased consciousness at onset, palpitations, and some topographic patterns, such as expressive aphasia or isolated hemianopia (4). Imaging features suggesting a cardioembolic mechanism include recent infarction in multiple cerebral or extracerebral arterial territories, a large ischaemic stroke which may harbour a haemorrhagic transformation, spontaneous recanalization of an intracranial artery, and evidence of prior systemic or cerebral embolism (5). Imaging for the detection of a cardioembolic source is described in Chapter 10. In young adults, ischaemic strokes can be related to a large panel of heart diseases, many of these being uncommon.

Valvular heart diseases

Rheumatic heart disease

Rheumatic fever is a major cause of valvular heart disease worldwide, although its incidence is low in industrialized countries. It may develop 2–4 weeks after an untreated group A streptococcal upper respiratory tract infection in childhood, and lead to arthritis, cutaneous manifestations, chorea, pericarditis, and valvular heart disease, most frequently involving the mitral and aortic valves

Box 5.1 Heart diseases predisposing to cerebral embolism in young adults

Valvular heart diseases

- Rheumatic valvular heart disease
- Prosthetic valve
- Mitral valve prolapse
- Congenital valvular heart disease (bicuspid aortic valve etc.)
- Infective endocarditis
- Libman–Sacks endocarditis
- Non-bacterial thrombotic endocarditis (marantic endocarditis)
- Calcific heart valves
- Strands.

Coronary artery disease

- Myocardial infarction; akinesia
- Left ventricular aneurysm.

Cardiomyopathies

- Dilated
- Hypertrophic
- Restrictive
- Arrhythmogenic right ventricular cardiomyopathy/dysplasia
- Unclassified.

Arrhythmias

- Atrial fibrillation
- Atrial flutter
- Sick sinus syndrome.

Intracardiac tumours

- Atrial myxoma
- Fibroelastoma
- Rhabdomyoma

- Sarcoma
- Metastasis
- Haemangioma
- Primary cardiac lymphoma
- Paraganglioma.

Septal defects

- Patent foramen ovale (with or without atrial septal aneurysm)
- Atrial septal defect
- Congenital heart diseases with right–left shunt.

Congenital heart diseases (Marelli classification)

- Group 1: common arterial trunk, transposition of great vessels, double-inlet ventricle, hypoplastic left heart syndrome, tetralogy of Fallot, atrio-ventricular septal defect
- Group 2: atrial septal defect, ventricular septal defect, patent ductus arteriosus, coarctation of aorta, Ebstein anomaly
- Group 3: unspecified congenital malformations of cardiac septum
- Group 4: congenital malformations of pulmonary artery, pulmonary valve, tricuspid valve, aortic valve, mitral valve, or great veins
- Group 5: other unspecified congenital malformations of aorta, other specified and unspecified congenital malformations of the heart, or unspecified.

Aortic arch atherosclerotic plaques

Iatrogenic

- Heart surgery
- Catheterization and electrophysiology studies
- Device or prosthetic valve-related embolism.

(6). In young patients, mitral stenosis almost exclusively occurs after rheumatic fever, and is characterized by a commissural fusion of mitral valve leaflets. This obstructs left ventricular (LV) diastolic filling and leads to elevated left atrial pressure, and subsequent left atrial dilatation which leads to increased risk of thrombus formation. Suspicion of mitral stenosis may arise if the patient reports symptoms of pulmonary congestion or during cardiac auscultation, revealing an opening snap after the second heart sound and a subsequent diastolic murmur localized at the apex. Transthoracic echocardiography (TTE) is needed to confirm the diagnosis, assess the severity of mitral stenosis (mean pressure gradient, mitral valve area, and pulmonary artery pressure), search for associated mitral or aortic regurgitation, and guide the therapeutic decision. A mitral valve area of 1.5 cm^2 or less corresponds to a severe mitral stenosis. Mitral stenosis is associated with a high risk of systemic embolization, approximately 1.5% per year (7). The risk of embolic ischaemic stroke increases with age and in the presence of AF or a history of a systemic embolization (8). Despite a lack of randomized controlled trials, oral anticoagulation with a vitamin K antagonist (VKA) with a target international normalized ratio (INR) of 2.0–3.0 is recommended in patients with mitral stenosis and AF, prior embolism, or in the presence of a left atrial thrombus (8). In patients experiencing a stroke despite well-controlled anticoagulation, the addition of low-dose aspirin may be considered. Intervention is indicated in symptomatic patients (exertional dyspnoea, palpitations) with a mitral valve area of 1.5 cm^2 or less. Percutaneous mitral balloon commissurotomy is the procedure of choice in cases of favourable valve anatomy and no left atrial thrombus (8). Alternatively, open heart surgery for mitral valve replacement is recommended if contraindications to percutaneous commissurotomy are present.

Prosthetic valves

Mechanical prosthetic valve replacement is often preferred to biological valve replacement in young patients due to high durability. However, mechanical valves carry an important risk of thrombogenicity. Indeed, the risk of systemic embolization in the absence of anticoagulation is 12% and 22% per year for aortic and mitral valves, respectively (7). Therefore, lifelong VKA anticoagulation with an INR in the target range is required, which reduces the annual risk of stroke to 2% and 4% for aortic and mitral valves, respectively (9). Of note, the target INR depends on the position and type of prosthetic valve, and associated risk factors for thromboembolism (Table 5.1) (8, 10). After the occurrence of an ischaemic stroke despite a well-controlled anticoagulation in a young patient with a mechanical prosthetic heart valve, the addition of low-dose aspirin (75–100 mg/day) is recommended (10).

In young patients, implantation of a bioprosthesis is recommended when long-term, good-quality anticoagulation is unlikely or contraindicated, and should be considered in women contemplating pregnancy (10). However, in patients aged 20 at the time of the implantation, the risk of structural deterioration of the bioprosthesis at the age of 35–40 is approximately 90% (8). The risk of systemic embolization is less frequent after biological prosthetic valve

Table 5.1 Target INR for mechanical prostheses according to the 2012 European Society of Cardiology Guidelines

Prosthesis thrombogenicity*	Patient-related risk factors**	
	No risk factor	At least 1 risk factor
Low	2.5	3.0
Medium	3.0	3.5
High	3.5	4.0

* Prosthesis thrombogenicity—low: Carbomedics, Medtronic Hall, St Jude Medical, ON-X; medium: other bileaflet valves; high: Lillehei–Kaster, Omniscience, Starr–Edwards, Bjork–Shiley, and other tilting-disc valves.

** Patient-related risk factors: mitral or tricuspid valve replacement; previous thromboembolism; atrial fibrillation; mitral stenosis of any degree; left ventricular ejection fraction <35%.

Reproduced from Eur Heart J, 33(19), ESC Committee for Practice Guidelines (CPG), Joint Task Force on the Management of Valvular Heart Disease of the European Society of Cardiology (ESC), European Association for Cardio-Thoracic Surgery (EACTS), Vahanian A, Alfieri O, Andreotti F, Antunes MJ, et al, Guidelines on the management of valvular heart disease (version 2012): the Joint Task Force on the Management of Valvular Heart Disease of the European Society of Cardiology (ESC) and the European Association for Cardio-Thoracic Surgery (EACTS), pp. 2451–96, Copyright (2012), with permission from Oxford University Press.

replacement, and most ischaemic strokes occur within the first months following surgery. Without anticoagulation therapy, the risks of ischaemic stroke at 3 months are approximately 2% and 6% for aortic and mitral valves, respectively (7). Hence, oral anticoagulation with VKA (target INR 2.5) is recommended during the first 3 months after implantation of a bioprosthesis in the mitral position (10). Aspirin or oral anticoagulation is recommended for 3 months after aortic bioprosthesis implantation (8, 10). For patients with a bioprosthetic aortic or mitral valve who experience a transient ischaemic attack (TIA) or ischaemic stroke despite antiplatelet therapy, infective endocarditis should be ruled out using the appropriate workup as described in Chapter 10. Thereafter, addition of VKA (INR 2.5) may be considered (11).

Infective endocarditis

Infective endocarditis may occur in the presence of ulceration and bacterial adherence of the valvular endothelial surface. Staphylococci and streptococci are the first and second most common causative organisms, respectively. The annual incidence of infective endocarditis is 2–6 cases per 100,000 inhabitants (12). Rates are higher in young adults with intravenous drug abuse or congenital heart disease (13). Other risk factors include prosthetic intracardiac material, valvular heart diseases (aortic and/or mitral regurgitation, rheumatic disease), poor hygiene, diabetes, HIV, and male sex. Presenting symptoms and signs are usually fever, chills, fatigue, weight loss, and heart murmur, but systemic emboli can indicate infective endocarditis. Classic signs (petechiae, Roth spots, Janeway lesions, Osler nodes) are nowadays uncommon. Diagnosis relies mostly on blood cultures, TTE, and transoesophageal echocardiography (8). However, blood cultures are negative in 10% of cases and a negative transoesophageal echocardiogram does not completely rule out infective endocarditis in the presence of a prosthetic valve (8). The use of the modified Duke criteria is recommended in patients with suspected infective endocarditis (Box 5.2) (8, 14). Neurological complications occur in 20–40% of patients and are associated with a poor outcome (15). They include ischaemic stroke, intracerebral haemorrhage, subarachnoid haemorrhage, subdural haemorrhage, seizures, meningitis, encephalitis, and brain abscess. Ischaemic strokes are mostly due to the migration of a fragment or the whole septic vegetation into the cerebral circulation, occur within the first 15 days of infective endocarditis in 70% of cases, and are located in the territory of the middle cerebral artery in more than 90% of cases (16). The risk of ischaemic stroke quickly decreases after commencing antimicrobial treatment. Transoesophageal echocardiography plays a key role in predicting the risk of systemic embolism. The risk of embolism is two times higher from a mitral valve location than an aortic valve location. Presence of large (>10 mm) or mobile vegetations predict embolism despite antibiotic therapy (17). Other predictors of cerebral embolism include an increasing size of the vegetation despite antibiotic therapy, presence of *Staphylococcus aureus*, multi-valvular involvement, and systemic inflammation (18).

Early and adapted antibiotic therapy is the cornerstone of treatment for infective endocarditis, but also for the prevention of cerebral embolism (13). In the only randomized controlled trial evaluating aspirin versus placebo to prevent stroke in infective endocarditis, aspirin did not reduce the risk of embolic events and seemed to be associated with an increased risk of bleeding (19). During the acute phase of an ischaemic stroke in patients with infective endocarditis, intravenous thrombolysis is associated with a high rate of symptomatic intracranial haemorrhage and is therefore not recommended (20). Due to an important risk of haemorrhagic transformation, it is considered reasonable to temporarily discontinue anticoagulation in patients with infective endocarditis and acute ischaemic stroke, regardless of the indication for anticoagulation (8). Cardiac surgery is recommended in case of valvular dysfunction causing heart failure, resistant micro-organisms, heart block or abscess, persistent infection, large mobile vegetation on a native valve, recurrent emboli with persistent vegetation despite appropriate antibiotics, or relapsing prosthetic valve endocarditis (8, 21). Early and complete removal of pacemakers or defibrillator systems is

Box 5.2 Modified Duke criteria

Pathological criteria

- Positive histology or microbiology of pathological material obtained at autopsy or cardiac surgery (valve tissue, vegetations, embolic fragments, or intracardiac abscess content)

Major criteria

- Two positive blood cultures showing typical organisms consistent with infective endocarditis, such as *Streptococcus viridans* and the HACEK group

  Or

- Persistent bacteraemia from 2 blood cultures taken >12 hours apart or ≥3 positive blood cultures where the pathogen is less specific, such as *Staphylococcus aureus* and *Staph epidermidis*

  Or

- Positive serology for *Coxiella burnetti*, *Bartonella* species, or *Chlamydia psittaci*

  Or

- Positive molecular assays for specific gene targets
- Positive echocardiogram showing oscillating structures, abscess formation, new valvular regurgitation, or dehiscence of prosthetic valves

Minor criteria

- Predisposing heart disease
- Fever >38°C
- Immunological phenomena such as glomerulonephritis, Osler's nodes, Roth spots, or positive rheumatoid factor
- Microbiological evidence not fitting major criteria
- Elevated C-reactive protein or erythrocyte sedimentation rate
- Vascular phenomena such as major emboli, splenomegaly, clubbing, splinter haemorrhages, petechiae, or purpura

Definite infective endocarditis

- Pathological criteria positive

  Or

- Two major criteria

  Or

- One major and two minor criteria

  Or

- Five minor criteria

Adapted from Clin Infect Dis, 30(4), Li JS, Sexton DJ, Mick N, Nettles R, Fowler VG, Jr., Ryan T, et al, Proposed modifications to the Duke criteria for the diagnosis of infective endocarditis, pp. 633–8, Copyright (2000), with permission from Oxford University Press.

indicated in patients with documented infection of the device or leads. Despite contemporary medical management, in-hospital mortality is approximately 20% in patients with infective endocarditis (8).

Libman–Sacks endocarditis

Libman–Sacks endocarditis is a rare non-infective endocarditis character-ized by verrucous valvular lesions, involving the mitral or aortic valves (22). It occurs in approximately one-third of patients with systemic lupus erythe-matosus. Immunoglobulin and complement deposition in the valvular struc-ture leads to Libman–Sacks vegetations and valve thickening, which may cause valvular regurgitation, or less frequently, stenosis. Presence of antiphospholipid antibodies favours the development of thrombi on the surface of cardiac valves, and is associated with ischaemic strokes (23). Treatment of Libman–Sacks endocarditis relies on VKA in the presence of an antiphospholipid syndrome (23). Target INR for patients with definite antiphospholipid syndrome and an arterial event is generally considered to be 3.5 (3.0–4.0) (24).

Arrhythmias

Atrial fibrillation

Although AF is a leading cause of stroke in the general population, it is an uncommon cause of stroke in young adults. The prevalence of AF is estimated to be less than 0.5% in those younger than 50 years, versus 1–2% in the general population and 5–15% in elderly people (25). In young adults, several condi-tions can contribute to the development of AF, including valvular and con-genital heart diseases and their surgical treatments, cardiomyopathies, septal defects, atrial tumours, licit and illicit drug intake, alcohol abuse, and hyper-thyroidism (26). As compared to patients in sinus rhythm, the risk of ischaemic stroke is estimated to be increased by 17- and 5-fold in patients with valvular and non-valvular AF, respectively (27). Four per cent of ischaemic strokes in young adults are attributable to AF (28). Ischaemic strokes associated with AF are more severe, and associated with a higher mortality, as compared to other stroke aetiologies. After an ischaemic stroke or a TIA due to AF, long-term oral anticoagulation is unambiguously recommended (26, 29). Compared with pla-cebo or aspirin, adjusted-dose warfarin (target INR 2–3) was associated with a 67% (95% confidence interval (CI), 54–77%) relative reduction in the risk of stroke (30). In patients aged 18 years and over with non-valvular AF, rivaroxa-ban and edoxaban were non-inferior to warfarin in the prevention of stroke and systemic embolism (31, 32), while apixaban and dabigatran were superior to warfarin (33, 34). These four direct oral anticoagulants were associated with a significantly lower risk of intracranial bleeding (31–34).

Therapeutic decision-making for primary stroke prevention in young patients with AF relies on risk estimation, for which the CHA_2DS_2-VASc score can be used. In young patients without a history of stroke or TIA and a CHA_2DS_2-VASc score of 2 or higher, oral anticoagulation is recommended (26). While no antithrombotic medication is considered to be reasonable in patients with a CHA_2DS_2-VASc score of 0 by both US and European guidelines, these recommendations slightly differ regarding patients with a score equal to 1 (26, 29). In such patients, no antithrombotic therapy, oral anticoagulation or aspirin are all considered valid options in US guidelines (26), while oral anticoagulant is recommended in European guidelines, except in young women with lone AF (29).

Atrial flutter

In the general population, the annual incidence of atrial flutter is estimated to be 0.05% in people younger than 50 years, versus 0.6% in elderly people (35). Stroke risk is considered similar for patients with AF or with atrial flutter. Antithrombotic therapy is recommended according to the same risk profile used for AF (26).

Septal defects

The prevalence of patent foramen ovale (PFO) is much higher in young adults with a cryptogenic stroke (approximately 50%) than in the general population (20–25%) (36, 37). The association between PFO and stroke is even stronger in patients with an atrial septal aneurysm (ASA), a severe right-to-left shunt, or a large PFO (37). Assuming that the relationship between PFO and stroke may be causal in some patients, mechanisms by which PFO may cause stroke remain uncertain. Although paradoxical embolism is usually considered the main mechanism of stroke in cases of PFO, in the vast majority of cases, a venous source of embolism cannot be detected (38). Other putative mechanisms include paroxysmal AF and direct embolization of thrombi formed in the PFO tunnel or in the ASA (39). As PFO is common in the general population, the association between PFO and cryptogenic stroke in a given patient may simply be due to chance. The Risk of Paradoxical Embolism (RoPE) score may be used to estimate the probability that a cryptogenic stroke is PFO related (Table 5.2) (40). Of note, patients who are the most likely to have stroke-related PFOs are also those with the lowest recurrence risk (Table 5.3) (41).

Table 5.2 The RoPE score (0–10 points)

Parameters	Points
No history of hypertension	1
No history of diabetes	1
No history of stroke of TIA	1
No smoking	1
Cortical infarct on imaging	1
Age (years)	
18–29	5
30–39	4
40–49	3
50–59	2
50–69	1
≥70	0

Reproduced from Neurology, 81(7), Kent DM, Ruthazer R, Weimar C, Mas JL, Serena J, Homma S, et al, An index to identify stroke-related vs incidental patent foramen ovale in cryptogenic stroke, pp. 619–25, Copyright (2013), with permission from Wolters Kluwer Health, Inc.

Table 5.3 Prevalence of PFO, PFO-attributable fraction, and risk of stroke recurrence, according to each value of the RoPE score

RoPE score	Patients with cryptogenic stroke (*N*=3023)		Patients with PFO and cryptogenic stroke (*N*=1324)
	Prevalence of PFO (95% CI)	PFO-attributable fraction (95% CI)	Estimated 2-year risk of stroke/ TIA recurrence (95% CI)
0–3	23% (19–26)	0% (0–4)	20% (12–28)
4	35% (31–39)	38% (25–48)	12% (6–18)
5	34% (30–38)	34% (21–45)	7% (3–11)
6	47% (42–51)	62% (54–68)	8% (4–12)
7	54% (49–59)	72% (66–76)	6% (2–10)
8	67% (62–73)	84% (79–87)	6% (2–10)
9	73% (66–79)	88% (83–91)	2% (0–4)

Adapted from Neurology, 81(7), Kent DM, Ruthazer R, Weimar C, Mas JL, Serena J, Homma S, et al, An index to identify stroke-related vs incidental patent foramen ovale in cryptogenic stroke, pp. 619–25, Copyright (2013), with permission from Wolters Kluwer Health, Inc.; Curr Opin Neurol., 27(1), Calvet D, Mas JL, Closure of patent foramen ovale in cryptogenic stroke: a never ending story, pp. 13–9, Copyright (2014), with permission from Wolters Kluwer Health, Inc.

Three published randomized controlled trials have compared PFO closure and medical treatment in patients 18–60 years of age who have had a cryptogenic stroke or TIA (41).

Patients in the medical group received aspirin or oral anticoagulants at the discretion of the investigator. All three trials failed to demonstrate superiority of device closure compared with medical therapy. However, a reduction in stroke risk after PFO closure was found in the per-protocol analysis of one study, although the number of events was low (42). An aggregated data meta-analysis of these randomized trials showed no significant difference in the risk of recurrent stroke in intention-to-treat analysis (risk ratio for stroke after PFO closure, 0.66; 95% CI, 0.37–1.19) (41). However, in an independent patient data meta-analysis of the same trials, PFO closure was marginally associated with the primary composite outcome, defined as stroke, TIA, or death (unadjusted hazard ratio (HR) 0.69 (0.47–1.01), $P=0.053$; adjusted HR 0.68 (0.46–1.00), $P=0.049$) (43). In this meta-analysis, PFO closure was associated with a lower risk of recurrent ischaemic stroke (HR 0.58 (0.34–0.98), $P=0.04$). An increased risk of AF was observed after PFO closure (HR 3.22 (1.76–5.90), $P=0.0002$) (43). The three published randomized clinical trials have several limitations, namely slow rates of enrolment, inclusion of a sizeable proportion of patients with potentially PFO-unrelated stroke, heterogeneous definitions of cryptogenic stroke, and lack of randomization between aspirin and oral anticoagulants, which may have different efficacies in recurrent stroke prevention in PFO patients (41, 42). Several other randomized controlled trials are ongoing (CLOSE, DEFENSE-PFO, and REDUCE) and are likely to shed new light on this topic. However, given the low annual stroke recurrence rate, namely 0.7% in patients treated by PFO closure and 1.3% in medically treated patients, an individual patient data meta-analysis of all randomized trials will probably be needed to reach a reliable conclusion.

Cardiomyopathies

Cardiomyopathies (CM) are defined as disorders 'characterized by morphologically and functionally abnormal myocardium in the absence of any other disease [i.e. coronary, hypertensive, valvular, or congenital heart disease] (44) that is sufficient, by itself, to cause the observed phenotype' (45). CM are usually associated with mechanical (diastolic or systolic dysfunction) or electrical myocardial failure, which may lead to life-threatening arrhythmias. Several classification systems have subsequently been proposed during the last 10 years, showing the complexity of CM and our incomplete understanding of their underlying pathological mechanisms (44–46). CM are usually classified as one of the five following phenotypic subtypes: dilated CM, which is the most frequent; hypertrophic CM; restrictive

CM; arrhythmogenic right ventricular CM/dysplasia; and unclassified CM (44). However, there is a notable overlap in clinical and molecular findings across sub-types, with the hypothesis of gene–environment interactions. Historically, CM have also been divided into primary CM, predominantly involving the heart, and secondary CM, which are part of systemic disorders (44). Primary CM which can be acquired (e.g. myocarditis; stress CM: takotsubo; peripartum CM; and tachycardia-induced CM), genetic, or mixed. A family history of CM is present in 30% of patients with dilated CM, with predominantly autosomal dominant inher-itance (45). Secondary CM include infiltrative diseases (amyloidosis, Gaucher disease), storage diseases (haemochromatosis; Fabry, Pompe, or Niemann–Pick diseases), endocrine disorders (diabetes mellitus, dysthyroidism), infectious dis-eases (Chagas disease), neurological diseases (Friedreich's ataxia, mitochondrial myopathies, muscular dystrophies, neurofibromatosis, tuberous sclerosis), sar-coidosis, systemic lupus erythematosus, dermatomyositis, rheumatoid arthritis, scleroderma, polyarteritis nodosa, nutritional deficiencies, and drug toxicity (anthracycline, cyclophosphamide) (44).

The main mechanisms underlying stroke in patients with cardiomyopathies are LV mural thrombus, mostly in patients with heart failure, and AF. Stroke incidence in patients with CM remains poorly known due to the heterogeneous nature of CM and of the scarce data in the literature, with likely publication bias. However, data can be extrapolated from the annual rate of ischaemic stroke in patients with chronic heart failure, ranging from 1% to 3.5% per year (47). In a cross-sectional review of the medical records of 790 patients with a car-diomyopathy, ischaemic stroke had occurred in 14% of patients (48). Factors independently associated with stroke were AF, pacemakers, coronary artery disease, hypertension, and Chagas disease (48). Other aetiologies, such as non-compaction CM, peripartum CM, infectious myocarditis, and amyloidosis, were reported to be associated with ischaemic stroke. The identification of a LV thrombus by echocardiography is an independent predictor of stroke in patients with dilated CM (adjusted odds ratio=3) (49). There are no randomized trials comparing oral anticoagulation versus aspirin in patients with a CM without AF. However, two randomized controlled trials showed that warfarin was not super-ior to aspirin in sinus rhythm patients with chronic heart failure (LV ejection fraction ≤35%) of various aetiologies (50, 51). Of note, in the Warfarin versus Aspirin in Reduced Cardiac Ejection Fraction (WARCEF) study, warfarin was associated with a reduced risk of ischaemic stroke as compared to aspirin (HR 0.52; 95% CI, 0.33–0.82), which was offset by an increased risk of major haemor-rhage (rate ratio 2.05; 95% CI, 1.36–3.12) (51). Although it remains debated, the risk–benefit ratio might be in favour of warfarin in selected patients with a high risk of ischaemic stroke and a low risk of major haemorrhage (52).

Myocardial infarction

Acute myocardial infarction

Stroke occurs within 4 weeks of acute myocardial infarction (MI) in 1–5% of patients (53). The main mechanism of ischaemic stroke is emboli from a left mural (often apical) ventricular thrombus, which usually appears between the first and tenth day after ST-elevation MI. Transmural MI of the anterior wall of the left ventricle is associated with an important increase in the risk of ventricular thrombus (approximately 35%) and ischaemic stroke (5% at 1 month). Other risk factors for ischaemic stroke are increasing age, history of AF, large MI, and LV dysfunction (54). Treatment with aspirin is not associated with a reduction in the incidence of ventricular thrombus, but reduces the risk of ischaemic stroke in the acute stage of MI by 50% (55). In sinus rhythm patients with ST-elevation MI with or at risk of LV thrombus (e.g. anteroapical akinesis or dyskinesis), anticoagulant therapy with a VKA limited to 3 months is reasonable, although randomized data are lacking (56).

Non-ST elevation acute coronary syndromes are associated with a low rate of ischaemic stroke, approximately 0.5% within the first 30 days (57). In these patients, independent predictors of stroke are age, history of stroke, and high heart rate.

Long-term stroke risk after myocardial infarction

The annual rate of ischaemic stroke after the acute phase of MI is approximately 1–2% (58). Risk factors include anterior wall MI, age, AF, LV dysfunction, history of stroke, and multiple MIs. In patients with LV thrombus persisting beyond 1 month post-MI, the risk of ischaemic stroke is estimated to be 5% per year. Although the risk of ischaemic stroke is lower in this situation than in patients with a LV thrombus during the acute stage of MI, oral anticoagulation may be reasonable.

LV aneurysms occur in less than 5% of patients after ST-elevation MI, and their incidence has decreased with reperfusion therapies (56). It is more frequent after anterior MI. Although ventricular thrombi occur frequently in patients with a LV aneurysm, the risk of systemic emboli is low, approximately 1% per year.

In patients with a prior MI who experience an ischaemic stroke, antithrombotic medication generally relies on aspirin or clopidogrel. To date, oral anticoagulation has not been compared to antiplatelet therapy in patients with a post-MI LV aneurysm. Observational data do not suggest that warfarin is superior to aspirin in such patients (59). Surgical treatment for a LV aneurysm with the risk of myocardial rupture may be considered in rare circumstances, such as recurrent thromboembolism despite anticoagulant therapy (56).

Tumours

Intracardiac tumours, such as atrial myxoma, fibroelastoma, and rhabdomyomas represent a rare cause of ischaemic stroke (<1% of cases) (60).

Intracardiac myxoma

Myxomas represent 80% of all primary tumours of the heart, and occur in the left atrium in 85% cases, near the fossa ovalis (61). Myxomas are most frequently seen between the third and sixth decades, with a 2:1 female predominance. Approximately one-third of patients with a myxoma experience systemic embolism, most frequently multiple ischaemic strokes (61). Emboli most often consist of myxomatous material. The mobility, but not the size of the myxoma seems to be associated with an increased risk of ischaemic stroke (61). Myxomatous emboli have the potential to invade the wall of cerebral arteries and keep growing within the subintima, inducing aneurysm formation. Intracranial aneurysms are frequently multiple, fusiform, and distal, and can rarely lead to intracranial haemorrhage. Intracranial metastatic myxoma is a rare complication of myxomatous tumour embolism.

Myxoma is often associated with constitutional symptoms, such as myalgia, elevated body temperature, asthenia, arthralgia, weight loss, and biological inflammation (61). Dyspnoea and obstructive cardiac symptoms are frequent. Echocardiography shows a heterogeneous, hyperechoic pedunculated mass, attached to the atrial septum. Despite surgical excision, recurrence of atrial myxoma can occur in 1–5% of cases (61).

Fibroelastoma

Cardiac papillary fibroelastomas are the most frequent primary valvular tumours, and are most frequently seen between the third and eighth decades (60). Fibroelastomas consist of multiple papillary fronds resembling a sea anemone and containing fibrous tissue, elastic fibres, and smooth muscle cells. The tumour is covered by endocardial cells. It is usually small (<2 cm), mobile, well-limited, and pedunculated. Its predominant location is the aortic valve, followed by the mitral, tricuspid, and pulmonary valves. The majority of patients are asymptomatic. The most common clinical presentations are TIA and ischaemic stroke. Embolism may occur from the frail papillary fronds or from a thrombus formed on the fibroelastoma. Stroke recurrence is frequent despite antithrombotic medication, but surgical excision is curative (60).

'Grown-up' congenital heart diseases

The improvement of survival in patients with congenital heart disease has led to an increasing number of young adults with so-called 'grown-up congenital heart disease' (GUCH), with an estimated prevalence of 2.8 cases per 1000 inhabitants (62). The cumulative risk of stroke over the course of adulthood in patients with GUCH was assessed in a large, retrospective, population-based cohort study (63). For an 18-year-old woman, the cumulative risk of ischaemic stroke up to 64 years old was 6.1% (95% CI, 5.0–7.0%) and for an 18-year-old man, 7.7% (95% CI, 6.4–8.8%). The rate of stroke was tenfold higher compared with a control group matched for age and sex, a finding consistent with another recent population-based study (64). Risk factors for stroke in GUCH patients include congestive heart failure, diabetes mellitus, recent MI, hypertension, and AF (63, 64). Underlying mechanisms for stroke include prosthetic valve/device-related thromboembolism, paradoxical embolism (intra- or extracardiac shunt), arrhythmia, septic embolism due to infective endocarditis, hypoxaemia and secondary erythrocytosis/hyperviscosity, and associated intracranial vascular abnormalities (aneurysms in patients with coarctation; Moyamoya syndrome) (65). Although GUCH represents a heterogeneous ensemble, all major subtypes of the Marelli classification (66) of congenital heart disease (Box 5.1) seem to be at increased risk of stroke, as compared to the general population (64). Although detailed guidelines for the management of each GUCH subtype have been published, no specific recommendations regarding the specific management of GUCH patients with stroke are provided (62, 67).

References

1. **Grau AJ**, **Weimar C**, **Buggle F**, **Heinrich A**, **Goertler M**, **Neumaier S**, et al. Risk factors, outcome, and treatment in subtypes of ischemic stroke: the German stroke data bank. Stroke. 2001;**32**(11):2559–66.

2. **Ferro JM.** Cardioembolic stroke: an update. Lancet Neurol. 2003;**2**(3):177–88.

3. **Hart RG**, **Albers GW**, **Koudstaal PJ.** Cerebrovascular Disease. Pathophysiology, Diagnosis and Treatment. Oxford: Blackwell Sciences; 1998.

4. **Kittner SJ**, **Sharkness CM**, **Price TR**, **Plotnick GD**, **Dambrosia JM**, **Wolf PA**, et al. Infarcts with a cardiac source of embolism in the NINCDS Stroke Data Bank: historical features. Neurology. 1990;**40**(2):281–84.

5. **Kittner SJ**, **Sharkness CM**, **Sloan MA**, **Price TR**, **Dambrosia JM**, **Tuhrim S**, et al. Features on initial computed tomography scan of infarcts with a cardiac source of embolism in the NINDS Stroke Data Bank. Stroke. 1992;**23**(12):1748–51.

6. **Wilson NJ**, **Voss L**, **Morreau J**, **Stewart J**, **Lennon D.** New Zealand guidelines for the diagnosis of acute rheumatic fever: small increase in the incidence of definite cases compared to the American Heart Association Jones criteria. N Z Med J. 2013;**126**(1379):50–59.

7. **Salem DN**, **O'Gara PT**, **Madias C**, **Pauker SG**, **American College of Chest Physicians**. Valvular and structural heart disease: American College of Chest Physicians Evidence-Based Clinical Practice Guidelines (8th Edition). Chest. 2008;**133**(6 Suppl):593S-629S.

8. **Nishimura RA**, **Otto CM**, **Bonow RO**, **Carabello BA**, **Erwin JP, 3rd**, **Guyton RA**, et al. 2014 AHA/ACC Guideline for the Management of Patients With Valvular Heart

Disease: a report of the American College of Cardiology/American Heart Association Task Force on Practice Guidelines. Circulation. 2014;**129**(23):e521–643.

9. **Vongpatanasin W, Hillis LD, Lange RA.** Prosthetic heart valves. N Engl J Med. 1996;**335**(6):407–16.

10. **Joint Task Force on the Management of Valvular Heart Disease of the European Society of C, European Association for Cardio-Thoracic S, Vahanian A, Alfieri O, Andreotti F, Antunes MJ**, et al. Guidelines on the management of valvular heart disease (version 2012). Eur Heart J. 2012;**33**(19):2451–96.

11. **Kernan WN, Ovbiagele B, Black HR, Bravata DM, Chimowitz MI, Ezekowitz MD,** et al. Guidelines for the prevention of stroke in patients with stroke and transient ischemic attack: a guideline for healthcare professionals from the American Heart Association/American Stroke Association. Stroke. 2014;**45**(7):2160–236.

12. **Beynon RP, Bahl VK, Prendergast BD.** Infective endocarditis. BMJ. 2006;**333**(7563):334–39.

13. **Chambers J, Sandoe J, Ray S, Prendergast B, Taggart D, Westaby S**, et al. The infective endocarditis team: recommendations from an international working group. Heart. 2014;**100**(7):524–27.

14. **Li JS, Sexton DJ, Mick N, Nettles R, Fowler VG, Jr., Ryan T**, et al. Proposed modifications to the Duke criteria for the diagnosis of infective endocarditis. Clin Infect Dis. 2000;**30**(4):633–38.

15. **Snygg-Martin U, Gustafsson L, Rosengren L, Alsio A, Ackerholm P, Andersson R**, et al. Cerebrovascular complications in patients with left-sided infective endocarditis are common: a prospective study using magnetic resonance imaging and neurochemical brain damage markers. Clin Infect Dis. 2008;**47**(1):23–30.

16. **Duval X, Iung B, Klein I, Brochet E, Thabut G, Arnoult F**, et al. Effect of early cerebral magnetic resonance imaging on clinical decisions in infective endocarditis: a prospective study. Ann Intern Med. 2010;**152**(8):497–504, W175.

17. **Anderson DJ, Goldstein LB, Wilkinson WE, Corey GR, Cabell CH, Sanders LL,** et al. Stroke location, characterization, severity, and outcome in mitral vs aortic valve endocarditis. Neurology. 2003;**61**(10):1341–46.

18. **Thuny F, Di Salvo G, Belliard O, Avierinos JF, Pergola V, Rosenberg V**, et al. Risk of embolism and death in infective endocarditis: prognostic value of echocardiography: a prospective multicenter study. Circulation. 2005;**112**(1):69–75.

19. **Chan KL, Dumesnil JG, Cujec B, Sanfilippo AJ, Jue J, Turek MA**, et al. A randomized trial of aspirin on the risk of embolic events in patients with infective endocarditis. J Am Coll Cardiol. 2003;**42**(5):775–80.

20. **Asaithambi G, Adil MM, Qureshi AI.** Thrombolysis for ischemic stroke associated with infective endocarditis: results from the nationwide inpatient sample. Stroke. 2013;**44**(10):2917–19.

21. **Habib G, Lancellotti P, Antunes MJ, Bongiorni MG, Casalta JP, Del Zotti F**, et al. 2015 ESC Guidelines for the management of infective endocarditis: The Task Force for the Management of Infective Endocarditis of the European Society of Cardiology (ESC). Endorsed by: European Association for Cardio-Thoracic Surgery (EACTS), the European Association of Nuclear Medicine (EANM). Eur Heart J. 2015;**36**(44):3075–128.

22. **Galve E, Candell-Riera J, Pigrau C, Permanyer-Miralda G, Garcia-Del-Castillo H, Soler-Soler J.** Prevalence, morphologic types, and evolution of cardiac valvular disease in systemic lupus erythematosus. N Engl J Med. 1988;**319**(13):817–23.

23. **Brey RL, Muscal E, Chapman J.** Antiphospholipid antibodies and the brain: a consensus report. Lupus. 2011;**20**(2):153–57.

24. **Ruiz-Irastorza G, Crowther M, Branch W, Khamashta MA.** Antiphospholipid syndrome. Lancet. 2010;**376**(9751):1498–509.

25. **Kannel WB, Wolf PA, Benjamin EJ, Levy D.** Prevalence, incidence, prognosis, and predisposing conditions for atrial fibrillation: population-based estimates. Am J Cardiol. 1998;**82**(8A):2N–9N.

26. **January CT, Wann LS, Alpert JS, Calkins H, Cigarroa JE, Cleveland JC, Jr.,** et al. 2014 AHA/ACC/HRS guideline for the management of patients with atrial fibrillation: executive summary: a report of the American College of Cardiology/ American Heart Association Task Force on practice guidelines and the Heart Rhythm Society. Circulation. 2014;**130**(23):2071–104.

27. **Wolf PA, Dawber TR, Thomas HE, Jr., Kannel WB.** Epidemiologic assessment of chronic atrial fibrillation and risk of stroke: the Framingham study. Neurology. 1978;**28**(10):973–77.

28. **Putaala J, Yesilot N, Waje-Andreassen U, Pitkaniemi J, Vassilopoulou S, Nardi K,** et al. Demographic and geographic vascular risk factor differences in European young adults with ischemic stroke: the 15 cities young stroke study. Stroke. 2012;**43**(10):2624–30.

29. **Camm AJ, Lip GY, De Caterina R, Savelieva I, Atar D, Hohnloser SH,** et al. 2012 focused update of the ESC Guidelines for the management of atrial fibrillation: an update of the 2010 ESC Guidelines for the management of atrial fibrillation. Developed with the special contribution of the European Heart Rhythm Association. Eur Heart J. 2012;**33**(21):2719–47.

30. **Hart RG, Pearce LA, Aguilar MI.** Meta-analysis: antithrombotic therapy to prevent stroke in patients who have nonvalvular atrial fibrillation. Ann Intern Med. 2007;**146**(12):857–67.

31. **Patel MR, Mahaffey KW, Garg J, Pan G, Singer DE, Hacke W,** et al. Rivaroxaban versus warfarin in nonvalvular atrial fibrillation. N Engl J Med. 2011;**365**(10):883–91.

32. **Giugliano RP, Ruff CT, Braunwald E, Murphy SA, Wiviott SD, Halperin JL,** et al. Edoxaban versus warfarin in patients with atrial fibrillation. N Engl J Med. 2013;**369**(22):2093–104.

33. **Granger CB, Alexander JH, McMurray JJ, Lopes RD, Hylek EM, Hanna M,** et al. Apixaban versus warfarin in patients with atrial fibrillation. N Engl J Med. 2011;**365**(11):981–92.

34. **Connolly SJ, Ezekowitz MD, Yusuf S, Eikelboom J, Oldgren J, Parekh A,** et al. Dabigatran versus warfarin in patients with atrial fibrillation. N Engl J Med. 2009;**361**(12):1139–51.

35. **Granada J, Uribe W, Chyou PH, Maassen K, Vierkant R, Smith PN,** et al. Incidence and predictors of atrial flutter in the general population. J Am Coll Cardiol. 2000;**36**(7):2242–46.

36. **Mas JL, Arquizan C, Lamy C, Zuber M, Cabanes L, Derumeaux G,** et al. Recurrent cerebrovascular events associated with patent foramen ovale, atrial septal aneurysm, or both. N Engl J Med. 2001;**345**(24):1740–46.

37. **Overell JR, Bone I, Lees KR.** Interatrial septal abnormalities and stroke: a meta-analysis of case-control studies. Neurology. 2000;**55**(8):1172–79.

38. **Ranoux D, Cohen A, Cabanes L, Amarenco P, Bousser MG, Mas JL.** Patent foramen ovale: is stroke due to paradoxical embolism? Stroke. 1993;**24**(1):31–34.

39. Berthet K, Lavergne T, Cohen A, Guize L, Bousser MG, Le Heuzey JY, et al. Significant association of atrial vulnerability with atrial septal abnormalities in young patients with ischemic stroke of unknown cause. Stroke. 2000;**31**(2):398–403.

40. Kent DM, Ruthazer R, Weimar C, Mas JL, Serena J, Homma S, et al. An index to identify stroke-related vs incidental patent foramen ovale in cryptogenic stroke. Neurology. 2013;**81**(7):619–25.

41. Calvet D, Mas JL. Closure of patent foramen ovale in cryptogenic stroke: a never ending story. Curr Opin Neurol. 2014;**27**(1):13–19.

42. Carroll JD, Saver JL, Thaler DE, Smalling RW, Berry S, MacDonald LA, et al. Closure of patent foramen ovale versus medical therapy after cryptogenic stroke. N Engl J Med. 2013;**368**(12):1092–100.

43. Kent DM, Dahabreh IJ, Ruthazer R, Furlan AJ, Reisman M, Carroll JD, et al. Device closure of patent foramen ovale after stroke: pooled analysis of completed randomized trials. J Am Coll Cardiol. 2016;**67**(8):907–17.

44. Maron BJ, Towbin JA, Thiene G, Antzelevitch C, Corrado D, Arnett D, et al. Contemporary definitions and classification of the cardiomyopathies: an American Heart Association Scientific Statement from the Council on Clinical Cardiology, Heart Failure and Transplantation Committee; Quality of Care and Outcomes Research and Functional Genomics and Translational Biology Interdisciplinary Working Groups; and Council on Epidemiology and Prevention. Circulation. 2006;**113**(14):1807–16.

45. Arbustini E, Narula N, Dec GW, Reddy KS, Greenberg B, Kushwaha S, et al. The MOGE(S) classification for a phenotype-genotype nomenclature of cardiomyopathy: endorsed by the World Heart Federation. J Am Coll Cardiol. 2013;**62**(22):2046–72.

46. Authors/Task Force m, Elliott PM, Anastasakis A, Borger MA, Borggrefe M, Cecchi F, et al. 2014 ESC Guidelines on diagnosis and management of hypertrophic cardiomyopathy: the Task Force for the Diagnosis and Management of Hypertrophic Cardiomyopathy of the European Society of Cardiology (ESC). Eur Heart J. 2014;**35**(39):2733–79.

47. Pullicino PM, Halperin JL, Thompson JL. Stroke in patients with heart failure and reduced left ventricular ejection fraction. Neurology. 2000;**54**(2):288–94.

48. da Matta JA, Aras R, Jr., de Macedo CR, da Cruz CG, Netto EM. Stroke correlates in chagasic and non-chagasic cardiomyopathies. PLoS One. 2012;**7**(4):e35116.

49. Crawford TC, Smith WTt, Velazquez EJ, Taylor SM, Jollis JG, Kisslo J. Prognostic usefulness of left ventricular thrombus by echocardiography in dilated cardiomyopathy in predicting stroke, transient ischemic attack, and death. Am J Cardiol. 2004;**93**(4):500–3.

50. Massie BM, Collins JF, Ammon SE, Armstrong PW, Cleland JG, Ezekowitz M, et al. Randomized trial of warfarin, aspirin, and clopidogrel in patients with chronic heart failure: the Warfarin and Antiplatelet Therapy in Chronic Heart Failure (WATCH) trial. Circulation. 2009;**119**(12):1616–24.

51. Homma S, Thompson JL, Pullicino PM, Levin B, Freudenberger RS, Teerlink JR, et al. Warfarin and aspirin in patients with heart failure and sinus rhythm. N Engl J Med. 2012;**366**(20):1859–69.

52. Ye S, Cheng B, Lip GY, Buchsbaum R, Sacco RL, Levin B, et al. Bleeding risk and antithrombotic strategy in patients with sinus rhythm and heart failure with reduced ejection fraction treated with warfarin or aspirin. Am J Cardiol. 2015;**116**(6):904–12.

53. **Maggioni AP, Franzosi MG, Santoro E, White H, Van de Werf F, Tognoni G.** The risk of stroke in patients with acute myocardial infarction after thrombolytic and antithrombotic treatment. Gruppo Italiano per lo Studio della Sopravvivenza nell'Infarto Miocardico II (GISSI-2), and The International Study Group. N Engl J Med. 1992;**327**(1):1–6.

54. **Vaitkus PT, Barnathan ES.** Embolic potential, prevention and management of mural thrombus complicating anterior myocardial infarction: a meta-analysis. J Am Coll Cardiol. 1993;**22**(4):1004–9.

55. **Randomised trial of intravenous streptokinase, oral aspirin, both, or neither among 17,187 cases of suspected acute myocardial infarction: ISIS-2.** ISIS-2 (Second International Study of Infarct Survival) Collaborative Group. Lancet. 1988;**2**(8607):349–60.

56. **O'Gara PT, Kushner FG, Ascheim DD, Casey DE, Jr., Chung MK, de Lemos JA,** et al. 2013 ACCF/AHA guideline for the management of ST-elevation myocardial infarction: a report of the American College of Cardiology Foundation/American Heart Association Task Force on Practice Guidelines. Circulation. 2013;**127**(4):e362–425.

57. **Westerhout CM, Hernandez AV, Steyerberg EW, Bueno H, White H, Theroux P,** et al. Predictors of stroke within 30 days in patients with non-ST-segment elevation acute coronary syndromes. Eur Heart J. 2006;**27**(24):2956–61.

58. **Loh E, Sutton MS, Wun CC, Rouleau JL, Flaker GC, Gottlieb SS,** et al. Ventricular dysfunction and the risk of stroke after myocardial infarction. N Engl J Med. 1997;**336**(4):251–7.

59. **Lee GY, Song YB, Hahn JY, Choi SH, Choi JH, Jeon ES,** et al. Anticoagulation in ischemic left ventricular aneurysm. Mayo Clin Proc. 2015;**90**(4):441–49.

60. **Gowda RM, Khan IA, Nair CK, Mehta NJ, Vasavada BC, Sacchi TJ.** Cardiac papillary fibroelastoma: a comprehensive analysis of 725 cases. Am Heart J. 2003;**146**(3):404–10.

61. **Lee VH, Connolly HM, Brown RD, Jr.** Central nervous system manifestations of cardiac myxoma. Arch Neurol. 2007;**64**(8):1115–20.

62. **Baumgartner H, Bonhoeffer P, De Groot NM, de Haan F, Deanfield JE, Galie N,** et al. ESC Guidelines for the management of grown-up congenital heart disease (new version 2010). Eur Heart J. 2010;**31**(23):2915–57.

63. **Lanz J, Brophy JM, Therrien J, Kaouache M, Guo L, Marelli AJ.** Stroke in adults with congenital heart disease: incidence, cumulative risk, and predictors. Circulation. 2015;**132**(25):2385–94.

64. **Mandalenakis Z, Rosengren A, Lappas G, Eriksson P, Hansson PO, Dellborg M.** Ischemic stroke in children and young adults with congenital heart disease. J Am Heart Assoc. 2016;**5**(2).

65. **Opotowsky AR, Webb GD.** Population-based data on congenital heart disease and stroke. J Am Heart Assoc. 2016;**5**(2).

66. **Marelli AJ, Mackie AS, Ionescu-Ittu R, Rahme E, Pilote L.** Congenital heart disease in the general population: changing prevalence and age distribution. Circulation. 2007;**115**(2):163–72.

67. **Warnes CA, Williams RG, Bashore TM, Child JS, Connolly HM, Dearani JA,** et al. ACC/AHA 2008 Guidelines for the Management of Adults with Congenital Heart Disease: a report of the American College of Cardiology/American Heart Association Task Force on Practice Guidelines (writing committee to develop guidelines on the management of adults with congenital heart disease). Circulation. 2008;**118**(23):e714–833.

Chapter 6

Special aetiologies

Katarina Jood and Turgut Tatlisumak

Introduction

The conventional aetiologies of ischaemic stroke, large artery atherosclerosis and small vessel disease, are relatively less common in young adults. The proportion of cardioembolic stroke is comparable to older patients, but is composed of other cardiac causes. In recent large series of young ischaemic stroke patients (<55 years of age) (1–3), other determined or special aetiologies accounted for 18–26% of the cases, making it the second largest aetiological group after cryptogenic stroke. However, this group is extremely diverse with about 200 different conditions reported as causative or associated with ischaemic stroke. Most of these conditions are very rare, and for some, the causal relationship to stroke remains to be established, as they are based on case reports or small series of patients only. In this chapter, we give an overview and briefly discuss the more common of these unusual aetiologies. Cardioembolic causes, however, are discussed in Chapter 5. A flowchart showing the aetiological diagnostic workup for young patients with ischaemic stroke is also provided.

Diagnostic workup

Diagnosing a special or rare aetiology in a young ischaemic stroke patient is essential as some of these conditions require specific treatments, genetic counselling, or follow-up programmes. For those conditions that lack specific treatments, diagnosis is still important as it may provide information about prognosis, and give some kind of explanation for being struck by a stroke at a young age. Given the broad spectrum of possible causes, diagnosis of the underlying aetiology in a young person with ischaemic stroke is challenging. Currently, there are no evidence-based diagnostic algorithms available and cost-effectiveness studies of different diagnostic approaches are lacking. Performing diagnostic tests for all possible underlying conditions in all patients is not an option as it would be extremely time-consuming, costly, and also

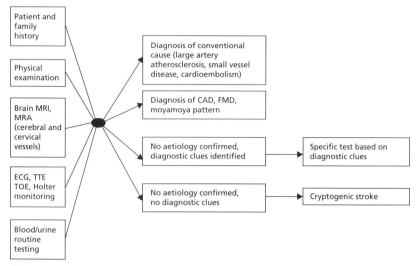

Fig. 6.1 Flowchart for exploring ischaemic stroke aetiology in young adults. CAD, cervical artery dissection; ECG, electrocardiogram; FMD, fibromuscular dysplasia; MRA, magnetic resonance angiography; MRI, magnetic resonance imaging; TTE, transthoracic echocardiogram; TOE, transoesophageal echocardiogram.

possibly harmful. A more attractive strategy would be to perform the diagnostic workup in a systematic stepwise manner as described in Fig. 6.1. A first-line group of tests are performed in all patients in order to (a) rule out or confirm the most common causes and (b) identify clues for how to proceed with specific tests for rare disorders. This enables a systematic patient-tailored diagnostic workup for each case.

First-line diagnostic evaluations

Patient and family history

A thorough clinical evaluation of family and patient medical history can deliver very useful aetiological hints (Table 6.1). A family history of stroke, dementia, other vascular events, or venous thromboembolism at a young age or in several family members, is suggestive of an inherited disorder. As some conditions are more prevalent in certain areas, useful clues may also come from ethnicity and geography. Moyamoya disease and Takayasu disease are more common among individuals of Asian origin, sickle cell disease in individuals of African origin, thalassemia in individuals from the Mediterranean, and Behçet's disease in individuals from Japan or the eastern Mediterranean (along the historical Silk Road). Prevalence of infectious disease associated with stroke differs

Table 6.1 Diagnosis of rare causes of ischaemic stroke guided by clinical signs and findings

Diagnosis	Clinical signs and findings/red flags	Diagnostic tests
Cervical artery dissection	Head or cervical trauma, facial or neck pain, Horner's syndrome, lower cranial nerve palsies	CTA/MRA, axial cervical MRI with T1-weighted suppression images
Moyamoya disease or syndrome	Headache, recurrent ischaemic events, events triggered by hypoperfusion, combination of ICH and cerebral infarcts, choreiform movements (children)	Brain MRI and MRA/DSA
Susac syndrome	Encephalopathy, focal deficits, sensorineural hearing loss, visual disturbances, lesions of the central corpus callosum on T2 MRI	Retinal fluorescein angiography
Primary angiitis of the central nervous system (PANCS)	Headache, subacute progressive cognitive impairment, encephalopathy, seizures, multifocal ischaemic, and/or haemorrhagic strokes. No signs of systemic involvement	MRI, DSA, CSF analysis, brain biopsy
Systemic vasculitis	Malaise, fever, weight loss, elevated ESR, CRP	
Takayasu disease	Headache, claudication of extremities, blood pressure differences between arms, decreased brachial pulse	CTA/MRA, aortic PET
Polyarteritis nodosa	Arthritis, polyneuropathy multiplex, myalgia, peripheral ischaemia, skin lesions	Skin, nerve, or muscle biopsy
Churg–Strauss syndrome (EGPA)	Late-onset allergic rhinitis, asthma	Blood eosinophilia, serum pANCA/MPO, lung, skin, or nerve biopsy
Granulomatosis with polyangiitis (Wegener's granulomatosis)	Necrotizing ulcerating inflammation of upper respiratory tract, lung infiltrates, nephritis	Serum cANCA/PR3, tissue biopsy
Behçet's disease	Brainstem involvement, sinus thrombosis. Recurrent oral and/or genital ulcerations, uveitis, retinal vasculitis, erythema nodosum, Mediterranean, Middle East, or Asian ethnic origin	Clinical criteria, no specific test aids diagnosis
RCVS	Recurrent thunderclap headaches, ischaemic and/or haemorrhagic strokes, reversible oedema	CTA/MRA, DSA
Migraine	Known migraine with aura, ischaemic stroke associated with, for that patient, a typical migrainous aura persisting >60 minutes	International Headache Society criteria, no specific test aids diagnosis

(continued)

Table 6.1 Continued

Diagnosis	Clinical signs and findings/red flags	Diagnostic tests
Antiphospholipid syndrome	Recurrent venous/and or arterial thrombosis, miscarriages, eclampsia, placental failure, prolonged APTT	Lupus anticoagulant, anticardiolipin and/or anti-β2-glycoprotein antibodies in serum on two or more occasions at least 12 weeks apart
Sneddon syndrome	Livedo racemosa, small ischaemic strokes in deep white matter and pons	Skin biopsy, DSA
CADASIL	Migraine with aura, recurrent subcortical ischaemic strokes, cognitive decline, mood disorders. MRI T2 white matter hyperintensities in the anterior temporal lobe and/or capsula externa	Molecular genetic testing, skin biopsy
CARASIL	Similar to CADASIL + premature alopecia, spondylosis	Molecular genetic testing
RVCL	Cerebral and retinal microvasculopathy, ischaemic stokes, mild kidney or liver dysfunction, migraine	Molecular genetic testing
COLA41 disorders	Cerebral small vessel disease, recurrent ICH and ischaemic strokes, cerebral aneurysms, porencephaly, retinal vascular tortuosity, kidney disease, muscular cramps	Molecular genetic testing
MELAS	Cortical ischaemic lesions not limited to vascular territories, short stature, sensorineural hearing loss, migraine-like headache, episodic vomiting, exercise intolerance, diabetes, cardiomyopathy, retinitis pigmentosa, diabetes	Lactate in serum/CSF, muscle biopsy, molecular genetic testing
Fabry	Painful acroparaesthesia, small fibre neuropathy, angiokeratoma, cardiomyopathy, renal dysfunction, retinitis pigmentosa	GLA activity, molecular genetic testing
Sickle cell disease	African ethnic origin, moyamoya syndrome, haemolytic anaemia, jaundice, retinal angioid streaks	Peripheral blood smear, haemoglobin electrophoresis, molecular genetic testing
Homocystinuria	Early onset of venous and/or arterial thrombosis, tall stature with Marfan-like features, lens dislocation, osteoporosis, decreased pigmentation of hair and skin	Urine analysis, plasma homocysteine, activity of cystathionine β-synthase in cultured fibroblasts

Table 6.1 Continued

Diagnosis	Clinical signs and findings/red flags	Diagnostic tests
Hereditary haemorrhagic telangiectasia (Osler –Weber – Rendu disease)	Nose bleeds, skin and mouth telangiectasia	CT thorax, molecular genetic testing
CVT	Progressive headache, papilloedema, venous infarction w/o haemorrhage with surrounding oedema	MRI and MR venography
Vascular Ehlers– Danlos syndrome	Arterial dissection, thin skin, blue sclera, easy bruising, poor wound healing, short stature, cerebral aneurysm, bowel and/or uterine rupture, joint hypermobility	Molecular genetic testing
Marfan syndrome	Arterial dissection, aortic aneurysm, lens dislocation, long and thin extremities, tall stature, pectus carinatum or excavatum, mitral valve prolapse, pneumothorax, dural ectasia	Molecular genetic testing
Pseudoxanthoma elasticum	Arterial dissection, elastic skin, redundant skin with cobblestone appearance in flexor areas, retinal angioid streaks	Molecular genetic testing
Loeys–Dietz syndrome	Arterial dissection, arterial tortuosities, tall stature, pectus carinatum or excavatum, joint laxity, craniosynostosis, widely spaced eyes, bifid uvula/cleft palate	Molecular genetic testing
Neurofibromatosis type 1	Café au lait skin spots, neurofibromas, Lisch nodules, optic glioma, intracranial aneurysms	Molecular genetic testing

between areas. HIV is more common in sub-Saharan Africa, Chagas disease in Latin America, syphilis and tuberculosis in the Indian subcontinent, and Lyme disease (borreliosis) in endemic areas mainly in the northern hemisphere temperate regions. Likewise, the use of illicit drugs differs widely, and in certain metropolitan regions of the United States, illicit drug use has been attributed to 5% of all young strokes.

A careful medical history is crucial. Malaise, fever, weight loss, or arthralgia indicates a systemic inflammatory disorder or infection. Hearing loss and visual disturbances are common in mitochondrial disease, Cogan syndrome, and Susac syndrome. Visual disturbances are also common in temporal arteritis and retinal vasculopathy with cerebral leucodystrophy (RVCL). Epistaxis is frequently the first symptom in Osler–Weber–Rendu disease. Recurrent oral and genital ulcers are important features of Behçet's disease, but also occur in systemic lupus erythematosus (SLE) and syphilis. Prior arterial or venous thrombotic events, especially when at unusual sites, indicate inherited or acquired thrombophilia. Recurrent spontaneous miscarriages should remind of the antiphospholipid syndrome. Peripheral neuropathy is a feature in systemic vasculitis and Fabry disease, and painful acroparaesthesias are typical for Fabry disease. Progressive cognitive dysfunction is common in cerebral autosomal dominant arteriopathy with subcortical infarcts and leucoaraiosis (CADASIL), Susac syndrome, and cerebral vasculitis, with a slow progressive course in CADASIL, and subacute in Susac syndrome and cerebral vasculitis. Presence of common vascular risk factors may indicate a conventional aetiology, but diabetes is also common in mitochondrial disease. Recent trauma may underlie cervical artery dissection or cerebral venous thrombosis, and a recently developed systolic bruit is common in cervical artery dissection. Intake of vasoactive or illicit drugs, late pregnancy, or postpartum period is suggestive of reversible cerebral vasoconstriction syndrome (RCVS).

Headache, especially migraine-like headache, is common in stroke patients and is a frequent symptom at admission. Migraine-like headache occurs in a number of conditions including mitochondrial myopathy, encephalopathy, lactic acidosis, and stroke-like episodes (MELAS), CADASIL, antiphospholipid syndrome, Moyamoya syndrome, Sneddon syndrome, and SLE. Headache with an insidious or subacute onset is a characteristic and early symptom of cerebral vasculitis and Susac syndrome, whereas attacks with thunderclap headache are characteristic for RCVS. Headache is also a common local symptom of cervical arterial dissection, typically with an onset hours or days before the ischaemic event. Progressive headache is typical for cerebral venous thrombosis (CVT); however, some CVT patients present with thunderclap headache.

Physical examination

A complete physical examination with attention to the cardiovascular system, skin, mucous membranes, and eyes is recommended. A tall stature and deformity of the chest wall may indicate Marfan syndrome, Loeys–Dietz syndrome or homocystinuria, while a short stature is common in mitochondrial disease. Lack of brachial pulse and/or blood pressure differences between arms is typical for Takayasu disease.

Examination of the skin may reveal clues indicating Sneddon syndrome (livedo racemosa), Fabry disease (angiokeratomas), neurofibromatosis type 1 (café au lait changes), Lyme borreliosis (erythema migrans), Osler–Weber–Rendu disease (widespread telangiectasias), pseudoxanthoma elasticum (extremely elastic skin and cobble-like skin lesions around neck and axillary regions), intravenous use of illicit drugs, and systemic disorders (erythema nodosum, butterfly erythema). Similarly, examination of the eyes is important. Bilateral ptosis is common in mitochondrial disease, while Horner syndrome may indicate carotid artery dissection. Dislocation of the lens is a common feature of Marfan syndrome and homocystinuria, and in patients with Ehlers–Danlos syndrome or osteogenesis imperfecta, the sclera may have a blueish appearance. Scleritis, uveitis, iritis, and keratitis are common in systemic inflammatory disease including Behçet's disease and Cogan syndrome. Hamartoma of the iris (Lisch nodules) is typical for neurofibromatosis type 1. Retinal changes with angioid streaks are found in pseudoxanthoma elasticum and sickle cell anaemia, retinitis pigmentosa in mitochondrial disease, and Fabry disease, while retinal haemorrhages may indicate vasculitis or septic emboli in infective endocarditis.

Imaging

Magnetic resonance imaging (MRI) is the method of choice for brain imaging as it provides important information about differential diagnosis as well as the pattern of vascular injury, which, in turn may give clues to the underlying aetiology. Multiple infarcts in different arterial territories indicate a central source of embolism (cardiac, pulmonary, or aortic), vasculitis, or moyamoya disease. Location of infarcts in watershed areas is a common finding in moyamoya, sickle cell disease, and RCVS. Haemorrhagic infarcts imply cardiac embolism or CVT, while a pattern with a combination of haemorrhage and infarcts of different ages suggests endocarditis, vasculitis, moyamoya, CVT, or RCVS. Multiple lacunar infarcts with widespread leucoaraiosis at a young age are hints of heritable small vessel disease, with a typical involvement of the anterior temporal pole and the capsula externa in CADASIL. In Behçet's disease and mitochondrial disease, lesions are more common in the posterior circulation, while lesions in the central corpus callosum are typical for Susac syndrome.

Magnetic resonance angiography (MRA) can be used for confirming or excluding atherosclerosis, arterial dissection, fibromuscular dysplasia (FMD), and moyamoya disease. MRA may also reveal other vascular changes, such as beading of cerebral arteries, intracranial aneurysms, dolichoectasias, and vascular tortuosities. These changes are less specific but may indicate an underlying disorder. For instance, beading of cerebral arteries may be caused by RCVS, vasculitis, mitochondrial arteriopathy, or intracranial atherosclerosis. Intracerebral aneurysms, dolichoectasias and vascular tortuosities are more prevalent in patients with FMD and inherited connective tissue disorders.

Laboratory investigations

Routine laboratory testing in young ischaemic stroke should include complete blood and platelet count, erythrocyte sedimentation rate (ESR),

C-reactive protein (CRP), electrolytes, glucose, lipid profile, renal and hepatic functions, activated partial thromboplastin time (APTT), international normalized ratio, thyroid stimulating hormone, heart enzymes, and pregnancy testing in women of child-bearing age. Findings from these tests may give clues to an array of different underlying disorders including infections, systemic vasculitides, lupus anticoagulant, connective tissue disease, anaemia, myeloproliferative disorders, and malignancy as well as conventional vascular risk factors.

Second-line evaluations

Second-line specific tests consist of a wide array of tests including digital subtraction angiography (DSA), magnetic resonance (MR) venography, thorax computed tomography (CT), retinal fluorescein angiography, cerebrospinal fluid (CSF) analysis, blood laboratory testing such as toxicology screen, autoantibodies, protein and haemoglobin electrophoresis, GLA activity, lactate, tests for inherited coagulopathies, and homocysteine, various tests for infectious diseases, genetic testing, tissue biopsies, and others. These tests should be considered in selected patients based on clinical clues and findings from imaging (Table 6.1 and Fig. 6.1). For instance, DSA should be considered when there are clinical hints of cerebral vasculitis as it is superior to MRA with respect to spatial and temporal resolution. Analysis of CSF is mainly indicated when there is a suspicion of vasculitis, central nervous system (CNS) infection or malignancy, and testing for inherited coagulopathies can be considered in patients with personal or family history of recurrent venous thrombosis or recurrent cryptogenic strokes.

Special aetiologies

Non-atherosclerotic non-inflammatory arteriopathies

The most common of the non-atherosclerotic non-inflammatory arteriopathies causing ischaemic stroke are cervical artery dissection, moyamoya, and FMD (Box 6.1). Cervical artery dissection accounts for about 15% of ischaemic strokes in young adults (1–3), is the most common single aetiology, and must be proven or excluded in every young stroke patient (Chapter 4).

Moyamoya is characterized by a chronic progressive stenosis or occlusion at the terminal intracranial portion of the internal carotid arteries and in the proximal portions of the anterior and middle cerebral arteries. Although less common, the basilar and posterior cerebral arteries may also be involved. Reduced blood flow in the stenosed or occluded arteries leads to development of a compensatory network of thin collaterals in the basal regions of the brain,

Box 6.1 Non-atherosclerotic non-inflammatory arteriopathic causes of ischaemic stroke

- Dissection of extracranial and intracranial arteries
- Fibromuscular dysplasia
- Moyamoya disease
- Radiation-induced angiopathy
- Dolichoectatic basilar artery, arterial kinking
- Coiling and hypoplasia of cervical arteries
- Cerebral amyloid angiopathies
- Tumoural encasement of cervicocerebral arteries
- Retinocochleocerebral arteriopathy (Susac syndrome)
- Divry–Van Bogaert syndrome (diffuse meningocerebral angiomatosis and leucoencephalopathy)
- Eosinophil-induced neurotoxicity
- Epidermal nevus syndrome
- Endovascular lymphoma
- Sturge–Weber syndrome (encephalotrigeminal angiomatosis)
- *SAMHD1* gene mutation associated cerebral vasculopathy.

appearing as a hazy 'puff of smoke' ('moyamoya' in Japanese) on angiographic imaging (4). The typical moyamoya pattern of angiopathy (Fig. 6.2) may be idiopathic ('moyamoya disease') or related to another underlying condition ('moyamoya syndrome'), such as atherosclerosis, neurofibromatosis type 1, Down's syndrome, cranial therapeutic irradiation, thyroid disease, sickle cell disease, and brain tumours.

Moyamoya disease is more common in East Asian populations than in Caucasians, affects females twice as often as males, with two incidence peaks, a first between 5 and 10 years of age, and a second around the mid 40s. Brain ischaemia is the most common clinical manifestation. Patients typically present with recurrent ischaemic stroke or transient ischaemic attack, or both, due to hypoperfusion in the territories of the affected vessels. Brain ischaemia may also manifest as seizures or progressive cognitive decline. Various situations contributing to reduced cerebral perfusion may trigger ischaemic events, including hyperventilation, crying, playing wind instruments, exertion, stress, dehydration, and induction of anaesthesia. Other manifestations of moyamoya

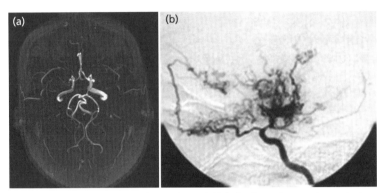

Fig. 6.2 Magnetic resonance angiography and digital subtraction angiography in a patient with moyamoya disease showing typical bilateral occlusion of the proximal middle cerebral arteries (a) and a compensatory network of thin collaterals in the basal regions of the brain (b).

are related to the compensatory mechanisms responding to arterial steno-occlusion. Migraine-like headache, possibly due to stimulation of dural noci-ceptors by dilated transdural collaterals, is frequent. Intracranial haemorrhage may occur as fragile vessels in the collateral networks rupture. Haemorrhage may also be caused by rupture of a saccular aneurysm developed at the apex of the basilar artery or posterior communicating artery secondary to the shift of blood flow. Choreiform movements have also been reported, probably reflect-ing basal ganglia damage due to moyamoya-associated collaterals in this area. Diagnosis is based on angiographic findings, with either MRA or DSA showing stenosis or occlusion of the terminal portion of the intracranial internal carotid artery or proximal portion of the anterior and/or middle cerebral arteries in combination with abnormal vascular networks near the occlusive or stenotic lesions.

FMD is a segmental vascular disease of small-to medium sized arteries of unknown pathophysiology that primarily affects middle-aged women. It is characterized by alternating thickening and thinning of the arterial wall with mural aneurysms resulting in a typical 'string-of-bead' pattern on angiography. The prevalence of FMD in the general population is not known. Renal arteries are the most prevalent location, followed by the cervical arteries (5) (Fig. 6.3). Cervical FMD typically affects the middle and distal portions of the internal carotid and vertebral arteries. The typical FMD string-of-beads pattern is rarely seen in intracranial arteries, but patients with cervical FMD have increased fre-quency of intracranial aneurysms (5).

The risk of cerebrovascular events in cerebrocervical FMD is considered rela-tively low, but data are very limited. However, there is a clear association with cervical artery dissection and intracranial aneurysms. When cervical FMD

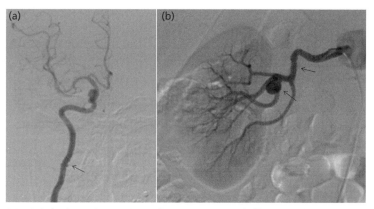

Fig. 6.3 Digital subtraction angiography in a patient with fibromuscular dysplasia showing a string-of-beads pattern in the internal carotid artery (a) and renal artery (b), along with a renal artery aneurysm (b).

is discovered in a stroke patient during diagnostic workup, screening of both renal and intracranial vessels for FMD involvement is recommended (5).

Susac syndrome (retinocochleocerebral arteriopathy) is a rare occlusive endotheliopathy affecting arterioles leading to microinfarcts in the brain, retina, and cochlea (6). Young and middle-aged females are predominately affected. The pathophysiology is unclear, but an autoimmune-mediated endothelial injury is presumed (7). Clinically, Susac syndrome is characterized by the triad of encephalopathy, visual disturbances, and sensorineural hearing loss. Few patients present with the complete triad and the disease usually starts with headache followed by encephalopathy characterized by focal, cognitive, and/or psychiatric features. Visual disturbances include scotoma, blurred vision, and photopsia reflecting multiple branch retinal artery occlusions. Hearing loss is usually bilateral and asymmetric; vertigo and tinnitus are also common features. In about half of the patients, the disease has a monophasic self-limiting course during less than 2 years, while in others the disease relapses and follows a polyphasic course. The diagnosis is based on clinical presentation, typical brain MRI findings with multifocal hyperintensive lesions in the central corpus callosum on T2-weighted imaging, and the demonstration of branch retinal occlusions on fluorescein angiography.

Non-atherosclerotic inflammatory arteriopathies

Vasculitis is a rare cause of stoke in young adults, accounting for about 1–2% of the cases (2, 3). It may occur as a manifestation of primary (isolated) angiitis of the central nervous system (PANCS), as cerebral involvement in the setting of systemic vasculitis, connective tissue disorders, or secondary to infections, neoplasms, drugs, or radiation (Box 6.2) (8, 9). The common characteristic

Box 6.2 Non-atherosclerotic inflammatory arterio-pathic causes of ischaemic stroke

Isolated CNS vasculitis

- Primary angiitis of the central nervous system.

Vasculitis in association with systemic disease

- Takayasu's arteritis
- Giant cell arteritis (temporal arteritis)
- Polyarteritis nodosa
- ANCA-associated vasculitis: granulomatosis with polyangiitis, microscopic polyarteritis, Churg–Strauss syndrome
- Cryoglobulinaemic vasculitis
- Behçet's disease
- Vasculitis associated with connective tissue disorders: SLE, rheumatoid arthritis, Sjögren's syndrome, dermatomyositis, mixed connective tissue disease, sarcoidosis, scleroderma
- Vasculitis associated with inflammatory bowel disease
- Eales disease
- Buerger disease (thromboangiitis obliterans)
- Kawasaki disease
- Cogan syndrome
- Sweet syndrome (acute febrile dermatosis)
- Kohlmeier–Degos disease (malignant atrophic papulosis)
- Acute posterior multifocal placoid pigment epitheliopathy
- Vogt–Koyanagi–Harada syndrome
- ADA2-associated polyarteritis nodosa vasculopathy.

Secondary vasculitis in association with infectious disease

- Viral: herpes zoster, HIV, hepatitis B and C, *Cytomegalovirus*, Coxsackie-9 virus, California encephalitis virus, mumps, Paramyxovirus, Epstein–Barr virus
- Bacterial: bacterial meningitis, syphilis, tuberculosis, *Mycoplasma pneumoniae, Borrelia burgdorferi*

- Parasitic: leptospirosis, cysticercosis, malaria
- Fungal infections: aspergillosis, mucormycosis, coccidioidomycosis, candidosis.

Other inflammatory arteriopathies

- Neoplastic and paraneoplastic vasculitis: lymphomas, malign histiocytosis, hairy cell leukaemia
- Radiation vasculitis
- Hypersensitive vasculitis: Henoch–Schönlein purpura, drug-induced, chemical.

feature is inflammation and sometimes necrosis of the vessel wall leading to stenosis, occlusion, aneurysmal dilatations, and occasionally rupture of the affected vessels. According to the calibre of the predominately affected vessel, vasculatures may be classified into three main groups; large, medium, and small vessel vasculitis.

Large vessel vasculitides include Takayasu's arteritis and temporal arteritis. Both conditions are characterized by a granulomatous vessel wall inflammation with giant cells, and affect women more frequently than men. They present with non-specific symptoms and signs of systemic illness such as fever, malaise, weight loss, and elevated CRP and ESR. However Takayasu's arteritis occurs earlier in life than temporal arteritis, usually before 50 years of age, while temporal arteritis is rare before the age of 50. Takayasu's arteritis affects the aorta and its major branches, eventually leading to stenosis and occlusion with ischaemic symptoms from the extremities or brain. Systolic blood pressure differences of more than 10 mmHg between both arms and decreased or absent brachial artery pulse are typical findings at physical examination. Temporal arteritis affects mainly temporal and ophthalmic arteries and may manifest as persisting headache, jaw claudication, visual symptoms including diplopia, amaurosis fugax, and blindness; and, rarely, as ischaemic stroke.

Medium vessel vasculitides include Kawasaki syndrome, polyarteritis nodosa, and PANCS, although the latter mainly affects small arteries. Cerebral involvement is unusual in Kawasaki syndrome, but polyarteritis nodosa may manifest as ischaemic stroke, haemorrhagic stroke, and/or progressive encephalopathy. The majority of these patients also display general symptoms and signs of systemic involvement including fever, malaise, weight loss, arthritis, polyneuropathy multiplex, acral necroses, and/or severe peripheral ischaemia.

Small vessel vasculitides include PANCS, ANCA-positive systemic vasculitides, and immune complex-associated vasculitides. PANCS is restricted to vessels of the brain and the spinal cord. Small arteries are primarily affected, but medium-sized arteries, arterioles, capillaries, venules, and veins may be involved as well. The median age of onset is 50 years; men and women are affected equally. As no other organs are involved, patients do not present with symptoms or signs of systemic disease. Acute-phase proteins (i.e. ESR, CRP) are seldom elevated, and serum auto-antibodies are negative. The clinical manifestations are restricted to the involvement of the brain and spinal cord, and include headache, encephalopathy, myelopathy, and ischaemic and haemorrhagic strokes. Onset may be acute, subacute, or slowly progressive with a relapsing–remitting course. Different subsets with respect to clinical features and prognosis have been identified. The most ominous variant is rapidly progressive PANCS presenting with repeated strokes, and angiogram showing multifocal involvement of cerebral arteries. Other subsets include variants restricted to small vessel involvement, often presenting with subacute or acute encephalopathy, headache, greatly raised concentrations of CSF proteins, meningeal or parenchymal enhancing lesions on MRI, and negative angiograms. These variants respond positively to treatment and have an overall favourable course. Intracerebral or subarachnoid haemorrhages are associated with necrotizing vasculitis and occur in about 10% of the cases with PANCS (8). Cognitive decline and MRI evidence of cerebral infarcts is less common in this subgroup.

In the ANCA-positive primary systemic vasculitides, Churg–Strauss syndrome, granulomatosis with polyangiitis (formerly known as Wegener's granulomatosis), and microscopic polyangiitis, the clinical cerebral manifestations are similar to PANCS. However, there are also signs and symptoms of extracranial involvement typically with asthma and eosinophilia in Churg–Strauss syndrome, and granulomas in the upper airways and/or renal involvement in granulomatosis with polyangiitis.

Cerebral small vessels may also be involved in immune complex-associated vasculitides in Behçet's disease, cryoglobulinaemic angiitis, or connective tissue diseases such as SLE, rheumatoid arthritis, and Sjögren's syndrome. However, connective tissue diseases may cause stroke by mechanisms other than vasculitis, as they may also be associated with antiphospholipid antibodies, heart valve disease, Libmann–Sacks endocarditis, thrombotic thrombocytopenic purpura, and accelerated atherosclerosis.

Behçet's disease is a multisystem, chronic relapsing vasculitis affecting predominately the venous system that is more prevalent along the route of the historical Silk Road in the Middle East, Central Asia, and Far East. Recurrent oral and genital ulcers and recurrent uveitides (Behçet's triad) are the most common clinical manifestations and frequently the only symptoms at onset. During the course of the disease, involvement of the CNS occurs in about 30% of the patients, usually as parenchymal neuro-Behçet's disease with headache and ischaemic lesions predominantly located in the brainstem, and more seldom as non-parenchymal neuro-Behçet's disease with cerebral venous thrombosis.

Diagnosing cerebral vasculitis is a challenge. It is a rare disease with a number of mimickers, and there is no single test that combines high sensitivity and specificity (10, 11). Diagnosis is based on a combination of clinical, laboratory, and imaging findings. Brain biopsy may be required in selected cases. Clinical hints for vasculitis are headache, multifocal ischaemic and/or haemorrhagic strokes, seizures, and subacute progressive cognitive impairments. Symptoms and signs of infection, systemic inflammatory or connective tissue disease, pulmonary or kidney involvement, elevated ESR, CRP, hypochromic anaemia, thrombocytosis, and low complement may indicate secondary cerebral vasculitis. Almost all patients with cerebral vasculitis show MRI abnormalities. These include ischaemic lesions of varying age, combinations of ischaemic and haemorrhagic lesions, and/or diffuse white matter lesions suggestive of small vessel involvement. MR or CT angiography may show vascular pathology, but conventional angiography should be used for confirmation when cerebral vasculitis is suspected. The typical findings are irregular alternating segments of arterial narrowing and dilatation and multilocular occlusions of intracranial vessels (Fig. 6.4). However, such findings are not pathognomonic for vasculitis. Similar angiographic changes may be seen in a broad range of conditions including RCVS, intracranial atherosclerosis, mitochondrial angiopathy, antiphospholipid syndrome, septic angiitis, and intravascular lymphoma.

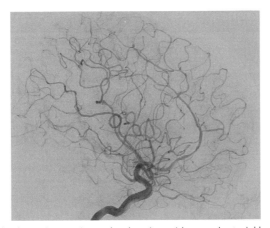

Fig. 6.4 Digital subtraction angiography showing widespread arterial beading in a patient with cerebral vasculitis.

Moreover, a normal angiogram cannot exclude vasculitis when small vessels are exclusively involved. In PANCS, about 25% of cases do not display any vessel changes on angiography despite repeated investigations. In contrast, CSF examinations disclose abnormal findings in 80–90% of the cases, usually with elevated protein levels and/or mild lymphocytic pleocytosis. Again, such findings are non-specific and common to CNS inflammatory conditions. However, a completely normal CSF examination makes cerebral vasculitis unlikely.

Brain biopsy is the only test that can definitely prove a diagnosis of cerebral vasculitis, and may be indicated when the combination of clinical, laboratory, and imaging features are suggestive but non-conclusive. Mortality and morbidity rates in stereotactic brain biopsies have been reported to be less than 1% and 3.5% respectively (11), and it can be argued that this risk is lower than blind treatment with aggressive immunotherapy. Other advantages of brain biopsy in uncertain cases are disclosure of an alternative diagnosis requiring specific treatment. However, given the segmental involvement of cerebral vasculitis, brain biopsy may also be falsely negative. In cases with clinical diagnosis of PANCS based on history, laboratory, imaging, and response to treatment, biopsy has a sensitivity of 53–74% (11).

Vasospastic syndromes

Vasospasm in cerebral arteries can occur in a number of different conditions (Box 6.3). If severe and longstanding, it may cause ischaemic or haemorrhagic strokes, or both. The most common conditions are RCVS and migraine.

Box 6.3 Vasospastic disorders associated with ischaemic stroke

- Migrainous infarction
- Paroxysmal hypertension
- Reversible cerebral vasoconstriction syndromes (RCVS)
- Subarachnoid haemorrhage
- Post-carotid endarterectomy syndrome
- Hypercalcaemia, hyperparathyroidism
- Neck procedures
- Cerebral angiography
- Systemic or specific infections
- Illicit drugs.

RCVS is a clinicoradiological syndrome characterized by thunderclap headache with or without focal neurological deficits and transient non-atherosclerotic non-inflammatory segmental constriction of cerebral arteries (12–14). It is not a uniform disease entity, but rather a common clinical presentation of a diverse group of disorders characterized by reversible but widespread constriction of the cerebral vasculature. RCVS may occur spontaneously, but is in most cases secondary to exogenous triggers (Table 6.2) of which vasoactive drugs and postpartum state are the most frequent. Dysregulation of the vascular tone leading to vasoconstriction is assumed to be a key pathophysiological mechanism, possibly induced by sympathetic overactivity, endothelial dysfunction, and/or oxidative stress. RCVS is often associated with concurrent posterior reversible encephalopathy syndrome (PRES), and the two syndromes overlap with similar triggers, clinical manifestations, and a monophasic self-limiting course. It is possible that the two syndromes represent clinical manifestations of a common pathophysiology involving altered cerebrovascular tone and endothelial dysfunction.

RCVS affects patients aged 20–50 years with a clear female predominance. The true incidence is not known. However, RCVS does not seem to be uncommon and is probably under-diagnosed. Typically, patients with RCVS present with recurrent thunderclap headaches, that is, attacks with 'worst-ever' headache with instant onset, like a clap of thunder. Concomitant marked blood pressure elevation is common. The headache is usually bilateral lasting 1–3 hours, but may last from minutes to several days. In most cases, the thunderclap headache recurs with several attacks over 1–4 weeks. Many patients report that the headache attacks are triggered by activities that induce sympathetic activation such as exertion, sexual activity, emotions, and Valsalva-triggering manoeuvres. Headache remains the sole clinical manifestation in up to 75% of the cases. Other clinical manifestations are seizures and focal neurological deficits related to ischaemic and/or haemorrhagic cerebrovascular events secondary to vasoconstriction. The clinical course is monophasic with initial progression within 1 month of onset, but no new symptoms after 1 month. Most neurological deficits are transient, but permanent lesions have been observed in about 10% of the patients. Convexity subarachnoid haemorrhage, PRES, and intracerebral haemorrhage mainly occur during the first week, while ischaemic events usually occur during the second or third week after onset. Other clinical patterns have also been described with stroke as the presenting manifestation without preceding thunderclap headache (15). The course is usually benign and self-limiting, but some cases have a fulminant course with multiple infarcts, haemorrhages, and massive brain oedema resulting in severe permanent deficits or even death.

Table 6.2 Potential triggers of the reversible cerebral vasoconstriction syndrome

Vasoactive drugs	Sympathomimetics
	Triptans
	Ergotamine
	Epinephrine
	Bromocriptine
	NSAIDs
	Selective serotonin reuptake inhibitors
	Serotonin noradrenaline reuptake inhibitors
	Cyclophosphamide
	Pseudoephedrine
	Amphetamine derivatives
	Interferon
	Others
Illicit drugs	Amphetamines
	Marijuana
	Cocaine
	Ecstasy
	Lysergic acid diethylamide (LSD)
Recreational drugs	Alcohol
	Nicotine
Pregnancy-related conditions	Late pregnancy
	Postpartum period
	Pre-eclampsia
	Eclampsia
Blood products	Red blood cell transfusion
	Erythropoietin
	Intravenous immunoglobulins
Tumours	Phaeochromocytoma
	Paraganglioma
	Bronchial carcinoid tumour
	Carotid glomus tumour
Medical conditions, interventions	Migraine
	Benign sexual headache
	Primary thunderclap headache
	Carotid artery dissection
	Unruptured saccular cerebral aneurysm
	Head trauma
	Thrombotic thrombocytopenic purpura
	Antiphospholipid antibody syndrome
	Systemic lupus erythematosus
	Hypercalcaemia
	Porphyria
	Haemolysis
	Post-bone marrow transplant
	Neurosurgery
	Carotid endarterectomy
	Neck surgery
	Others

Diagnosis of RCVS is based on the clinical presentation in combination with reversible widespread segmental cerebral artery vasoconstriction on repeated angiograms. Typically, cerebral angiograms show a bilateral string-of-beads pattern reflecting segmental vasoconstriction involving both the posterior and anterior circulation. DSA remains the gold standard; the sensitivity of CT or MR angiography is about 70%. In about one-third of the patients, angiograms may be negative during the first week, and repeated investigations may therefore be required for diagnosis. It must be emphasized that the string-of-beads pattern is not specific for RCVS. A similar pattern may be seen in atherosclerosis, infectious arteritis, and inflammatory vasculitis. Moreover, aneurysmal subarachnoid haemorrhage, cerebral artery dissection, and cerebral venous thrombosis may have a similar clinical presentation with thunderclap headache and focal neurological deficits and must be ruled out. In RCVS, the angiographic findings disappear within 12 weeks of disease onset. CSF analysis is normal which helps to distinguish RCVS from vasculitis. High-resolution MR vessel wall imaging may also be helpful in distinguishing RCVs from inflammatory vasculitis (13).

Migraine roughly doubles the risk of ischaemic stroke (16). This risk seems to be confined to migraine with aura, correlates to the number of migraine attacks, affects mainly women and young adults, and is modified by other risk factors. The combination of smoking and oral contraceptive use confers a particularly high risk as it increases the risk of stroke by a factor of ten in young females with aural migraine. The mechanisms explaining the association between migraine with aura and stroke are not clear and probably complex. The International Headache Society criteria for migrainous infarction require that a patient with a history of aural migraine has, for that patient, a typical aura that persists for longer than 60 minutes, with neuroimaging evidence of infarct in a relevant area, and that the infarct cannot be attributed to another cause. Applying these criteria, migrainous infarction accounts for less than 1% of the cases in large series of ischaemic stroke (2, 3, 17). Thus, vasospastic migrainous infarctions may only explain a minor part of the association between migraine and stroke. Other possible mechanisms include increased prevalence of vascular risk factors among patients with migraine, a shared genetic susceptibility, and use of vasoconstrictor medication in sensitive individuals. Moreover, focal brain ischaemia may trigger a symptomatic migraine attack with aura, and migraine with aura is more prevalent in a number of conditions that themselves increase the risk of stroke, such as CADASIL, brain arteriovenous malformations, leptomeningeal angiomatosis, Moyamoya syndrome and disease, hereditary haemorrhagic telangiectasia, Sneddon syndrome, MELAS, disorders related to the *COL4A1* and *TREX1* gene mutations, patent foramen ovale (PFO), cervical artery dissection, cardiac myxoma, antiphospholipid antibody syndrome, SLE, essential thrombocythaemia, and polycythaemia (16). As migraine is common, it is important not to over-diagnose migrainous infarction as the underlying cause in any patient with active migraine with aura and concurrent stroke, as other conditions requiring specific treatments may be missed.

Haematological disorders

Various haematological disorders may alter blood rheological or clotting properties and thereby increase the risk of ischaemic stroke (Box 6.4). Blood hyperviscosity may occur in any condition associated with increased cellularity, decreased deformability of red blood cells, or plasma abnormalities. Severe anaemia is associated with increased risk for thrombosis and severe thrombocytosis causes hypercoagulability. All these conditions are easily detected by routine laboratory blood tests including serum and urine protein electrophoresis. Although most of these conditions, except sickle cell anaemia, lack well-documented causality to ischaemic stroke, ischaemic stroke may be the first clinical manifestation, and are important to identify as they may require specific treatment.

The inherited thrombophilias, protein C deficiency, protein S deficiency, antithrombin deficiency, and the factor V Leiden and the prothrombin gene mutations are all firmly associated with increased risk of venous thrombosis but only weakly associated with arterial thrombosis (18). Routine screening for these conditions in young adults with ischaemic stroke is not recommended, as positive findings are likely to be coincidental (19). However, inherited thrombophilia appear to be strongly associated with arterial ischaemic stroke in neonates and children (20), indicating that these factors do contribute to ischaemic stroke in certain situations. Thus, in selected young ischaemic stroke patients with a history of venous thrombosis, a family history of venous thrombosis, or recurrent cryptogenic strokes, testing for the inherited thrombophilias can be motivated, as anticoagulation may be considered in these settings. Moreover, if PFO is involved in stroke mechanisms in a young adult, factors associated with venous thrombosis may well be involved, as PFO is found in 50% of young stroke patients compared to 25% of general populations.

Antiphospholipid antibodies are a group of acquired autoantibodies leading to a hypercoagulative state (21). They are also associated with cardiac valvular abnormalities which may lead to cerebral embolization. Antiphospholipid antibodies are more prevalent in females, in patients with SLE, and can be demonstrated in about half of the patients with Sneddon syndrome. They are well-established risk factors for both venous and arterial thrombosis, with a higher risk for stroke than for myocardial infarction, and can be found in about one of six young stroke patients (22). However, the risk of recurrent vascular

Box 6.4 Haematological disorders associated with ischaemic stroke

Hyperviscosity states

- Plasma abnormalities (paraproteinaemia, Waldenström's macroglobulinaemia, congenital hyperfibrinogenaemia)
- Increased cellularity (polycythaemia vera, stress polycythaemia, erythrocytosis, myeloproliferative syndromes, hyperleucocytic leukaemias)
- Decreased deformability (sickle cell anaemia, spherocytosis, methaemoglobinopathies).

Coagulopathies

- Homocysteinuria
- Sneddon syndrome
- Antiphospholipid syndrome
- Systemic lupus erythematosus
- Nephrotic syndrome
- Deficiencies of protein S, C, antithrombin III, plasminogen, prekallikrein, factors VIII and XII, heparin cofactor II
- Platelet hyperaggregability
- Fibrinolytic insufficiency
- Factor V Leiden mutation
- Prothrombin G202010A mutation
- Vitamin K treatment
- Antifibrinolytic therapy
- Disseminated intravascular coagulation
- Essential thrombocytosis
- Paroxysmal nocturnal haemoglobinuria
- Thrombotic thrombocytopenic purpura
- Snakebite.

Anaemias

- Microcytic anaemias (iron deficiency, thalassaemias, chronic disease, sideroblastic anaemias)

- ◆ Normocytic anaemias (acute haemorrhage or haemolysis, anaplastic anaemia, chronic disease, combined iron and folate deficiencies)
- ◆ Macrocytic anaemias (vitamin B12 deficiency, folic acid deficiency, alcohol-induced, chronic disease.

events seems to be associated with persistent antiphospholipid antibodies as found in the antiphospholipid syndrome. This syndrome is characterized by recurrent thrombosis and pregnancy complications, mainly recurrent miscarriage. According to the laboratory criteria for this syndrome, antiphospholipid antibodies should be present in plasma on two or more occasions at least 12 weeks apart. Thus, a single positive test is not sufficient to indicate increased risk of recurrent vascular events due to phospholipid antibodies. In recent large series of young ischaemic stroke, about 1% of the cases were attributed to the antiphospholipid syndrome (2, 3). Laboratory tests for phospholipid antibodies in plasma include the coagulation inhibitor lupus anticoagulant, anticardiolipin, and anti-β2-glycoprotein antibodies. In patients with lupus anticoagulant, APTT is often prolonged. According to current evidence, presence of lupus anticoagulant seems to be the strongest predictor for recurrent clinical manifestations.

Sneddon syndrome is a rare, non-inflammatory thrombotic vasculopathy involving small- and medium-sized arteries characterized by the combination of cerebrovascular disease and livedo racemose, mainly affecting females between the ages of 20 and 40 (23). The aetiology is unknown, but about half of the patients are positive for antiphospholipid antibodies. Typically, the first clinical manifestation is livedo racemose, a persistent, irregular, net-like bluish pattern in the skin located on limbs, trunk, and buttocks followed by cerebrovascular events, mainly minor ischaemic strokes located in the deep white matter and pons. The course is slowly progressive and repeated ischaemic events may lead to cognitive decline and eventually dementia.

Monogenic and metabolic disorders

Ischaemic stroke has been linked to a large number of monogenic and metabolic disorders, as listed in Table 6.3 and Box 6.5. Most of these disorders are very rare, involve multiple organs, and usually present early in childhood with clinical manifestations other than stroke. However, in some, ischaemic stroke in childhood or early adulthood may be the first major clinical manifestation leading to diagnosis (MELAS, Fabry disease, sickle cell disease), and in others (CADASIL, cerebral autosomal recessive arteriopathy with subcortical infarcts

Table 6.3 Monogenic diseases associated with ischaemic stroke

	Gene region, inheritance
Monogenic disorders with ischaemic stroke as the primary manifestation	
Cerebral autosomal dominant arteriopathy with subcortical infarcts and leucoencephalopathy (CADASIL)	*NOTCH3* mutation, AD
Cerebral autosomal recessive arteriopathy with subcortical infarcts and leucoencephalopathy (CARASIL)	*HTRA1* mutation, AR
Autosomal dominant retinal vasculopathy with cerebral leucodystrophy (RVCL)	*TREX* mutation, AD
COL4A1-related disorders	*COL4A1* mutation, AD
Familiar moyamoya	*ACTA* 2, *MTCP1*, or *RNF213* mutation, AD or AR
ADA2-associated polyarteritis nodosa vasculopathy	*CERC1* mutation, AR
Monogenic disorders with ischaemic stroke as a recognized but not primary manifestation	
Sickle cell disease	*HBB* mutation, AR
Fabry disease	*GLA* mutation, X-linked recessive
Familiar hemiplegic migraine	*CACNA1A, ATP1A2*, or *SCAN1* mutation, AD
Hereditary haemorrhagic telangiectasia (Osler–Weber syndrome)	Several, *ACVRL1, ENG*, or *SMAD4* mutations most common, AD
Vascular Ehlers–Danlos syndrome	*COL3A1* mutation, AD
Marfan syndrome	Fibrillin 1 mutation, AD
Pseudoxanthoma elasticum	*ABCC6* mutation, AR
Loeys–Dietz syndrome	*TGFBR1* or *TGFBR2* mutation, AD
Arterial tortuosity syndrome	*SLCA10* mutation, AR
Neurofibromatosis type 1 (von Recklinghausen disease)	*NF1* mutation, AD
Carney syndrome (facial lentiginosis and myxoma)	*PRKAR1A* gene, AD
MELAS	Several, mitochondrial tRNA-Leu mutation most common
SAMHD1 gene mutation-associated cerebral vasculopathy	*SAMHD1* mutation, AD
Adult progeria	*LMNA* gene

Box 6.5 Metabolic disorders associated with ischaemic stroke

- Mitochondrial disorders
  - Mitochondrial encephalopathy, lactic acidosis, and stroke-like episodes (MELAS)
  - Myoclonic epilepsy with ragged-red fibres (MERRF)
  - Leigh's disease (subacute necrotizing encephalomyelopathy)
  - Kearns–Sayre syndrome
  - Mitochondrial recessive ataxia syndrome (MIRAS)
  - Hyperornithinaemia-hyperammonaemia-homocitrullinuria syndrome (HHH)
- Homocystinuria
- Menkes disease
- Tangier disease
- Branched chain organic acidurias (isovaleric-, propionic-, and methylmalonic-aciduria)
- Glutaric aciduria type 1 and type 2
- Urea cycle disorders (ornithine transcarbamylase deficiency, carbamoyl phosphate synthetase 1 deficiency, citrullinaemia, argininosuccinic aciduria, argininaemia)
- Purine nucleoside phosphorylase deficiency.

and leucoencephalopathy (CARASIL), RVCL, familiar moyamoya), cerebrovascular disease is the primary clinical manifestation (Table 6.3). A brief summary of the most important clinical features of these conditions are given later in this section. A more detailed overview of monogenic disorders linked to ischaemic stroke is given in Chapter 11.

CADASIL is the most common monogenic disorder involving the cerebral small arteries and is caused by mutations in the *NOTCH3* gene on chromosome 19q13 (24). The clinical picture is progressive with recurrent subcortical ischaemic strokes and vascular cognitive decline, with about two-thirds of patients developing dementia at 65 years of age. Migraine with aura occurs in about one-third of the cases, and is frequently the initial symptom. Other manifestations include mood disorders, most commonly depression, and acute reversible encephalopathy. Although the mode of inheritance is autosomal dominant, a family history may not be present as the age of onset is highly variable between the second and seventh decade (25). Brain MRIs show multiple lacunar infarcts and widespread white matter hyperintensities on T2 imaging, typically involving the anterior temporal pole and the capsula externa. Diagnosis is confirmed by molecular genetic testing and may also be based on a skin biopsy showing the pathognomonic granular osmiophilic material around vascular smooth muscle cells and basal membranes in dermal arterioles.

CARASIL, RVCL, and the COL4A1-related disorders also involve the cerebral small vessels but are much rarer (25, 26). The clinical picture and imaging findings in CARASIL resembles CADASIL, but is more severe with earlier onset, faster progression of cognitive decline, and is also characterized by premature alopecia and spondylosis. In RVCL and the COL4A1-related disorders, the arteriopathy also involves other organs, mainly the retina and kidney. In COL4A-related disorders, haemorrhagic strokes are more common than ischaemic strokes.

Sickle cell disease is most prevalent in individuals of African descent and is caused by a point mutation in the haemoglobin β-gene leading to changes in red blood cell shape and rheology (27). Sickled red cells tend to adhere to the endothelium which favours thrombus formation, vascular occlusion, and remodelling. In some patients, this leads to a slowly progressive large artery arteriopathy resembling moyamoya with bilateral stenosis and gradual occlusion of the proximal cerebral arteries with compensatory collaterals. Ischaemic stroke may occur in early childhood and are typically located in border zones. Haemorrhagic stroke occurs in the third decade, related to fragile collaterals and aneurysm formation. Other clinical manifestations include vaso-occlusive crises with chest, back, and extremity pain, haemolytic anaemia, and jaundice. Diagnosis can be confirmed by peripheral blood smear, haemoglobin electrophoresis, and molecular genetic testing.

Fabry disease is a rare X-linked lysosomal storage disorder that can be found in about 1% of young patients with ischaemic strokes (1). It is caused by an α-galactosidase A (*GLA*) gene defect that leads to progressive accumulation of glycosphingolipids in vascular endothelium, smooth muscle cells, and autonomic and dorsal root ganglia. The clinical spectrum in females ranges from asymptomatic carriers to severe disease (28). Multiple organs may be involved and the clinical manifestations include painful acroparaesthesia, hypohydrosis, impaired temperature sensation and intestinal dysmotility, angiokeratoma, hearing impairment, corneal dystrophy, cognitive dysfunction, cardiac conduction disturbance, cardiomyopathy, renal failure, cerebral venous thrombosis, and ischaemic and haemorrhagic strokes. However, in a recent large series of young ischaemic strokes, patients with Fabry disease were surprisingly oligosymptomatic, with no or few clinical clues for the diagnosis and mostly no family history for clinical manifestation of the disease. Ischaemic strokes are more common than haemorrhagic strokes, and occur in both large and small vessel levels, and all vascular territories. Brain MRI findings are not disease specific and fail to distinguish patients with Fabry disease from other young stroke patients (29). The diagnosis is based on measurements of GLA activity in plasma, peripheral blood leucocytes, or cultivated fibroblasts and molecular genetic testing.

MELAS is the most common mitochondrial disorder associated with stroke or stroke-like episodes and is associated with mutations in the mitochondrial DNA (mtDNA). It is a genetically and phenotypically heterogeneous disorder that can affect every energy-dependent process and organ in the human body. Inheritance is maternal (30). Symptoms occur before 40 years of age and the course may be relapsing–remitting with progressive disability. Stroke or stroke-like episodes usually manifest clinically as hemiparesis, hemianopia, or cortical blindness. MRI commonly shows involvement of the cortex with a predilection for the posterior areas of the brain, and the lesions may cross vascular territories (Fig. 6.5). The underlying pathophysiologic mechanisms are suggested to

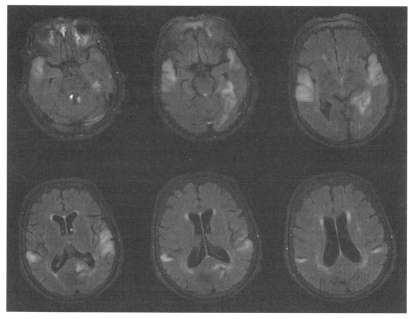

Fig. 6.5 Brain magnetic resonance imaging (FLAIR sequence) in a patient with MELAS showing multiple acute ischaemic lesions.

include failure of neuronal oxidative metabolism, disturbance of the blood–brain barrier, and impaired autoregulation of the cerebral blood flow.

Other clinical manifestations associated with MELAS include encephalopathy, cognitive impairment and seizures, developmental delay, short stature, sensorineural hearing loss, episodic vomiting, diabetes, migraine-like headache, muscle weakness, exercise intolerance, cardiomyopathy, and gastrointestinal disturbance. However, most patients are oligosymptomatic, displaying only one or a few of these symptoms. Most patients have elevated lactate in serum or CSF, or both. Diagnosis of MELAS can be confirmed with a skeletal muscle biopsy showing ragged red fibres or by mitochondrial DNA mutation analysis on blood, skeletal muscle, hair follicles, urinary sediment, or buccal mucosa.

Homocystinuria is a rare disorder, characterized by high plasma concentrations of homocysteine (>100 µmol/L) and increased urinary excretion of the oxidized form of homocysteine, homocystine, early-onset venous thrombosis, atherosclerosis, mental retardation, long stature with Marfan-like features, downward lens dislocation, osteoporosis, and decreased pigmentation of hair and skin (31). This multisystem disorder must be separated from mild hyperhomocysteinaemia (15–100 µmol/L) associated with deficient dietary vitamin B. Homocystinuria is most commonly caused by mutations in the gene encoding cystathionine β-synthase, a key enzyme in the degradation of homocysteine. About half of the patients respond to vitamin B6 treatment. In untreated patients, the hyperhomocysteinaemia causes endothelial dysfunction, promotes atherosclerosis, and enhance coagulation and platelet activation. About half of the patients have a thromboembolic event before the age of 30. The diagnosis can be confirmed by urine analysis, plasma homocysteine, and assessment of cystathionine β-synthase in cultured fibroblasts.

Other causes

A number of miscellaneous disorders are associated with ischaemic stroke (Box 6.6). These include CVT, use of illicit drugs, surgical procedures, pulmonary disease, external mechanical compression interfering with vessel blood flow, and unconventional embolic phenomena. Except for CVT, use of illicit drugs, and iatrogenic stroke, these conditions are very rare and seldom encountered in clinical practise. Virtually all illicit drugs have been reported to increase stroke risk, mainly by causing vasospasm in cerebral arteries. However, other mechanisms may also be involved, including foreign body embolism, infective endocarditis, increased platelet aggregation, and vasculitis. Iatrogenic stokes occur mostly during or directly after cardiac or vascular procedures.

CVT predominantly affects young individuals and may account for about 0.5–1% of ischaemic strokes. Women are affected three times more often than

Box 6.6 Miscellaneous causes of ischaemic stroke

- Cerebral venous thrombosis
- Illicit drugs.

Pulmonary disease

- Arteriovenous fistulas
- Arteriovenous malformations
- Pulmonary tumours.

Mechanical or systemic

- Traumas
- Mediastinal mass
- Cervical rib or atlanto-axial subluxation
- Iatrogenic (cardiac or vascular procedures, transplantation)
- Decompression sickness
- Eagle syndrome (styloid process compressing internal carotid artery)
- Unconventional embolic phenomena
- Fat embolism
- Air embolism
- Fibrocartilaginous embolism
- Aneurysm-borne embolus.

Rare syndromes

- Malignant neuroleptic syndrome
- Stroke-like migraine attacks after radiation therapy (SMART).

men, probably related to gender-specific risk factors such as oral contraceptives, hormonal replacement therapy, pregnancy, and puerperium (32). Other risk factors for CVT include genetic and acquired thrombophilia, local and systemic infection, haematological disorders, inflammatory disease, surgical procedures of the head, cancer, and dehydration. The spectrum of clinical manifestation is wide and may be associated with increased intracranial pressure (progressive headache, papilloedema, and coma) and secondary parenchymal oedema, haemorrhage, or venous infarction (focal symptoms and seizures). Occasionally, patients also present with diffuse encephalopathy or a cavernous sinus syndrome. However, in many patients, the symptoms are limited to mild or moderate headache. Onset may be acute or subacute with slowly progressing symptoms. Diagnosis is based on the visualization of clot material within a sinus or cerebral vein, preferably by MRI and contrast-enhanced MR venography or CT angiography.

Conclusion

The broad spectrum of rare causes in young adults with ischaemic stroke constitutes a major diagnostic challenge. Despite the fast moving technical developments, a thorough clinical evaluation of family and patient medical history, and a careful physical examination combined with neuroimaging and routine laboratory tests remains the basis for identifying these aetiologies.

References

1. **Rolfs A, Fazekas F, Grittner U, Dichgans M, Martus P, Holzhausen M**, et al. Stroke in Young Fabry Patients (sifap) Investigators. Acute cerebrovascular disease in the young: the Stroke in Young Fabry Patients study. Stroke. 2013;**44**:340–49.

2. **Yesilot Barlas N, Putaala J, Waje-Andreassen U, Vassilopoulou S, Nardi K, Odier C**, et al. Etiology of first-ever ischaemic stroke in European young adults: the 15 cities young stroke study. Eur J Neurol. 2013;**20**:1431–39.

3. **Putaala J, Metso AJ, Metso TM, Konkola N, Kraemer Y, Haapaniemi E**, et al. Analysis of 1008 consecutive patients aged 15 to 49 with first-ever ischemic stroke: the Helsinki young stroke registry. Stroke. 2009;**40**:1195–203.

4. **Scott RM, Smith ER.** Moyamoya disease and moyamoya syndrome. N Engl J Med. 2009;**36**:1226–37.

5. **Olin JW, Gornik HL, Bacharach JM, Biller J, Fine LJ, Gray BH**, et al. Fibromuscular dysplasia: state of the science and critical unanswered questions: a scientific statement from the American Heart Association. Circulation. 2014;**129**:1048–78.

6. **Dörr J, Krautwald S, Wildemann B, Jarius S, Ringelstein M, Duning T**, et al. Characteristics of Susac syndrome: a review of all reported cases. Nat Rev Neurol. 2013;**9**:307–16.

7. **Greco A, De Virgilio A, Gallo A, Fusconi M, Turchetta R, Tombolini M**, et al. Susac's syndrome—pathogenesis, clinical variants and treatment approaches. Autoimmun Rev. 2014;**13**:814–21.

8. **Salvarani C, Brown RD Jr, Hunder GG.** Adult primary central nervous system vasculitis. Lancet. 2012;**380**:767–77.

9. **Berlit P.** Diagnosis and treatment of cerebral vasculitis. Ther Adv Neurol Disord. 2010;**3**:29–42.

10. **Berlit P, Kraemer M.** Cerebral vasculitis in adults: what are the steps in order to establish the diagnosis? Red flags and pitfalls. Clin Exp Immunol. 2014;**175**:419–24.

11. **Bhattacharyya S, Berkowitz AL.** Primary angiitis of the central nervous system: avoiding misdiagnosis and missed diagnosis of a rare disease. Pract Neurol. 2016;**16**:195–200.

12. **Miller TR, Shivashankar R, Mossa-Basha M, Gandhi D.** Reversible cerebral vasoconstriction syndrome, part 1: epidemiology, pathogenesis, and clinical course. AJNR Am J Neuroradiol. 2015;**36**:1392–99.

13. **Miller TR, Shivashankar R, Mossa-Basha M, Gandhi D.** Reversible cerebral vasoconstriction syndrome, part 2: diagnostic work-up, imaging evaluation, and differential diagnosis. AJNR Am J Neuroradiol. 2015;**36**:1580–88.

14. **Ducros A, Wolff V.** The typical thunderclap headache of reversible cerebral vasoconstriction syndrome and its various triggers. Headache. 2016;**56**:657–73.

15. **Wolff V, Ducros A.** Reversible cerebral vasoconstriction syndrome without typical thunderclap headache. Headache. 2016;**56**(4):674–87.

16. **Kurth T, Chabriat H, Bousser MG.** Migraine and stroke: a complex association with clinical implications. Lancet Neurol. 2012;**11**:92–100.

17. **Kurth T, Diener HC.** Migraine and stroke: perspectives for stroke physicians. Stroke. 2012;**43**:3421–26.

18. **Morris JG, Singh S, Fisher M.** Testing for inherited thrombophilias in arterial stroke: can it cause more harm than good? Stroke. 2010;**41**:2985–90.

19. **Kalaria C, Kittner S.** The therapeutic value of laboratory testing for hypercoagulable states in secondary stroke prevention. Neurol Clin. 2015;**33**:501–13.

20. **Kenet G, Lütkhoff LK, Albisetti M, Bernard T, Bonduel M, Brandao L**, et al. Impact of thrombophilia on risk of arterial ischemic stroke or cerebral sinovenous thrombosis in neonates and children: a systematic review and meta-analysis of observational studies. Circulation. 2010;**121**:1838–47.

21. **Ruiz-Irastorza G, Crowther M, Branch W, Khamashta MA.** Antiphospholipid syndrome. Lancet. 2010;**376**:1498–509.

22. **Sciascia S, Sanna G, Khamashta MA, Cuadrado MJ, Erkan D, Andreoli L**, et al. The estimated frequency of antiphospholipid antibodies in young adults with cerebrovascular events: a systematic review. Ann Rheum Dis. 2015 Nov;**74**:2028–33.

23. **Wu S, Xu Z, Liang H.** Sneddon's syndrome: a comprehensive review of the literature. Orphanet J Rare Dis. 2014;**9**:215.

24. **Chabriat H, Joutel A, Dichgans M, Tournier-Lasserve E, Bousser MG.** CADASIL. Lancet Neurol. 2009;**8**:643–53.

25. **Tikka S, Baumann M, Siitonen** et al. CADASIL and CARASIL. Brain Pathol. 2014;**24**:525–44.

26. **Choi JC.** Genetics of cerebral small vessel disease. J Stroke. 2015;**17**:7–16.

27. **Switzer JA, Hess DC, Nichols FT, Adams RJ.** Pathophysiology and treatment of stroke in sickle-cell disease: present and future. Lancet Neurol. 2006;**5**:501–12.

28. **Ranieri M, Bedini G, Parati EA, Bersano A.** Fabry disease: recognition, diagnosis, and treatment of neurological features. Curr Treat Options Neurol. 2016;**18**:33.

29. **Fazekas F, Enzinger C, Schmidt R, Grittner U, Giese AK, Hennerici MG**, et al. Brain magnetic resonance imaging findings fail to suspect Fabry disease in young patients with an acute cerebrovascular event. Stroke. 2015;**46**:1548–53.

30. **Sproule DM, Kaufmann P.** Mitochondrial encephalopathy, lactic acidosis, and stroke like episodes: basic concepts, clinical phenotype, and therapeutic management of MELAS syndrome. Ann N Y Acad Sci. 2008;**1142**:133–58.

31. **Testai FD, Gorelick PB.** Inherited metabolic disorders and stroke part 1: Fabry disease and mitochondrial myopathy, encephalopathy, lactic acidosis, and strokelike episodes. Arch Neurol. 2010;**67**(1):19–24.

32. **Coutinho JM.** Cerebral venous thrombosis. J Thromb Haemost. 2015;**13**:S238–44.

Chapter 7

Brain imaging (CT/MRI)

Thomas Gattringer, Christian Enzinger,
Stefan Ropele, and Franz Fazekas

Introduction

In the acute phase of a clinically evident stroke, the exclusion of brain haemorrhage is one of the main goals of neuroimaging to rapidly initiate reperfusion therapies. This information can be sufficiently and rapidly derived from non-contrast cerebral computed tomography (CT), which is not only widely available but also allows other types of intracranial bleeding and gross morphologic brain changes such as mass lesions to be ruled out. In fact, this approach is very efficient and practicable given the 'time is brain' concept and the proven therapeutic efficacy of intravenous thrombolysis within only a short time window of currently 4.5 hours (1–3).

However, stroke patients do not always present with classical symptoms and a variety of other neurologic disorders may present with a stroke-like appearance. These diagnostic uncertainties are especially critical and challenging in young individuals and can often be clarified by magnetic resonance imaging (MRI) using the appropriate sequences. Along these lines, the high sensitivity of diffusion-weighted imaging (DWI) for acute ischaemic lesions has also impacted on the concept of transient ischaemic attacks (TIA), that is, patients with evidence of an acute ischaemic lesion should be considered as having suffered from stroke and not from TIA even when clinical symptoms resolve within 24 hours. MRI also helps to better elucidate the often quite wide range of covert vascular damage encompassing old silent infarcts, white matter hyperintensities, and old microbleeds (4–10). Such findings are not infrequent already in younger stroke patients (11) and highlight the need for an extensive search for aetiological causes including risk factors for stroke and their close control and treatment. Furthermore, the often devastating effects of stroke also justify concentrating all efforts on an optimal use of the increasing armamentarium of stroke treatment, especially in the young, and sophisticated neuroimaging may help in this endeavour. Despite still open questions, we already have some useful hints on how to select those patients who may profit from vessel reopening beyond the 4.5-hour time window or with unclear symptom onset, what treatment strategies to offer patients with large vessel occlusion, or even when a large ischaemic infarct has already developed such as by decompressive hemicraniectomy.

In this chapter, we therefore discuss the role of brain CT and MRI in the diagnosis/differential diagnosis and management (including treatment guidance) of ischaemic stroke patients in general but will focus especially on stroke imaging in the young, which is faced with specific demands and challenges. As information on the blood vessels supplying the brain is a further prerequisite for the adequate management of patients with ischaemic stroke and overlaps in part with morphologic imaging, this chapter should also be seen as complementary to the following Chapter 8 on 'Vascular imaging (CTA/MRA)'.

Computed tomography

With large areas of focal ischaemic damage, CT changes follow a well-recognized temporal pattern as also described elsewhere (Table 7.1) (12). Commonly, three main stages of infarction have been described with CT, which are an initial (acute) stage, a developmental (subacute) stage, and a late or sequellar stage (13). Historically, the initial stage was considered to consist of about the first 24 hours after the acute event with a usually normal or near normal CT. Thus, the main purpose of obtaining a CT scan at that time was primarily to exclude cerebral haemorrhage. The 'developmental stage', which spans the period of the following day up to 4–5 weeks, shows the fundamental characteristics of ischaemic infarction including tissue hypodensity, mass effect, and contrast enhancement which develop to different grades depending on several factors such as size, location, and vascular supply of the area of ischaemic tissue damage. Contrast enhancement usually does not occur before a few days. In the second and third weeks, areas of infarction may also revert back to 'false normal' density. This phenomenon of 'fogging' has been attributed to the resolution of oedema, small petechial haemorrhages, and infiltration of the infarcted tissue with macrophages, which can mask the actual extent of ischaemic damage. In the late or sequelar stage (i.e. approximately after the fourth to sixth weeks of infarction), an area of definite hypodensity or a cystic cavity remains, which is often associated with signs of focal atrophy, that is, a widening of local cerebrospinal fluid (CSF) spaces. The late stage of infarction has been also termed chronic but it appears preferable to rather talk about old infarcts as this residual deficit constitutes a final stage rather than a chronic process.

With the therapeutic option of intravenous thrombolysis, attention in CT interpretation has shifted strongly to the initial stage of infarction and subtle

Table 7.1 CT characteristics of acute ischaemic lesions and their evolution

Stages	Morphologic changes	Time
Initial (acute)	Vague blurring of grey–white matter boundaries, slight attenuation of the insular ribbon, slight indistinctness of basal ganglia grey matter	First hours
	Suggestion of crowding sulci (subtle mass effect)	
	'Dense artery' sign Changes become increasingly distinct	
Developmental (subacute)	Distinctly hypodense area within territory of vascular supply	> Day 1 to 2–4 weeks
	focal swelling/mass effect (sulcal and/or ventricular effacement)	
	Contrast enhancement (especially of grey matter structures)	
	'Fogging' (area of ischaemia becomes poorly recognizable—rare)	2–3 weeks
Late (old infarct)	Demarcated area of pronounced hypodensity (close to CSF), cystic cavity	4–6 weeks
	Focal atrophy	

Reproduced from Fazekas F, Ropele S, Enzinger C, Stroke. In: Filippi M (ed), Oxford Textbook of Neuroimaging, p. 185–199, Copyright (2015), with permission from Oxford University Press.

morphologic changes that may indicate an acute ischaemic infarct quite early (14). These changes mainly consist of a blurring of anatomic borders such as of the grey/white matter interface with slight sulcal effacement and may appear already within the first 3 hours after stroke. However, they are expected to be seen predominantly with larger infarcts and cannot fully compensate for the undisputedly lower sensitivity of CT for ischaemic tissue changes when compared to MRI (2). Such increased sensitivity is especially desirable for patients with minor symptoms, suspected brainstem or recent small subcortical infarcts (formerly termed acute lacunar infarcts) and especially when there are diagnostic challenges.

Magnetic resonance imaging

MRI findings of infarction also vary with time (Table 7.2) (12). Similar to CT, volume changes accompany the evolution of infarction, at least if sufficiently large, which consist of swelling in the acute phase and of volume loss/focal atrophy after brain tissue has undergone necrosis. These changes may be seen directly involving large portions of the brain, but can also be restricted to only small areas or compartments such as the cortical ribbon. Mass effect and atrophy can be appreciated from changes in the widths of the cortical sulci or the ventricles. Signal changes on conventional MRI per se, such as CT hypodensity, are not very specific. Thus the shape and location of signal abnormalities are important aspects. As for many types of pathology, ischaemic lesions appear hyperintense on T2-weighted sequences. Heavily T2-weighted sequences are most sensitive and focal increases in signal intensity may occur as early as 90 minutes after symptom onset, but usually become apparent only within 2–3 hours. An obvious disadvantage of T2-weighted MRI is the overlap in signal intensity of the acute lesion with that of CSF spaces, which also appear bright on this sequence. This problem is avoided by using fluid-attenuated inversion recovery (FLAIR) sequences, which suppress the signal from CSF and thus increase the conspicuity of ischaemic lesions particularly at the brain–CSF interfaces. On T1-weighted images, most acute infarcts are first barely or not seen at all. With time, the ischaemic lesion becomes increasingly hypointense until it reaches isointensity with CSF, if complete necrosis occurs and a cystic defect remains. Table 7.2 summarizes the characteristics of lesion evolution on conventional MRI.

While MRI already excels in terms of sensitivity for tissue changes over CT when using conventional sequences, a decisive further step forward comes from using DWI (15, 16). This technique is sensitive to the motion of water protons which

Table 7.2 MRI characteristics of acute ischaemic lesions and their evolution

Stage	Signal changes	Time
Internal (acute)	DWI hyperintensity (reduced ADC)	45–90 minutes
	T2 hyperintensity (T2-weighted sequences, FLAIR), often early on vague and indistinct	60 minutes to first hours
	No or minimal T1 hypointensity	
	Subtle mass effect	
	Absence of 'flow void', 'vessel signs'	
Developmental (subacute)	Bright lesion on DWI (reduced ADC), 'light bulb'	> Day 1 to
	Well-defined area of T2 hyperintensity (T2-weighted sequences, FLAIR)	2–4 weeks > 3–7 days
	T1 hypointensity	
	Mass effect (sulcal and/or ventricular effacement)	
	Gyriform contrast enhancement	
Late (old infarct)	Demarcated lesion with central isointensity to CSF on all sequences, i.e. cystic cavity	4–6 weeks
	Focal atrophy	

Reproduced from Fazekas F, Ropele S, Enzinger C, Stroke. In: Filippi M (ed), Oxford Textbook of Neuroimaging, pp. 185–199, Copyright (2015) with permission from Oxford University Press.

differs between tissues/compartments and starts to change almost immediately after the onset of ischaemia due to the development of intracellular oedema. The shift in water from the extracellular to the intracellular compartment(s) obviously causes a reduction in the diffusivity of the water protons, which can be appreciated on a map of the apparent diffusion coefficient (ADC). On DWI, this translates into high signal intensity of the ischaemic tissue against a background of medium to low signal intensity that makes it light up ('light bulb phenomenon'). Thus DWI abnormalities are the first morphologic evidence for ischaemic damage to appear and are quite easily detected. Furthermore, the reduction of diffusivity is also rather specific for ischaemic damage, which helps in differential diagnosis and to identify acute lesions among pre-existing morphologic abnormalities both in the very acute setting as well as over the first few days (17). In rare cases and most likely due to successful reperfusion of incomplete ischaemic damage, the DWI lesion may revert to normal within hours. Otherwise it takes 3–10 days—and sometimes even longer—before the ADC reverts back to a stage of pseudonormalization and subsequently increases to a level of the CSF as a consequence of tissue necrosis (18).

It is of note that the development of signal changes from acute ischaemia including DWI may take longer in infra- rather than supratentorial brain structures and especially in the brainstem. Thus, acute brainstem infarcts can remain invisible on MRI for several hours after the acute event (19). Higher b-values and thin sagittal sections may help to overcome this problem. Otherwise a follow-up MRI should be considered (Fig. 7.1). Further evolution of ADC changes appears also delayed which is probably a consequence of the structural properties of the brainstem (20).

For some time, concerns existed regarding the sensitivity and specificity of MRI for haematoma detection in the acute setting of stroke, that is, CT was needed to rule out intracerebral bleeding. The introduction of T2*-weighted gradient-echo images and subsequently of DWI put an end to this debate. Acute bleeding appears hypointense at least at the periphery of the haematoma on both sequences, which is clearly different from an acute ischaemic lesion. Thus acute bleeds often have mixed signal intensity on both sequences with a 'target-like' appearance (21). Using these sequences, a similar sensitivity and specificity for the detection of intracerebral bleeding was confirmed in a large head-to-head comparison with CT (22). However, this is certainly not true for detecting blood in the CSF and CT remains the preferred imaging technique for patients with suspected subarachnoid haemorrhage.

In regard to intracerebral bleeding, however, the sensitivity of MRI for iron and the resulting ability to detect residues of haemorrhage provides unprecedented insights. The paramagnetic effects of haemosiderin cause a loss of signal on T2-weighted images, which allows lasting identification of defects from prior intracerebral bleeds by their hypointense rim. Susceptibility-sensitive

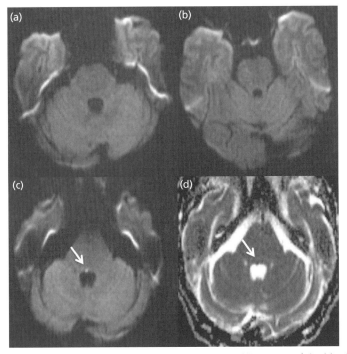

Fig. 7.1 A 45-year-old male patient complained about sudden onset of double vision. In the clinical examination he had internuclear ophthalmoplegia in the right eye. Initial MRI a few hours after symptom onset did not depict any abnormalities (a, b). Follow-up MRI scans 5 days later showed the small corresponding ischaemic infarct in the right medial longitudinal fasciculus (DWI (c) and ADC (d) scans, arrows).

sequences, such as T2*-weighted images, are even more sensitive and can detect already very small amounts of haemosiderin deposition by a kind of 'blooming' artefact. This has led to the recognition of microbleeds. Several lines of evidence indicate their association especially with hypertensive microangiopathy, cerebral amyloid angiopathy, but also hereditary angiopathies such as 'cerebral autosomal dominant arteriopathy with subcortical infarcts and leucoencephalopathy' (CADASIL) and they are now an accepted hallmark finding of cerebral small vessel diseases (10, 23, 24).

Table 7.3 summarizes the advantages and limitations of brain CT and MRI in the evaluation of patients with suspected acute stroke (25).

Patterns of ischaemic changes and their relation to aetiology

The acute ischaemic lesion(s) vary strongly in number, size, and location in the brain between different stroke patients. Major contributing factors to this

Table 7.3 Advantages of brain CT and MRI in the setting of acute stroke

Advantages of brain CT	Advantages of brain MRI
Organizational aspects	
Wide availability	
Rapid image acquisition	
Lower costs	
Patient-related aspects	
Robust against motion artefacts	No ionizing radiation
Ease for patient monitoring	Less renal toxicity of contrast agent
Scanning of ventilated patients	
Accessibility for patients with metallic implants	
Diagnostic aspects	
Detection of acute subarachnoid haemorrhage	Depiction of acute ischaemic lesions
	Detection of small ischaemic infarcts and infratentorial lesions
	Differentiation between acute and chronic infarcts
	Detection of chronic haemorrhage (e.g. microbleeds, superficial haemosiderosis)
	Diagnosis of central nervous system disorders mimicking acute stroke

Source: data from AJNR Am J Neuroradiol., 34(11), Wintermark M, Sanelli PC, Albers GW, Bello JA, Derdeyn CP, Hetts SW, et al, Imaging Recommendations for Acute Stroke and Transient Ischemic Attack Patients, E117–27, Copyright (2013), American Journal of Neuroradiology.

variability are the affected vascular territories including the individual formation of the extra- and intracranial vasculature and the source and aetiology of the perfusion deficit. This may give rise to some infarct patterns, which suggest specific stroke aetiologies whereby coexisting morphologic changes such as old infarcts or lacunes, white matter hyperintensities, and microbleeds should be included in this consideration.

Thus, multiple acute ischaemic lesions throughout the brain are suggestive of a proximal (heart or aortic arch) embolic mechanism, especially when cortical areas are affected. The same suggestion will come from one acute and one old cortical infarct in vascular territories supplied by different extracranial vessels. In young stroke patients, other less common stroke aetiologies such as central nervous system vasculitis or metastatic cancer also have to be considered with multiple ischaemic lesions throughout the brain (Fig. 7.2) (26, 27) and they may occur even in patients with pronounced small vessel disease (28–30).

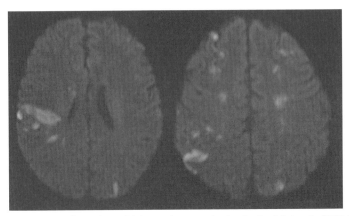

Fig. 7.2 Ischaemic infarcts in multiple cerebrovascular territories bilaterally (DWI MRI scans) in a 47-year-old male patient with metastatic pancreatic cancer in the absence of any cardioembolic source.

Multiple, unilateral, deep border zone infarcts (often of different ages) have been closely linked to artery-to-artery embolism from an ulcerated or high-grade carotid stenosis although some have also speculated that this pattern may be a consequence of haemodynamic impairment rather than embolism. In young individuals, craniocervical artery dissection with arterio-arterial embolization or severe flow-reducing stenosis may also produce this pattern (Fig. 7.3) (31).

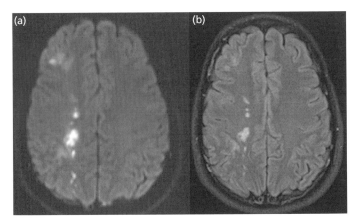

Fig. 7.3 Right hemispheric border zone infarct pattern on DWI (a) and FLAIR (b) MRI scans in a 31-year-old male patient with right internal carotid artery dissection and high-grade stenosis. The patient had fluctuating weakness and numbness of his left arm and leg.

There is also quite good evidence that recent small subcortical infarcts (earlier termed lacunar infarcts in expectation of a lacune to develop) are indicative of small vessel disease (10). The probability of such aetiology certainly increases with the presence of coexisting lacunes of presumed vascular origin, white matter hyperintensities, and microbleeds.

The multiplicity of possibly underlying causes and limited distinction between patterns make it clear that aetiological assumptions just on the basis of brain imaging findings are dangerous and do not obviate a thorough clinical workup (28, 29). With this precaution in mind, however, brain imaging findings certainly offer important clues to the actual cause of the acute ischaemic event and are successfully used as elements of more novel classification schemes of ischaemic stroke (32).

Neuroimaging and treatment selection

Algorithms of how to employ available techniques must be strongly driven by the actual impact of imaging findings on patient management and therapy.

Identification of patients for thrombolysis beyond approved criteria

Assessment of morphologic and functional changes after stroke by multimodal MRI suggests some patients still have salvageable tissue as long as 24 hours after stroke onset. This assumption comes from the observation of areas of the brain with a reduction in perfusion threatening tissue viability much larger than the region with visible ischaemic damage. This mismatch between morphologic and perfusion changes, that is, the zone of purely functional changes or 'penumbra' around the core of an infarct, may indicate the potential for successful therapeutic intervention beyond the 4.5-hour time window.

Support for the feasibility and efficacy of treating acute stroke patients with systemic thrombolysis based on the presence of a 'penumbra' as defined by a mismatch between diffusion/perfusion abnormalities has come from non-randomized studies (33).

The Diffusion and perfusion imaging Evaluation For Understanding Stroke Evolution (DEFUSE) study investigated patients receiving systemic thrombolysis within 3–6 hours after stroke and found favourable results after the administration of recombinant tissue plasminogen activator only in patients with a clear diffusion/perfusion mismatch. Individuals without evidence for any DWI/perfusion-weighted imaging mismatch showed no favourable response to systemic thrombolysis. A group of patients with very large DWI lesions and corresponding perfusion deficits even appeared to deteriorate following vessel recanalization and this pattern of MRI abnormalities was thus considered as consistent with a malignant profile (34).

The DEFUSE 2 trial largely replicated these results over a 12-hour time window in 100 patients scheduled to have endovascular treatment. Reperfusion was associated with more favourable clinical outcomes in the presence of a target DWI/perfusion-weighted imaging mismatch identified by an automated system while no association between reperfusion and outcome was seen in patients without target mismatch (35).

Unfortunately, placebo-controlled trials have come up with controversial results and did not confirm that delayed thrombolysis in patients selected by mismatch improved clinical outcome (36). Thus, mismatch selection currently cannot be recommended as part of routine care, but may be used in clinically questionable cases as a supportive argument in the decision for or against intravenous thrombolysis or mechanical thrombectomy. It is important to consider that the optimal perfusion-weighted imaging maps and their levels still have to be defined.

Workup of patients with unclear onset time of stroke

Approximately 25% of ischaemic strokes occur during sleep which precludes knowledge of the time of symptom onset (37). According to current guidelines, which indicate a strict time window, these wake-up stroke patients are not eligible for thrombolysis, although many of them might be good candidates to receive thrombolytic therapy. It has thus been suggested to use imaging information to estimate the duration of pre-existing cerebral ischaemia. In a first study of 94 consecutive patients with stroke who underwent an MRI within 12 hours after known symptom onset, negative FLAIR had a sensitivity of 46% and a specificity of 79% for allocating patients to a time window of less than 4.5 hours (38). A subsequent multicentre observational study repeated this evaluation in 543 patients (39). Ischaemic lesions were identified on DWI in 95% and on FLAIR in 50% of these patients. A DWI–FLAIR mismatch (i.e. the presence of only DWI signal abnormality), identified patients within 4.5 hours of symptom onset with 62% sensitivity and 78% specificity. Taken together these findings indicate some variability in the evolution of signal abnormalities, but suggest that patients with an acute ischaemic lesion detected with DWI but not seen on FLAIR are likely to be in a time window for which thrombolysis is safe (39). In addition, it could also be argued that a negative FLAIR scan may indicate a greater benefit from systemic thrombolysis and/or a lower risk for haemorrhage irrespective of the time interval. These hypotheses are currently tested in prospective studies (40).

Imaging prediction of malignant cerebral infarction

Approximately 5% of all ischaemic strokes have a so-called malignant course in which space-occupying cerebral oedema develops. This is the most frequent cause of death within the first days of stroke. Malignant cerebral infarction typically occurs in patients with persistent middle cerebral or internal carotid artery occlusion and young and middle-aged individuals are at especially high risk. The term malignant refers to mortality rates of up to 80% despite modern neurointensive care management. Early decompressive hemicraniectomy within 48 hours of stroke symptom onset has been found very effective in lowering both mortality and moderate and severe disability in randomized controlled trials. To offer this treatment, it is necessary to rapidly and reliably identify those patients who will need early surgery. Besides clinical predictors, neuroimaging markers are valuable in this setting. Infarction of more than 50% on CT and a perfusion deficit of more than 66% of the middle cerebral artery territory have been identified as determinants of a malignant course. Using MRI may allow an even more accurate and earlier prediction with DWI volumes of more than 145 mL within 14 hours and more than 82 mL within 6 hours as cut-off values (41–43).

Large cerebellar infarction with developing space-occupying oedema is another stroke subtype that needs special attention. In younger individuals it occurs mainly as a consequence of vertebrobasilar artery dissection and often requires sub-occipital decompressive surgery. Due to often unspecific clinical symptoms and the low sensitivity of CT in the early phase of infratentorial stroke, large cerebellar infarctions are often not recognized until severe complications become clinically evident as oedema formation is especially critical. Therefore, MRI with DWI, which also accurately depicts associated brainstem infarction, is recommended in the early diagnosis of patients with suspected cerebellar ischaemia (43, 44).

Identification of patients with high risk for subsequent attacks

Accumulating evidence suggests a strong impact of neuroimaging, and especially of MRI, on the management of patients with TIA, which has traditionally been defined clinically by a resolution of focal neurologic deficits within 24 hours from symptom onset. While CT can just serve to exclude rare non-ischaemic causes of transient focal neurologic episodes, MRI findings actually predict the reoccurrence of ischaemia. Studies using conventional MRI have shown the frequent occurrence of infarcts in patients who had suffered from a clinical TIA (45). Consistent with the notion of transient symptoms, they were often seen not in an area corresponding to the patient's neurologic symptoms, but rather in clinically silent regions of the brain.

The introduction of DWI has further increased the recognition of acute ischaemic lesions in TIA. Importantly it has been consistently shown that patients with transient symptoms and the presence of DWI lesions have an increased risk for a recurrent stroke compared to patients with clinically defined TIA without DWI abnormalities. This risk is further increased with concomitant vessel stenosis/occlusion. Therefore, it has been proposed to add DWI MRI and MRA findings to clinical scores in order to improve risk stratification in TIA patients (46–49). These findings also led to the recommendation of a tissue-based diagnosis of TIA. Patients with evidence for an acute ischaemic lesion should be considered as having suffered from stroke irrespective of the duration of symptoms (9, 50).

Along these lines we have performed a sub-analysis of the MRI data of the Stroke in Young Fabry Patients (sifap1) study which enrolled 5023 young patients with stroke and TIA aged 55 years or younger. We found an unexpectedly high rate of silent old infarcts of 21.7% in patients with ischaemic stroke and 9.9% in patients with a clinical TIA. We also found that morphologic findings in patients with a clinical TIA but with acute infarction on DWI were much more like those in stroke patients than in patients with a clinical TIA and no DWI abnormality (11, 51). Our observations thus support the move towards a tissue-based diagnosis of TIA but also alert for the obvious subtlety of clinical signs and symptoms associated with focal cerebral ischaemia, which often may be overlooked.

Neuroimaging in the differential diagnosis of ischaemic stroke in young adults

Early diagnosis of ischaemic stroke in young individuals is clinically challenging. This is due to a lack of awareness and often atypical clinical presentations. Age younger than 35 years and posterior circulation stroke have been identified as predictors of a missed diagnosis among young ischaemic stroke patients. This is specifically important in view of the predominance of posterior circulation strokes in the younger age group shown by the sifap1 study (11, 52).

Young stroke patients also more often have heterogeneous and uncommon stroke aetiologies and a high frequency of diseases that mimic brain ischaemia (52, 53). Many of these disorders can only be sufficiently detected or ruled out by brain MRI. Figs. 7.4–7.7 illustrate some selected cases of central nervous system disorders which must be considered in the differential diagnosis of young stroke and which can be diagnosed with a thorough interpretation

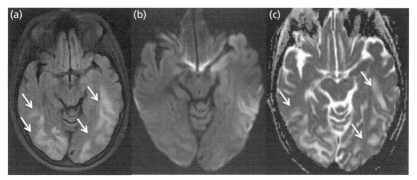

Fig. 7.4 A 27-year-old pregnant female patient (34th gestational week) complained about acute onset of headache and increasing bilateral visual disturbance. A few minutes later she presented with generalized tonic–clonic seizures. Brain MRI revealed FLAIR signal hyperintensities in temporal, parietal, and occipital lobes (a). The white matter is predominately affected. Together with (b) DWI (no significant signal changes) and (c) ADC (hyperintensities) findings this pattern is indicative for vasogenic oedema in the setting of posterior reversible encephalopathy syndrome (PRES), which is an important differential diagnosis of infratentorial stroke. A follow-up MRI 1 week later showed nearly complete remission of signal abnormalities and confirmed the diagnosis (not shown).

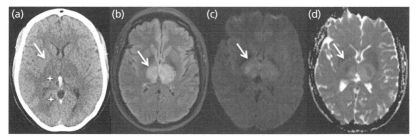

Fig. 7.5 A 32-year-old female patient presented with an acute confusional state and alternating reduced consciousness. Initial non-contrast-enhanced brain CT shows bilateral thalamic hypodensities with swelling (a, arrow) and a hyperdense signal in projection to the straight sinus, vena cerebri magna Galeni and the inner cerebral veins (a, stars), indicative of deep cerebral venous thrombosis with venous thalamic infarction. Subsequent MRI confirms the diagnosis and shows oedema formation in the thalamus bilaterally (b, FLAIR; c, DWI; and d, ADC). Top of the basilar artery thrombosis and artery of Percheron cerebral ischaemia are important other differential diagnoses of bithalamic lesions.

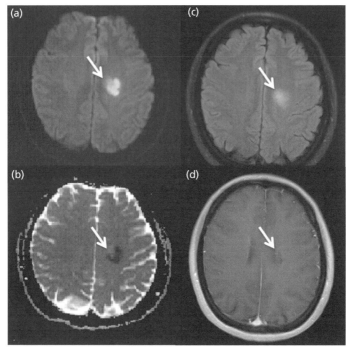

Fig. 7.6 A brain MRI of a 34-year-old female patient with progressive leg-dominant right-sided hemiparesis. DWI (a) depicts bright signal hyperintensity with incomplete ADC restriction (b) in the supraventricular white matter. On FLAIR MRI (c) this lesion shows an atypical configuration with a patchy border. No significant contrast enhancement was seen on gadolinium-weighted T1 scans (d). This is an example of an atypical (very) acute demyelinating lesion, which is sometimes difficult to distinguish from recent subcortical infarcts.

of neuroimaging. Figure legends give explanations to differential diagnostic clues. The respective entities are discussed in more detail in other chapters of this book.

Conclusion and proposed algorithm

Both CT and MRI have important roles in the diagnosis of ischaemic stroke. CT is usually sufficient to indicate thrombolysis in the approved time window, but often does not provide other information than ruling out intracranial haemorrhage. MRI has advantages in the detection of small and infratentorial brain infarcts, the diagnosis of stroke mimics, and the identification of special stroke aetiologies. MRI is therefore the modality of choice in younger individuals with a presumed cerebrovascular attack. All imaging information (with the

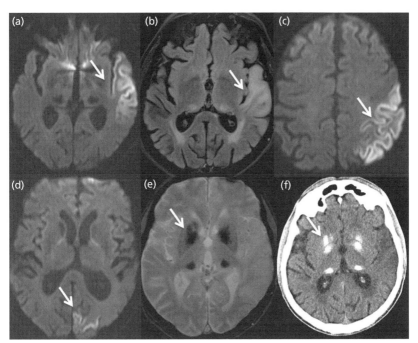

Fig. 7.7 A 42-year-old male patient presented with headache, aphasia, and visual neglect to the right. His medical history was remarkable for type 1 diabetes mellitus and bilateral sensorineural deafness. Brain MRI reveals mainly cortical DWI (a) and FLAIR (b) signal hyperintensities, which were not confined to vascular territories and showed a spreading over the next days (c and d, DWI). Additionally, basal ganglia calcification was present (e, T2*-weighted MRI; and f, CT). Such a constellation is highly indicative of mitochondrial encephalopathy (MELAS syndrome).

use of selected sequences (6)) needs integration with the clinical findings and appropriate neurological expertise. The potential information gained must be weighed against the burden to the patient and disadvantages such as a delay in treatment in the very acute setting of stroke. Therefore it is recommended that the neuroimaging units for the workup of acute stroke patients are located near to the emergency department.

Table 7.4 summarizes our recommendations including the consideration of several specific aspects in the management of young patients with suspected acute focal cerebral ischaemia. These recommendations will certainly have to be modified by advancements in imaging technology and treatment options and have to be adapted to the local situation. All this needs a very close interaction of involved specialists on the basis of a profound understanding of available options.

Table 7.4 Proposed neuroimaging algorithm for young patients with suspected stroke with regard to different clinical scenarios

Clinical settings	Diagnostic goals	Imaging tools
Candidates for systemic thrombolysis ≤4.5 hours	Exclude intracranial bleeding or other contraindications for intravenous rtPA	CT or MRI (FLAIR, DWI, T_2*-GRE)
Acute ischaemic stroke patients >4.5–9 hours	Selection for intravenous rtPA beyond 4.5 hours	MRI (DWI, PWI)
(Presumed) non-responders to systemic thrombolysis	Selection for interventional recanalization (e.g. thrombectomy)	CT + CTA or MRI (DWI) + IC MRA (EC MRA optional)
Unclear stroke onset (e.g. wake-up stroke)	Identification of candidates for thrombolysis	MRI (FLAIR/DWI mismatch)
Transient ischaemic attack	Identify patients at high risk for recurrence	MRI (DWI) + IC MRA (EC MRA optional)
Atypical clinical presentation	Confirm ischaemic stroke/rule out stroke mimics	MRI (FLAIR, DWI, T_2*-GRE, further sequences according to the individual situation)

CT, computed tomography; CTA, computed tomography angiography; DWI, diffusion-weighted imaging; EC, extracranial; GRE, gradient-echo imaging; IC, intracranial; MRA, magnetic resonance angiography; MRI, magnetic resonance imaging; PWI, perfusion-weighted imaging; rtPA, recombinant tissue plasminogen activator.

References

1. **Lövblad K**, **Baird A.** Actual diagnostic approach to the acute stroke patient. Eur Radiol. 2006;**16**(6):1253–69.

2. **Lövblad K-O**, **Baird AE.** Computed tomography in acute ischemic stroke. Neuroradiology. 2010;**52**:175–87.

3. **Hacke W**, **Kaste M**, **Bluhmki E**, **Brozman M**, **Dávalos A**, **Guidetti D**, et al. Thrombolysis with alteplase 3 to 4.5 hours after acute ischemic stroke. N Engl J Med. 2008;**359**(13):1795–806.

4. **Muir KW**, **Buchan A**, **von Kummer R**, **Rother J**, **Baron J-C.** Imaging of acute stroke. Lancet Neurol. 2006;**5**(9):755–68.

5. **Merino JG**, **Warach S.** Imaging of acute stroke. Nat Rev Neurol. 2010;**6**(10):560–71.

6. **Wintermark M**, **Albers GW**, **Broderick JP**, **Demchuk AM**, **Fiebach JB**, **Fiehler J**, et al. Acute stroke imaging research roadmap II. Stroke. 2013;**44**(9):2628–39.

7. **Kloska SP**, **Wintermark M**, **Engelhorn T**, **Fiebach JB.** Acute stroke magnetic resonance imaging: current status and future perspective. Neuroradiology. 2010;**52**:189–201.

8. **Young JY**, **Schaefer PW.** Acute ischemic stroke imaging: a practical approach for diagnosis and triage. Int J Cardiovasc Imaging. 2016;**32**(1):19–33.

9. **Easton JD**, **Saver JL**, **Albers GW**, **Alberts MJ**, **Chaturvedi S**, **Feldmann E**, et al. Definition and evaluation of transient ischemic attack: a scientific statement for

healthcare professionals from the American Heart Association/American Stroke Association Stroke Council; Council on Cardiovascular Surgery and Anesthesia; Council on Cardiovascular Radiology and Intervention; Council on Cardiovascular Nursing; and the Interdisciplinary Council on Peripheral Vascular Disease: The American Academy of Neurology affirms the value of this statement as an educational tool for neurologists. Stroke. 2009;**40**:2276–93.

10. **Wardlaw JM, Smith EE, Biessels GJ, Cordonnier C, Fazekas F, Frayne R**, et al. Neuroimaging standards for research into small vessel disease and its contribution to ageing and neurodegeneration. Lancet Neurol. 2013;**12**:822–38.

11. **Fazekas F, Enzinger C, Schmidt R, Dichgans M, Gaertner B, Jungehulsing RMGJ**, et al. MRI in acute cerebral ischemia of theyoung the stroke in young fabry patients (sifap1) study. Neurology. 2013;**81**:1914–21.

12. **Fazekas F, Ropele S, Enzinger C.** Stroke. In: Filippi M, ed. Oxford Textbook of Neuroimaging. Oxford: Oxford University Press; 2015, 185–99.

13. **Bories J, Derhy S, Chiras J.** CT in hemispheric ischaemic attacks. Neuroradiology. 1985;**27**(6):468–83.

14. **von Kummer R, Allen KL, Holle R, Bozzao L, Bastianello S, Manelfe C**, et al. Acute stroke: usefulness of early CT findings before thrombolytic therapy. Radiology. 1997;**205**(2):327–33.

15. **Warach S, Gaa J, Siewert B, Wielopolski P, Edelman RR.** Acute human stroke studied by whole brain echo planar diffusion-weighted magnetic resonance imaging. Ann Neurol. 1995;**37**(2):231–41.

16. **Bammer R, Stollberger R, Augustin M, Simbrunner J, Offenbacher H, Kooijman H**, et al. Diffusion-weighted imaging with navigated interleaved echo-planar imaging and a conventional gradient system. Radiology. 1999;**211**:799–806.

17. **Augustin M, Bammer R, Simbrunner J, Stollberger R, Hartung HP, Fazekas F.** Diffusion-weighted imaging of patients with subacute cerebral ischemia: comparison with conventional and contrast-enhanced MR imaging. AJNR Am J Neuroradiol. 2000;**21**(9):1596–602.

18. **Schlaug G, Siewert B, Benfield a, Edelman RR, Warach S.** Time course of the apparent diffusion coefficient (ADC) abnormality in human stroke. Neurology. 1997;**49**(1):113–19.

19. **Toi H, Uno M, Harada M, Yoneda K, Morita N, Matsubara S**, et al. Diagnosis of acute brain-stem infarcts using diffusion-weighed MRI. Neuroradiology. 2003;**45**(6):352–56.

20. **Axer H, Gräßel D, Brämer D, Fitzek S, Kaiser WA, Witte OW**, et al. Time course of diffusion imaging in acute brainstem infarcts. J Magn Reson Imaging. 2007;**26**(4):905–12.

21. **Fiebach JB, Schellinger PD, Gass A, Kucinski T, Siebler M, Villringer A**, et al. Stroke magnetic resonance imaging is accurate in hyperacute intracerebral hemorrhage: a multicenter study on the validity of stroke imaging. Stroke. 2004;**35**(2):502–506.

22. **Chalela J a, Kidwell CS, Nentwich LM, Luby M, Butman J a, Demchuk AM**, et al. Magnetic resonance imaging and computed tomography in emergency assessment of patients with suspected acute stroke: a prospective comparison. Lancet. 2007;**369**(9558):293–98.

23. **Fazekas F, Kleinert R, Roob G, Kleinert G, Kapeller P, Schmidt R**, et al. Histopathologic analysis of foci of signal loss on gradient-echo T2*-weighted

MR images in patients with spontaneous intracerebral hemorrhage: evidence of microangiopathy-related microbleeds. Am J Neuroradiol. 1999;**20**(4):637–42.

24. **Charidimou A, Krishnan A, Werring DJ, Rolf Jäger H.** Cerebral microbleeds: a guide to detection and clinical relevance in different disease settings. Neuroradiology. 2013;**55**(6):655–74.

25. **Wintermark M, Sanelli PC, Albers GW, Bello JA, Derdeyn CP, Hetts SW**, et al. Imaging recommendations for acute stroke and transient ischemic attack patients. J Am Coll Radiol. 2013;**10**(11):828–32.

26. **Kneihsl M, Enzinger C, Wünsch G, Khalil M, Culea V, Urbanic-Purkart T**, et al. Poor short-term outcome in patients with ischaemic stroke and active cancer. J Neurol. 2016;**263**(1):150–56.

27. **Mustanoja S, Putaala J, Haapaniemi E, Strbian D, Kaste M, Tatlisumak T.** Multiple brain infarcts in young adults: clues for etiologic diagnosis and prognostic impact. Eur J Neurol. 2013;**20**(2):216–22.

28. **Chowdhury D, Wardlaw JM, Dennis MS.** Are multiple acute small subcortical infarctions caused by embolic mechanisms? J Neurol Neurosurg Psychiatry. 2004;**75**(10):1416–20.

29. **Seifert T, Enzinger C, Storch MK, Pichler G, Niederkorn K, Fazekas F.** Acute small subcortical infarctions on diffusion weighted MRI: clinical presentation and aetiology. J Neurol Neurosurg Psychiatry. 2005;**76**(11):1520–24.

30. **Wolf ME, Sauer T, Kern R, Szabo K, Hennerici MG.** Multiple subcortical acute ischemic lesions reflect small vessel disease rather than cardiogenic embolism. J Neurol. 2012;**259**(9):1951–57.

31. **Del Sette M, Eliasziw M, Streifler JY, Hachinski VC, Fox AJ, Barnett HJM.** Internal borderzone infarction : a marker for severe stenosis in patients with symptomatic internal carotid artery disease. Stroke. 2000;**31**(3):631–36.

32. **Amarenco P, Bogousslavsky J, Caplan LR, Donnan GA, Hennerici MG.** New approach to stroke subtyping: the A-S-C-O (phenotypic) classification of stroke. Cerebrovasc Dis. 2009;**27**(5):502–508.

33. **Köhrmann M, Jüttler E, Fiebach JB, Huttner HB, Siebert S, Schwark C**, et al. MRI versus CT-based thrombolysis treatment within and beyond the 3 h time window after stroke onset: a cohort study. Lancet Neurol. 2006;**5**(8):661–67.

34. **Albers GW, Thijs VN, Wechsler L, Kemp S, Schlaug G, Skalabrin E**, et al. Magnetic resonance imaging profiles predict clinical response to early reperfusion: the diffusion and perfusion imaging evaluation for understanding stroke evolution (DEFUSE) study. Ann Neurol. 2006;**60**(5):508–17.

35. **Lansberg MG, Straka M, Kemp S, Mlynash M, Wechsler LR, Jovin TG**, et al. MRI profile and response to endovascular reperfusion after stroke (DEFUSE 2): a prospective cohort study. Lancet Neurol. 2012;**11**(10):860–67.

36. **Mishra NK, Albers GW, Davis SM, Donnan GA, Furlan AJ, Hacke W**, et al. Mismatch-based delayed thrombolysis: a meta-analysis. Stroke. 2010;**41**(1).

37. **Rimmele DL, Thomalla G.** Wake-up stroke: clinical characteristics, imaging findings, and treatment option—an update. Front Neurol. 2014;**5**:35.

38. **Ebinger M, Galinovic I, Rozanski M, Brunecker P, Endres M, Fiebach JB.** Fluid-attenuated inversion recovery evolution within 12 hours from stroke onset: a reliable tissue clock? Stroke. 2010;**41**(2):250–55.

39. **Thomalla G, Cheng B, Ebinger M, Hao Q.** DWI-FLAIR mismatch for the identification of patients with acute ischaemic stroke within 4.5 h of symptom onset (PRE-FLAIR): a multicentre observational study. Lancet. 2011;**10**(11):978–86.

40. **Thomalla G, Fiebach JB, Østergaard L, Pedraza S, Thijs V, Nighoghossian N**, et al. A multicenter, randomized, double-blind, placebo-controlled trial to test efficacy and safety of magnetic resonance imaging-based thrombolysis in wake-up stroke (WAKE-UP). Int J Stroke. 2014;**9**(6):829–36.

41. **Wartenberg KE.** Malignant middle cerebral artery infarction. Curr Opin Crit Care. 2012;**18**(2):152–63.

42. **Neugebauer H, Jüttler E.** Hemicraniectomy for malignant middle cerebral artery infarction: Current status and future directions. Int J Stroke. 2014;**9**(4):460–7.

43. **Wijdicks EFM, Sheth KN, Carter BS, Greer DM, Kasner SE, Kimberly WT**, et al. Recommendations for the management of cerebral and cerebellar infarction with swelling: a statement for healthcare professionals from the American Heart Association/American Stroke Association. Stroke. 2014;**45**(4):1222–38.

44. **Neugebauer H, Witsch J, Zweckberger K, Jüttler E.** Space-occupying cerebellar infarction: complications, treatment, and outcome. Neurosurg Focus. 2013;**34**(5):E8.

45. **Fazekas F, Fazekas G, Schmidt R, Kapeller P, Offenbacher H.** Magnetic resonance imaging correlates of transient cerebral ischemic attacks. Stroke. 1996;**27**(4):607–11.

46. **Coutts SB, Simon JE, Eliasziw M, Sohn C-H, Hill MD, Barber PA**, et al. Triaging transient ischemic attack and minor stroke patients using acute magnetic resonance imaging. Ann Neurol. 2005;**57**(6):848–54.

47. **Purroy F, Montaner J, Rovira A, Delgado P, Quintana M, Alvarez-Sabin J.** Higher risk of further vascular events among transient ischemic attack patients with diffusion-weighted imaging acute ischemic lesions. Stroke. 2004;**35**:2313–19.

48. **Prabhakaran S, Chong JY, Sacco RL.** Impact of abnormal diffusion-weighted imaging results on short-term outcome following transient ischemic attack. Arch Neurol. 2007;**64**(8):1105–109.

49. **Merwick Á, Albers GW, Amarenco P, Arsava EM, Ay H, Calvet D**, et al. Addition of brain and carotid imaging to the ABCD2 score to identify patients at early risk of stroke after transient ischaemic attack: a multicentre observational study. Lancet Neurol. 2010;**9**(11):1060–69.

50. **Albers GW, Caplan LR, Easton JD, Fayad PB, Mohr JP, Saver JL**, et al. Transient ischemic attack--proposal for a new definition. N Engl J Med. 2002;**347**(21):1713–16.

51. **Rolfs A, Fazekas F, Grittner U, Dichgans M, Martus P, Holzhausen M**, et al. Acute cerebrovascular disease in the young: The Stroke in Young Fabry patients study. Stroke. 2013;**44**(2):340–49.

52. **Singhal AB, Biller J, Elkind MS, Fullerton HJ, Jauch EC, Kittner SJ**, et al. Recognition and management of stroke in young adults and adolescents. Neurology. 2013;**81**:1089–97.

53. **Ji R, Schwamm LH, Pervez MA, Singhal AB.** Ischemic stroke and transient ischemic attack in young adults: risk factors, diagnostic yield, neuroimaging, and thrombolysis. JAMA Neurol. 2013;**70**(1):51–57.

Chapter 8

Vascular imaging (CTA/MRA)

Thomas Gattringer, Christian Enzinger,
Stefan Ropele, and Franz Fazekas

Introduction

As outlined in Chapter 7 on 'Brain imaging (CT/MRI)', information on the condition and patency of the blood vessels supplying the brain has increasingly become another prerequisite for the adequate management of ischaemic stroke (1). Often, the occlusion of larger vessels can already be suspected on plain images. On T2-weighted magnetic resonance imaging (MRI), the lumen of vessels usually appears dark especially when perpendicular to the imaging plane because of the outflow of excited protons. Absence of this 'flow void sign' is a sensitive and rather specific marker of no or very slow flow such as from a more proximal high-grade stenosis. Therefore occlusions of the internal carotid artery, basilar artery, or vertebral arteries are usually quite conspicuous already on axial MRI (Fig. 8.1).

Non- or slow-flowing blood is also seen as hyperintensity in the peripheral vessels on fluid-attenuated inversion recovery (FLAIR) images. To what extent such abnormalities provide relevant pathophysiologic information in association with large vessel occlusion is still under examination. Furthermore, iron-sensitive MRI sequences such as gradient echo or susceptibility-weighted images can be used to increase the conspicuity of an intravascular thrombus. Erythrocyte-rich thrombi appear hypointense and are characterized by some 'blooming', that is, hypointensity extending beyond the vessel wall, because of the effects of iron content in the clotted erythrocytes on magnetic susceptibility (Fig. 8.2). On computed tomography (CT), occluded intracranial vessels also appear bright, that is, hyperdense due to the clotted blood and a dense middle cerebral artery on plain CT is already a robust indicator of middle cerebral artery occlusion in a patient with acute stroke and appropriate clinical findings (Fig. 8.2). However, vessel calcification may also cause a dense vessel appearance and lead to false-positive findings and the bony skull base prohibits appreciating the content of the carotid arteries on plain CT (2, 3). Blood flow in the extra- and intracranial vessels and the condition of the vessel walls can also be

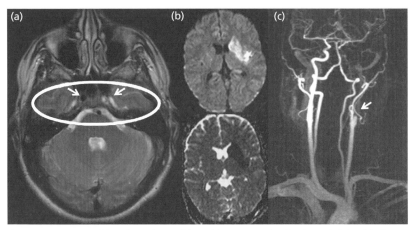

Fig. 8.1 A 32-year-old male patient with sudden onset of aphasia and right-sided hemiparesis. T2-weighted MRI shows absence of the flow void sign in the left intracranial internal carotid artery suggestive of proximal high-grade flow reducing stenosis or occlusion (a). The respective acute ischaemic infarct can be seen on diffusion-weighted MRI (b). Image (c) depicts the corresponding steno-occlusive process at the origin of the left internal carotid artery.

visualized rapidly and cost-effectively by duplex sonography. However, ultrasound examination cannot access the vessels at the base of the skull and a thick skull may prohibit performing transcranial Doppler sonography, which in addition suffers from limited spatial resolution.

Nowadays, both computed tomography angiography (CTA) and magnetic resonance angiography (MRA) provide the most accurate and comprehensive information on the cerebral vasculature in a non-invasive manner. A further

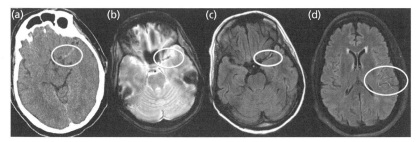

Fig. 8.2 A 52-year-old male patient with a complete left middle cerebral artery syndrome. Correspondingly, plain CT (a) shows a hyperdense middle cerebral artery sign, suggestive of a thrombotic vessel occlusion. The thrombus is also visualized on T2* gradient echo-weighted sequences (b) and fluid-attenuated inversion recovery scans (FLAIR) (c). Image (d) shows peripheral FLAIR vessel signs, indicative of slow flow.

significant advantage of CTA and MRA is the possibility to immediately add them to plain imaging. Thus, information on the brain and its supplying vessels can be obtained in one examination. This is especially crucial in the acute phase of ischaemic stroke when all information needed for therapeutic decision-making should be obtained as fast as possible in order not to delay time-dependent treatment (1, 4–6).

Vascular imaging also plays an important role in differential diagnosis. In young patients, specific vascular changes such as arterial dissection, other vasculopathies, and various types of vasculitis are frequent and have to be considered as possible causes of stroke (7). Combining MRI and MRA allows imaging of the vessel lumen, the vessel wall, and the perivascular space and thus is very sensitive and specific for identifying vessel dissection. Technical advances also allow investigating intracranial artery stenoses and changes in the vessel walls with increasing sensitivity. The detection of alterations in the end branches of the cerebral arteries such as in primary cerebral angiitis, however, still remains the domain of digital subtraction angiography (DSA).

After considering some important technical aspects, we concentrate on the diagnostic role of CTA and MRA in the acute phase of stroke, their therapeutic implications, and their contribution to the clarification of stroke aetiology, with a focus on disorders that are especially relevant in young stroke patients.

Computed tomography angiography

Advanced helical multidetector CT scanners with the possibility to obtain large numbers of image slices within a very short time period have made CTA an extensively used technique for the non-invasive evaluation of the neurovascular circulation (6). Together with MRA, CTA has thus replaced conventional catheter DSA as the initial examination for most neurovascular indications. Advances in three-dimensional post-processing techniques have contributed to this development. In essence, CTA is performed by acquiring data during the passage of an iodine-based contrast agent through the blood vessels, which elevates their 'density'. The contrast material is applied preferentially by injection into the right antecubital vein. Synchronizing scan acquisition with peak opacification of the targeted vasculature is one of the main challenges of CTA and several techniques can be used to achieve this goal (6). Thus, imaging protocols have to vary according to the area of angiographic interest and depending on the indication for CTA.

Advantages of CTA are the high spatial resolution and the speed of the examination. Some limitation comes from the need to use iodinated contrast material. While this has been shown to be generally safe in the setting of cerebral ischaemia, there is some risk of contrast-induced nephropathy (CIN), which is increased in patients with diabetes and pre-existing renal dysfunction. Importantly for the acute stroke setting, large studies of patients with acute ischaemic and haemorrhagic stroke have shown a rather low incidence of acute CIN in the range from 2% to 7% and this risk was not higher in patients whose baseline creatinine value was unknown at the time of scanning (8, 9). In young stroke patients, this complication is presumably less frequent. Adequate pre-procedure and post-procedure hydration are considered to be the most important factors in preventing CIN and CTA protocols need to be tailored to use the smallest amount of contrast material possible. The exposure to ionizing radiation also needs to be considered. This deserves special attention in patients, who may repeatedly undergo such examinations and CTA therefore has to be performed only for a valid medical reason and with the minimum exposure that provides an image quality necessary for adequate diagnostic information (10). Also, radiation exposure with CTA is markedly lower than when undergoing DSA (16). Other limitations come from image obscuration and artefacts due to adjacent bony structures and a limited sensitivity for very small vascular changes.

Magnetic resonance angiography

MRA draws on a wealth of available contrast mechanisms, which can be based just on specific excitation of the flowing blood protons or on contrast material. Among the various techniques, time-of-flight (TOF) imaging for evaluation of the intracranial vasculature and contrast-enhanced MRA for the extracranial vessels have become the most frequently used techniques in acute ischaemic stroke. Phase contrast (PC) imaging is commonly used to assess the intracranial venous system.

Time-of-flight imaging

In TOF (as with other MRA techniques), visualization of the blood vessels comes from the difference in signal intensities between the stationary background tissues and that of the flowing blood (11). Repeatedly applied radiofrequency pulses serve to achieve a steady-state magnetization and signal saturation (reduction) of the brain and other stationary tissues. Blood that flows into the excited volume has not been affected by these pulses (i.e. is unsaturated), and thus gives considerably more MR signal than the background tissue. TOF imaging uses a gradient echo sequence with a short repetition time and is inherently T1-weighted. A higher field-strength and the use of gadolinium-containing contrast agents can both serve to increase the vessel contrast.

The size of the flip angle also has an important effect as a higher flip angle increases the level of saturation in both tissue and blood. In such instances, the slower-flowing venous blood will become more saturated. Thus higher flip angles are effective at visualizing the faster moving blood in the arterial system whereas lower flip angles can be used to visualize both veins and arteries (11). Suppression of the veins in TOF can also be achieved by application of saturation pulses to regions superior to the imaging slab. MRI TOF techniques are inherently good for imaging the macroscopic intracranial arteries and veins but cannot serve to image the microcirculation. In addition, the extracranial cerebral vessels are not displayed with adequate quality.

Contrast-enhanced MRA

Contrast material can also be used with MRI to increase the intravascular signal from blood and is specifically used to assess the extracranial brain-supplying vessels. For this purpose, gadolinium-containing contrast agents are injected intravenously and a fast three-dimensional T1-weighted gradient echo image is collected before and after the contrast injection. Subtraction of the pre- and post-contrast injection images serves to highlight the enhanced signals from the desired vessels. Contrast-enhanced MRA can be timed to acquire images in different phases of the passage of the contrast material, which allows focusing on specific vascular systems. Normally, the acquisition of the second volume is timed in a manner that just the arteries but not the veins are enhanced. Mid-phase imaging is collected when the contrast agent is in both arteries and veins, and late-phase imaging is collected with the contrast agents predominantly in the veins. Therefore the timing of the image acquisition is of paramount importance for the adequate display of the vessels of interest (12). Apart from rare instances of allergic reactions, gadolinium may cause nephrogenic systemic fibrosis in patients with renal disease (13). This risk, like the accumulation of gadolinium in the brain, increases with repeated applications (14). For assessing acute stroke, the benefits mostly outweigh these potential risks.

Phase contrast imaging

PC imaging relies on the fact that a gradient magnetic field will affect the phase of the MR signal from moving blood differently to that from static tissue. PC imaging is typically developed from a gradient echo sequence by adding a bipolar velocity-encoding gradient pulse to encode blood velocity. This encoding process can be applied in three orthogonal directions to measure velocity but in practice only the velocity magnitude is displayed and used to form projection angiograms mostly of the intracranial venous system (11).

The contribution of CTA and MRA to treatment selection

Identifying the need for endovascular treatment

Recently, several randomized trials have shown that mechanical thrombectomy with stent retrievers improves the clinical outcome of patients with large vessel occlusion in the anterior cerebral circulation compared to treatment with intravenous thrombolysis alone. The number needed to treat to achieve one additional patient with independent functional outcome was in the range of 3.2 to 7.1 and exceeded the known efficacy of intravenous thrombolysis (15). The rate of procedural complications was low and no increase in symptomatic intracerebral haemorrhage was noted. These results were confirmed in respective meta-analyses (15–18) and led the European Stroke Organization to recommend mechanical thrombectomy in addition to intravenous thrombolysis within 4.5 hours (when eligible) as the preferred treatment modality of acute stroke patients with large artery occlusions in the anterior circulation up to 6 hours after symptom onset (19).

A consequence of this shift in treatment paradigm is the need to identify intracranial vessel occlusion, which was also a prerequisite of the successful thrombectomy trials. Furthermore, meta-analysis of the thrombectomy trials has confirmed that the improvement in functional outcomes associated with endovascular therapy was significantly greater when CTA or MRA was used to confirm proximal arterial occlusion prior to trial enrolment (Fig. 8.3) (16). This is conceivable since this strategy prohibits catheterization of patients without a proximal occlusion who are unlikely to benefit from the procedure. For clinical practice, this raises the question in whom to perform angiography. The Safe Implementation of Treatments in Stroke (SITS) registry showed that National Institutes of Health Stroke Scale (NIHSS) scores of 11 and 12 points were good predictors for baseline vessel occlusion (20). However, if imaging was performed 3 hours after stroke onset, the NIHSS score threshold predicting baseline occlusion decreased to 9. This is in line with a large monocentric study, which found an NIHSS score of 9 or greater within the first 3 hours and 7 or greater between 3 and 6 hours strongly suggestive of an occlusion of a major intracranial artery (21). However, patients with good collaterals may for at least some time have an even lower NIHSS score despite large vessel occlusion. Thus, the same authors recently concluded that a sizeable number of patients with major vessel occlusion are missed whatever thresholds of clinical scores are applied (22). Fortunately, none of the concerns related to CTA apply to intracranial MRA. Intracranial MRA can be performed without contrast material and takes only 2–3 minutes to show patency or occlusion of the major intracerebral

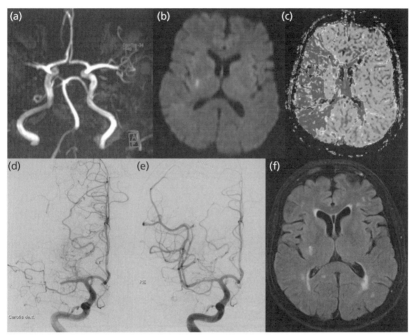

Fig. 8.3 A 47-year-old female patient was admitted with a dense left-sided hemiparesis and hemineglect. Acute brain MRI/MRA shows a right middle cerebral artery occlusion (a, time-of-flight MRA), a small ischaemic infarct in the internal capsule (b, DWI MRI) and a huge perfusion deficit in the right MCA territory (mean transit time map) (c). Intravenous thrombolysis was initiated and the patient was transferred to the angio suite for mechanical thrombectomy. Digital subtraction angiography confirms the MCA occlusion (d). After thrombectomy with a stent-retriever system the right MCA was recanalized (e). On day 2 post-intervention, the patient had only a minor weakness of her left arm. The final infarct is shown on figure (f) (FLAIR MRI).

vessels. Intracranial MRA can thus be added to the evaluation of every patient even with transient or minor ischaemic symptoms in order not to overlook an occluded large vessel. Otherwise, infarction and clinical deficits may progress once collateral flow becomes insufficient. The vessel occlusion is the culprit event and thus may precede visible morphologic abnormalities in the very acute phase of stroke. This can happen especially in the brainstem, where morphologic changes often need several hours to develop (23, 24). In this context, CTA or MRA is helpful to rule out basilar artery occlusion.

Imaging of the extracranial arteries is not a prerequisite for endovascular stroke treatment, but information about vessel patency can certainly be helpful in planning the procedure. Such comprehensive information can be provided by

CTA when it covers the neurovascular tree from the aortic arch up to the intracranial arteries. Because of the loss of time, an additional examination of the extracranial arteries such as with contrast-enhanced MRA should not be routinely performed. The condition of the extracranial vessels will anyway become apparent during the interventional procedure and internal carotid artery occlusion or stenosis does not represent a contraindication for thrombectomy.

There are also suggestions that CTA could provide important insights regarding viability of brain tissue as indicated by the presence or absence of collaterals via the external carotid artery (25). In specific cases, such information could help to better select responders to thrombectomy and to extend the time interval for intervention. However, patient selection on the basis of collateral image processing cannot yet be recommended (5).

Identification of patients with high risk for subsequent attacks

As outlined in Chapter 7, the presence of an acute diffusion-weighted imaging (DWI) lesion on MRI is indicative of a higher risk of stroke recurrence in patients with TIA or minor ischaemic stroke. Plain CT has less predictive capacity because of the much lower sensitivity for detecting acute and small ischaemic infarcts. The additional use of CTA may compensate for this. In a prospective study of 510 patients with transient ischaemic attack (TIA) or minor ischaemic stroke, the presence of acute ischaemia on CT and/or of intracranial or extracranial vessel occlusion or stenosis greater or equal to 50% on CTA were equally predictive for a recurrent stroke than the presence of an acute ischaemic lesion on MRI (26).

Prevention of stroke recurrence, however, is certainly even more important than prediction. Regarding vascular imaging, this refers especially to the identification of high-grade carotid artery stenosis, which conveys a risk for further ischaemic events. This risk is especially high during the first days after the first cerebrovascular attack (27). As CTA and contrast-enhanced MRA can be easily added to the morphologic brain imaging, it should be considered to perform both examinations together when morphologic imaging shows abnormalities suggestive of extracranial vascular pathology such as watershed infarcts of different age except in the very acute setting as outlined previously. If carotid stenosis is suspected from duplex sonography, CTA or contrast-enhanced MRA serve as complementary diagnostic tools to plan thromboendarterectomy or endovascular stenting and eliminate the need to perform catheter angiography (DSA) for such a purpose (Fig. 8.4). In addition to duplex sonography, both techniques can detect more distally located vessel stenosis, which may be important in the choice of recanalization procedure.

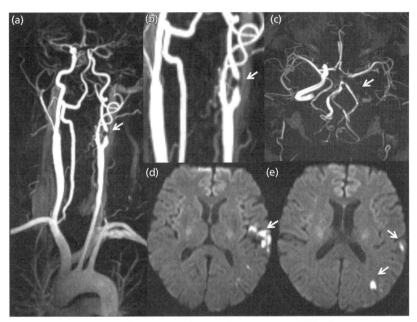

Fig. 8.4 A 53-year-old male patient with stuttering symptoms (difficulty to speak, weakness of the right arm, transient monocular blindness on the left eye). Contrast-enhanced MRA depicts a high-grade left internal carotid artery stenosis (a, b). The left intracranial internal carotid artery is nearly missing on TOF-MRA (c) suggestive of a severe haemodynamic compromise of the stenosis. Images (d) and (e) show the corresponding ischaemic infarcts in the left middle cerebral artery and posterior border zone territory (DWI MRI).

In comparison to extracranial carotid artery stenosis, more uncertainty exists in relation to intracranial cerebral vessel stenosis, apart from the fact that a stenosis also is associated with a higher risk of recurrent stroke. In younger stroke patients, the incidence of intracranial vessel stenosis or occlusion may even be higher than that of the extracranial cerebral vessels, as suggested by the results of the Stroke in Young Fabry Patients (sifap1) study (28). Supratentorial vessel stenosis or occlusions were found in 11.8% of 1612 patients and were especially frequent in individuals between 45 and 55 years (13%). As the sifap1 study was based on ultrasonography, similar and even more specific findings can be expected with CTA or MRA (Fig. 8.5). However, it has to be acknowledged that the therapeutic consequences are much less clear than for extracranial arteriosclerosis. This is due to the controversial results of therapeutic approaches including the uncertainty of the aetiological causes.

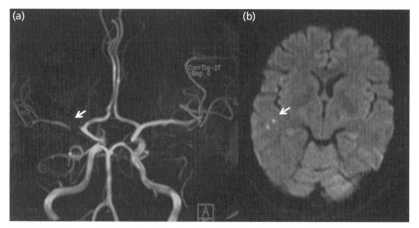

Fig. 8.5 A 47-year-old female patient with multiple atherosclerotic risk factors presented with recurrent left-sided hemiparesis. Corresponding to the clinical symptoms, TOF-MRA (a) demonstrates a proximal high-grade right middle cerebral artery stenosis. DWI MRI shows the respective ischaemic infarction (b).

Vascular imaging in the differential diagnosis of ischaemic stroke in young adults

To allow for specific treatment, it would be desirable to identify the actual cause(s) for vessel wall changes beyond establishing just the presence of a stenosis or occlusion. Extracranial vessel wall changes and stenosis due to atherosclerosis are localized typically at the carotid bifurcation. Symptomatic vessels often show irregular vessel walls with ulceration. The stenosed segment is mostly short and may be associated with an ectatic enlargement of the blood vessel before and after the stenosis and vessel tortuosity. While the high risk of stroke recurrence with higher-grade stenosis is well established, there often remains uncertainty about a causal relationship of moderate-grade stenosis with a distal ischaemic infarct. Attempts are made to better characterize such vessel changes with vessel wall imaging using MRI. Intraplaque haemorrhage, lipid-rich necrotic core, and thinning/rupture of the fibrous cap have been identified as MRI carotid plaque features that are associated with an increased risk for future stroke or TIA (29, 30). However such investigations have not yet entered clinical routine and it is unclear if and how they can add to patient management.

Another disorder is craniocervical artery dissection (CAD), which can be identified as the cause of vessel stenosis or occlusion by MRI and MRA. CAD has been reported to be the single most common cause of ischaemic stroke in young adults. It is responsible for up to 15% of strokes in patients below 55 years of age. CAD appears to develop from an intimal tear, which allows the blood to extend into and along the vessel wall. An alternative mechanism is direct bleeding within the arterial wall caused by ruptured vasa vasorum (31). This usually results in a longitudinal and smooth narrowing of the vessel lumen up to complete occlusion. Direct evidence for dissection can be obtained with axial T1-weighted MRI sequences perpendicular to the blood vessel, which show the extravasated blood as a semicircular rim of high signal intensity. To avoid confusion with other tissues, fat suppression should be used and the investigation has to be performed before the application of contrast material (Fig. 8.6). Due to the high sensitivity of this approach, it sometimes also reveals dissection in other asymptomatic vessels without stenosis. Of note, ischaemic stroke in CAD often appears to come not from a haemodynamic compromise due to severe stenosis or occlusion but rather from thrombotic emboli favoured by the intimal tear and changing flow dynamics (31, 32).

Aetiological classification of intracranial stenosis or occlusions is more demanding and can often just be made in the context of additional clinical and laboratory findings. In the anterior circulation, the absence of a main vessel on CTA or MRA always suggests occlusion. In the posterior circulation, however, it is not unusual that one of the vertebral arteries is hypoplastic. In such instances, the combined interpretation of the morphologic image on MRI, which shows the signal of an occluded vessel and the absence of that vessel on MRA, can serve to unequivocally identify vessel occlusion. The presence of a vessel occlusion without concomitant vascular changes throughout the neuro-vascular tree indicates a proximal (cardio-aortic) embolic origin and this likelihood increases with multiple vessel occlusions.

Narrowing of intracranial vessels in the context of an ischaemic infarct is difficult to interpret as this may indicate a local process, but also a resolving thrombus. Multiple stenosed vessels suggest a systemic process and research efforts are made to help in the differentiation between atherosclerosis and inflammatory causes (i.e. vessel wall imaging; Fig. 8.7). Primary cerebral angiitis, however, mostly cannot be detected by CTA or MRA as it commonly affects the distal intracerebral branches. A suspicion of angiitis is therefore an indication for catheter angiography (DSA). Finally, multiple stenoses may also arise from spasms due to subarachnoid haemorrhage, drug abuse (such as cannabis or cocaine), or a reversible cerebral vasoconstriction syndrome. In the latter condition it has to be considered that vasoconstriction occurs usually only a few days after the acute onset of thunderclap headache. The restitution of vasoconstriction is an important differential diagnostic clue to distinguish reversible cerebral vasoconstriction syndrome (that is often associated with posterior

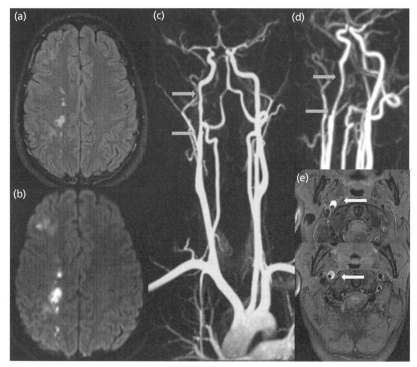

Fig. 8.6 A 37-year-old male patient with stuttering left-sided hemiparesis and neck pain on the right side. FLAIR (a) and DWI (b) MRI show right hemispheric ischaemic infarcts in a border zone pattern. Extracranial contrast-enhanced MRA depicts long-segmental irregularities of the right extracranial internal carotid artery extending to the high cervical/intracranial level (c, d). Axial T1 fat-suppressed sequences show a corresponding intramural haematoma indicative of arterial dissection (e).

reversible encephalopathy syndrome) and central nervous system vasculitis (33–35).

Conclusion and proposed algorithm

Vascular imaging has become of paramount importance in the management of acute ischaemic stroke given the option of intravenous thrombolysis and especially endovascular thrombectomy in case of large vessel occlusion. For practical reasons and in order to not delay treatment, either CTA or MRA should be included in the hyperacute imaging protocol of young stroke patients.

Vascular imaging is also needed to identify causes of stroke that necessitate rapid action to avoid recurrence such as high-grade internal carotid artery stenosis. In this context, both CTA and contrast-enhanced extracranial MRA

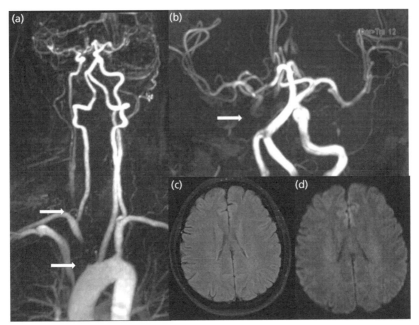

Fig. 8.7 A 33-year-old woman with fever, general weakness and fatigue, persistent headache, and painful claudication of the right arm. Contrast-enhanced MRA reveals stenoses of the brachiocephalic and the proximal right common carotid artery (a). TOF MRA shows decreased signal in the right internal carotid artery (b). The patient had no ischaemic lesions on brain MRI (FLAIR (c), and DWI (d)). Such a finding is indicative of Takayasu's arteritis, which typically affects the aorta and its large proximal branches (most often quite asymmetrically).

may be used as primary tools or to confirm duplex sonography findings before carotid revascularization. Suspected cerebral artery dissection can be reliably detected using MRI by combining morphologic and vessel imaging. Thus only a few questions such as a suspicion for primary cerebral angiitis still necessitate invasive DSA. With technical advances, however, the characterization of intracranial vascular pathologies by MRI/MRA becomes increasingly possible.

References

1. **Kurz KD, Ringstad G, Odland A, Advani R, Farbu E, Kurz MW.** Radiological imaging in acute ischaemic stroke. Eur J Neurol. 2016;23 Suppl 1:8–17.
2. **Liebeskind DS, Sanossian N, Yong WH, Starkman S, Tsang MP, Moya AL**, et al. CT and MRI early vessel signs reflect clot composition in acute stroke. Stroke. 2011;**42**:1237–43.

3. Schellinger PD, Chalela JA, Kang D-W, Latour LL, Warach S. Diagnostic and prognostic value of early MR imaging vessel signs in hyperacute stroke patients imaged. AJNR Am J Neuroradiol. 2005;**26**:618–24.

4. Fazekas F, Niederkorn K, Ebner F, Díez-Tejedor E. Relevance of neuroimaging in the evaluation of cerebral ischemia. Cerebrovasc Dis. 2009;**27** Suppl 1:1–8.

5. Fiehler J, Cognard C, Gallitelli M, Jansen O, Kobayashi A, Mattle HP, et al. European Recommendations on Organisation of Interventional Care in Acute Stroke (EROICAS). Int J Stroke. 2016;**11**:701–16.

6. Mohan S, Agarwal M, Pukenas B. Computed tomography angiography of the neurovascular circulation. Radiol Clin North Am. 2016;**54**:147–62.

7. Ferro JM, Massaro AR, Mas J-L. Aetiological diagnosis of ischaemic stroke in young adults. Lancet Neurol. 2010;**9**:1085–96.

8. Luitse MJA, Dauwan M, van Seeters T, Horsch AD, Niesten JM, Kappelle LJ, et al. Acute nephropathy after contrast agent administration for computed tomography perfusion and computed tomography angiography in patients with acute ischemic stroke. Int J Stroke. 2015;**10**:E35–6.

9. Dittrich R, Akdeniz S, Kloska SP, Fischer T, Ritter MA, Seidensticker P, et al. Low rate of contrast-induced nephropathy after CT perfusion and CT angiography in acute stroke patients. J Neurol. 2007;**254**:1491–97.

10. Kramer M, Ellmann S, Allmendinger T, Eller A, Kammerer F, May MS, et al. Computed tomography angiography of carotid arteries and vertebrobasilar system: a simulation study for radiation dose reduction. Medicine (Baltimore). 2015;**94**:e1058.

11. MacDonald ME, Frayne R. Cerebrovascular MRI: a review of state-of-the-art approaches, methods and techniques. NMR Biomed. 2015;**28**:767–91.

12. Chandra T, Pukenas B, Mohan S, Melhem E. Contrast-enhanced magnetic resonance angiography. Magn Reson Imaging Clin N Am. 2012;**20**:687–98.

13. Ramalho J, Semelka RC, Ramalho M, Nunes RH, AlObaidy M, Castillo M. Gadolinium-based contrast agent accumulation and toxicity: an update. AJNR Am J Neuroradiol. 2016;**37**:1192–98.

14. Stojanov D, Aracki-Trenkic A, Benedeto-Stojanov D. Gadolinium deposition within the dentate nucleus and globus pallidus after repeated administrations of gadolinium-based contrast agents-current status. Neuroradiology. 2016;**58**:433–41.

15. Campbell BCV, Donnan GA, Lees KR, Hacke W, Khatri P, Hill MD, et al. Endovascular stent thrombectomy: the new standard of care for large vessel ischaemic stroke. Lancet Neurol. 2015;**14**:846–54.

16. Badhiwala JH, Nassiri F, Alhazzani W, Selim MH, Farrokhyar F, Spears J, et al. Endovascular thrombectomy for acute ischemic stroke: a meta-analysis. JAMA. 2015;**314**:1832–43.

17. Goyal M, Menon BK, van Zwam WH, Dippel DWJ, Mitchell PJ, Demchuk AM, et al. Endovascular thrombectomy after large-vessel ischaemic stroke: a meta-analysis of individual patient data from five randomised trials. Lancet. 2016;**387**:1723–31.

18. Campbell BCV, Hill MD, Rubiera M, Menon BK, Demchuk A, Donnan GA, et al. Safety and efficacy of solitaire stent thrombectomy: individual patient data meta-analysis of randomized trials. Stroke. 2016;**47**:798–806.

19. Wahlgren N, Moreira T, Michel P, Steiner T, Jansen O, Cognard C, et al. Mechanical thrombectomy in acute ischemic stroke: consensus statement by ESO-Karolinska

Stroke Update 2014/2015, supported by ESO, ESMINT, ESNR and EAN. Int J Stroke. 2016;**11**:134–47.

20. **Cooray C, Fekete K, Mikulik R, Lees KR, Wahlgren N, Ahmed N.** Threshold for NIH stroke scale in predicting vessel occlusion and functional outcome after stroke thrombolysis. Int J Stroke. 2015;**10**:822–29.

21. **Heldner MR, Zubler C, Mattle HP, Schroth G, Weck A, Mono M-L,** et al. National Institutes of Health stroke scale score and vessel occlusion in 2152 patients with acute ischemic stroke. Stroke. 2013;**44**:1153–57.

22. **Heldner MR, Hsieh K, Broeg-Morvay A, Mordasini P, Bühlmann M, Jung S,** et al. Clinical prediction of large vessel occlusion in anterior circulation stroke: mission impossible? J Neurol. 2016;**263**:1633–40.

23. **Frey LC, Sung GY, Tanabe J.** Early false-negative diffusion-weighted imaging in brainstem infarction. J Stroke Cerebrovasc Dis. 2002;**11**:51–53.

24. **Sylaja PN, Coutts SB, Krol A, Hill MD, Demchuk AM, VISION Study Group.** When to expect negative diffusion-weighted images in stroke and transient ischemic attack. Stroke. 2008;**39**:1898–900.

25. **Berkhemer OA, Jansen IGH, Beumer D, Fransen PSS, van den Berg LA, Yoo AJ,** et al. Collateral status on baseline computed tomographic angiography and intra-arterial treatment effect in patients with proximal anterior circulation stroke. Stroke. 2016;**47**:768–76.

26. **Coutts SB, Modi J, Patel SK, Demchuk AM, Goyal M, Hill MD,** et al. CT/CT angiography and MRI findings predict recurrent stroke after transient ischemic attack and minor stroke: results of the prospective CATCH study. Stroke. 2012;**43**:1013–17.

27. **Balami JS, Chen R-L, Grunwald IQ, Buchan AM.** Neurological complications of acute ischaemic stroke. Lancet Neurol. 2011;**10**:357–71.

28. **Sarnowski von B, Schminke U, Tatlisumak T, Putaala J, Grittner U, Kaps M,** et al. Prevalence of stenoses and occlusions of brain-supplying arteries in young stroke patients. Neurology. 2013;**80**:1287–94.

29. **Mono M-L, Karameshev A, Slotboom J, Remonda L, Galimanis A, Jung S,** et al. Plaque characteristics of asymptomatic carotid stenosis and risk of stroke. Cerebrovasc Dis. 2012;**34**:343–50.

30. **Gupta A, Baradaran H, Schweitzer AD, Kamel H, Pandya A, Delgado D,** et al. Carotid plaque MRI and stroke risk: a systematic review and meta-analysis. Stroke. 2013;**44**:3071–77.

31. **Debette S, Leys D.** Cervical-artery dissections: predisposing factors, diagnosis, and outcome. Lancet Neurol. 2009;**8**:668–78.

32. **Lucas C, Moulin T, Deplanque D, Tatu L, Chavot D.** Stroke patterns of internal carotid artery dissection in 40 patients. Stroke. 1998;**29**:2646–48.

33. **Ducros A.** Reversible cerebral vasoconstriction syndrome. Lancet Neurol. 2012;**11**:906–17.

34. **Fugate JE, Rabinstein AA.** Posterior reversible encephalopathy syndrome: clinical and radiological manifestations, pathophysiology, and outstanding questions. Lancet Neurol. 2015;**14**:914–25.

35. **Wolff V, Lauer V, Rouyer O, Sellal F, Meyer N, Raul JS,** et al. Cannabis use, ischemic stroke, and multifocal intracranial vasoconstriction: a prospective study in 48 consecutive young patients. Stroke. 2011;**42**:1778–80.

Chapter 9

Vascular imaging: Ultrasound

Ulrike Waje-Andreassen and Nicola Logallo

Basic principles

Ultrasound is a non-invasive technique that can be applied at the bedside for nearly any patient after first-line acute computed tomography angiography (CTA) or magnetic resonance angiography (MRA), or both. The technology is based on the Doppler effect (Christian Doppler, 1803–1853), and transcranial and extracranial ultrasound are therefore also called transcranial Doppler (TCD) and extracranial Doppler ultrasound, respectively. However, the first medical ultrasound was not used before the 1960s. In the late 1980s, brightness mode (B-mode) scanning and colour-coded sonography (CCS) were introduced to improve diagnostics for extracranial and intracranial arterial disease.

The first ultrasound probe able to record blood flow velocity through the skull was introduced in 1982 (1). The TCD machines in use today do not differ considerably from the first prototype, and still use probes which depict moving blood and display the Doppler spectrum on the screen (Fig. 9.1).

Since TCD does not provide anatomical information about intracranial vessels, identification of a specific artery in the skull is deduced by flow direction, depth of the recording sample volume, and position of the transducer. In CCS, the recorded Doppler shift frequencies are used to create a spatial colour map of blood velocity overlaid onto the B-mode image, which provides visualization of both anatomy and blood flow, and improves the examination of cerebral haemodynamics (Fig. 9.2) and artery wall disease.

Both with TCD and transcranial CCS (TCCS), the skull is insonated through areas where the ultrasound beam penetrates without being excessively dampened, the so-called acoustic window. The transtemporal, transorbital, and transforaminal (or transnuchal) windows allow insonation of the circle of Willis and the other major intracranial arteries. Inadequacy of transtemporal window occurs in 5–20% of stroke patients. Older age and female gender are the major predictive factors for a poor acoustic window. Use of microbubble contrast may, however, enable satisfactory examination in almost all patients. Both transcranial and extracranial ultrasound have important diagnostic, prognostic, and

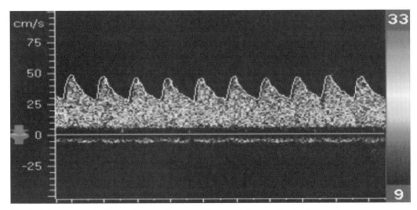

Fig. 9.1 Transcranial Doppler spectrum of the middle cerebral artery.

therapeutic applications in stroke patients at all ages. The safety profile of ultrasound allows monitoring of both extracranial and intracranial haemodynamics over time and at several time points. This chapter will provide a brief overview of the major applications of both ultrasound technologies after acute stroke at a young age (Box 9.1).

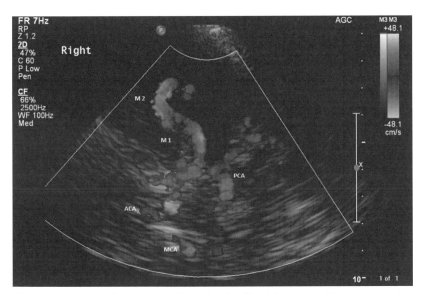

Fig. 9.2 Colour-coded overview of the circle of Willis with transcranial colour-coded sonography. ACA: anterior cerebral artery; M1, proximal segment of the MCA; M2, distal segment of the MCA; MCA, middle cerebral artery; PCA, posterior cerebral artery.

> ## Box 9.1 Possible clinical use of transcranial and extracranial cerebrovascular ultrasound
>
> - Detection of site and degree of stenosis or occlusion of extra- and intra-cranial vessels
> - Assessment of collateral flow
> - Detection of minor extracranial wall disease as supplementary information to angiography
> - Detection of microemboli
> - Detection and quantification of right-to-left shunt
> - Assessment of cerebral vasoreactivity
> - Monitoring of patients with sickle cell disease
> - Educational tool
> - Sonothrombolysis.

Transcranial ultrasound

Intracranial steno-occlusive disease

Both TCD and TCCS have high sensitivity, specificity, and positive and negative predictive values for detection of large intracranial artery occlusion. Such diagnosis is based on the absence of a Doppler signal in the insonated artery and the detection of at least one ipsilateral cerebral artery proving an adequate acoustic window. Concomitant blood flow changes in other intracranial arteries may increase diagnostic accuracy. For instance, high velocities in the ipsilateral anterior and posterior cerebral arteries may be seen in case of proximal middle cerebral artery (MCA, M1 segment) occlusion as a sign of collateral flow through leptomeningeal arteries (a haemodynamic pattern known as *flow diversion*).

Detection of an acute intracranial occlusion is crucial in acute stroke treatment and is a major stroke prognostic factor. A normal flow pattern at 6 hours after stroke independently predicts early improvement whereas persistent occlusion at the same time point is associated with haemorrhagic transformation (2, 3). Transcranial ultrasonography should therefore be repeated at several time points during the first days after large artery occlusion stroke.

Both TCD and TCCS have high diagnostic accuracy in detection of intracranial stenosis. A focal increase in blood flow velocities at the site of luminal narrowing is the characteristic haemodynamic sign of stenosis, often with low turbulent flow immediately distal to the lesion. However, low velocities with low pulsatility may be found downstream in case of a near-occlusive stenosis. Transcranial ultrasonography has also shown high diagnostic accuracy in determining the degree of stenosis, compared to other angiographic modalities. Traditionally, stenosis is dichotomized into more or less than 50% based on threshold velocity values (Table 9.1). The percentage of stenosis may be evaluated more exactly by comparing peak systolic velocities (PSVs) measured before and into the stenosis according to the formula derived from the continuity equation: $[1 - (PSV_{prestenotic}/PSV_{intrastenotic}) \times 100]$. This method is more easily performed by TCCS which enables accurate assessment of haemodynamics through the stenosis by visualization of the target vessel (4).

Transcranial ultrasonography may help in the aetiological workup of intracranial stenosis, and its diagnostic value increases with repetitive examinations.

In case of focal increase in flow velocity, complete normalization or greater than 50% reduction in PSV at follow-up suggests the diagnosis of recanalized embolus, whereas persistence of the haemodynamic abnormalities indicates atherosclerotic disease. A multifocal or diffuse increase in flow velocity combined with a clinical context of sudden, intense headache, with or without

Table 9.1 Diagnostic performance of threshold values in detection of 50% or greater stenosis in different intracranial arteries

	TCCS[a]	Sensitivity	Specificity	TCD	Sensitivity	Specificity
	PSV (cm/s)	%	%	MV (cm/s)	%	%
MCA	≥220[a]	100	100	≥100[c]	100	97
ACA	≥155[a]	100	100	≥80[b]	–	–
ICA	≥120[d]	87	83	≥80[d]	93	76
PCA	≥145[a]	100	91	≥50[b]	–	–
Basilar	≥140[a]	100	100	≥80[e]	69	69
Vertebral	≥120[a]	100	100	≥80[d]	69	69

ACA, anterior cerebral artery; ICA, internal cerebral artery; MCA, middle cerebral artery; MV, mean velocity; PCA, posterior cerebral artery; PSV, peak systolic velocity; TCCS, transcranial colour-coded sonography; TCD, transcranial Doppler.

[a] Baumgartner RW, Stroke. 1999;30:87–92.

[b] Alexandrov AV, Cerebrovascular Ultrasound in Stroke Prevention and Treatment. Wiley; 2011.

[c] Navarro JC, Cerebrovasc Dis. 2007;23:325–30.

[d] You Y, J Neuroimaging. 2010;20:234–39.

[e] Zhao L, Stroke. 2011;42:3429–34.

neurological deficit, may either be suggestive of reversible cerebral vasoconstriction syndrome, if flow velocity normalizes at follow-up, or vasculitis, in case of no resolution. Repetitive ultrasonographic examination should therefore be part of the aetiological evaluation of young stroke patients with intracranial stenosis.

Ultrasound imaging alone may sometimes provide a probable diagnosis. For instance, the combination of high-pulsatility flow in the extracranial carotid arteries, low velocities with low pulsatility in both the intracranial internal carotid and the middle cerebral arteries, and visualization of the leptomeningeal collateral network is pathognomonic of moyamoya disease.

Assessment of intracranial collateral flow

Transcranial ultrasound provides accurate evaluation of collateral circulation in carotid and intracranial steno-occlusive conditions by real-time assessment of the intracranial haemodynamics (5). The major collateral pathways are the anterior and the posterior communicating arteries (ACoA and PCoA), the ophthalmic artery (OA), and the leptomeningeal arteries. Reliable direct visualization and blood flow measurement of the ACoA is not possible because of its short length and small calibre. Indirect signs of a patent and functioning ACoA are flow inversion in A1 with sufficient blood flow in the ipsilateral MCA after compression of the ipsilateral common carotid artery. The PCoA may be reliably visualized by TCCS, whereas identification by TCD may be challenging. Collateralization through the PCoA is suggested by increased blood flow velocity in the basilar artery and in the ipsilateral P1. Patients with MCA occlusion may show high-velocity and low-pulsatility flow in the ipsilateral anterior cerebral artery and/or posterior cerebral artery (flow diversion), which is a sign of collateralization from the leptomeningeal arteries. In case of proximal internal carotid artery occlusion or severe stenosis, reversed flow in the ipsilateral OA suggests insufficient collateral function of the communicating arteries.

The presence of intracranial collateral flow predicts infarct volume and stroke outcome. Assessment of intracranial collateral flow and haemodynamics should be repeated daily in the first days after stroke to detect recanalization, progression, or instability of steno-occlusive disease (6). Evaluation of collateral status is also of crucial importance before procedures in the extracranial or intracranial vessels, or both.

Ultrasound treatment: sonothrombolysis and targeted drug delivery

Ultrasound as an adjunct to thrombolytic therapy (i.e. sonothrombolysis) may improve the recanalization rate of occluded intracranial arteries. Microbubbles may further potentiate the effect of sonothrombolysis. Some of the proposed underlying mechanisms of sonothrombolysis are acceleration of enzymatic fibrinolysis and increased local tissue perfusion by peripheral vasodilatation. The oscillation and rupture of microbubbles when intercepted by the ultrasound beam add mechanical energy in proximity of the clot and may further increase the effect of sonothrombolysis. According to a meta-analysis of phase II trials (7), patients with visible intracranial occlusion treated with sonothrombolysis have more than a twofold higher likelihood of achieving both complete recanalization at 2 hours and favourable functional outcome at 3 months compared to patients not receiving sonothrombolysis. No safety issues have been reported for probes within 1.8–4 MHz frequencies, whereas an increased rate of spontaneous intracerebral haemorrhage has been observed when probes with lower frequency were used. The major limitations of the pooled trials are small sample size and no double blindness in randomization and clinical follow-up. The CLOTBUST-ER study (NCT#01098981), a phase III trial which aimed to investigate efficacy and safety of sonothrombolysis vs recombinant tissue plasminogen activator (rt-PA) alone in moderate to severe acute ischaemic stroke patients (baseline National Institutes of Health Stroke Scale (NIHSS) score >9), showed that sonothrombolysis is safe but does not improve functional outcome at 90 days compared to rt-PA alone. However, trends towards a beneficial effect of sonothrombolysis were observed in patients with proven large artery occlusion and in patients treated in high-volume centres, showing promise of efficacy worth being explored (8).

In animal models, microbubble-enhanced sonothrombolysis has been shown to significantly improve microvascular patency (9). Ongoing research is further investigating if microbubble-enhanced sonothrombolysis may potentiate the effect of rt-PA by ameliorating microcirculation also in ischaemic stroke patients without visible occlusion (10), and thereby improve the efficacy of acute stroke treatment for the majority of patients.

Microbubbles may also be used as carriers of therapeutic agents. Drugs may be attached to the membrane of microbubbles and later released when the ultrasound energy cavitates the microbubbles. In ischaemic stroke patients, targeted drug delivery with ultrasound may be applied to tissue plasminogen activator (t-PA). The targeted delivery and release of t-PA at the thrombus site may potentiate the effect of thrombolytics and reduce risk for bleeding complications. Studies have shown that targeted drug delivery with t-PA and ultrasound is feasible but its therapeutic efficacy remains to be explored in clinical trials.

Emboli monitoring in acute stroke

TCD may detect microembolic signals (MES) in the intracranial vessels. Compared to angiography, ultrasound has the advantage of simultaneously recording both visual and acoustic information. Microemboli have different acoustic properties compared to the circulating erythrocytes and appear randomly in the cardiac cycle as high- and short-intensity signals with a characteristic 'chirp' sound. Emboli monitoring (EM) should be performed by bilateral insonation of the target vessels, usually the middle cerebral arteries. The 2 MHZ probes should be secured by a headband and monitoring should last at least 30 minutes. MES may be detected also by extracranial cerebrovascular ultrasound. This is an option during extracranial examination in case of a poor transtemporal acoustic window. The rate of MES in acute stroke varies from 10% to 70% according to the time frame, concomitant therapies, and criteria for MES detection (11). The earlier the EM is started after stroke onset, the higher the detection rate (12). Potential applications of EM are stroke risk stratification, aetiological workup, and follow-up of antiplatelet/antithrombotic therapy efficacy. MES detection is an independent predictor of new stroke events. Unilateral MES distal to an extracranial or intracranial stenosis, either symptomatic or asymptomatic, indicate active embolization from an unstable plaque or a dissection. Instability of plaques in coronary arteries is more predictive for myocardial infarction than the degree of stenosis. Such knowledge has also been confirmed for extracranial arteries by contrast-enhanced extracranial ultrasound studies showing vasa vasorum (neovascularization) in the carotid plaque to be a sign of inflammation and degeneration in atherosclerosis (13).

In stroke patients with unknown aetiology, EM may help to identify potential embolic sources. Bilateral MES most likely indicate a cardioembolic origin or a source in the ascending aorta or the aortic arch, whereas unilateral MES are often a sign of artery-to-artery embolism. In the post-acute phase of stroke, EM may measure efficacy of secondary prevention. Persistent detection of MES may indicate therapy failure and need for therapy optimization (14).

Detection and quantification of right-to-left shunts

Patent foramen ovale (PFO) and other right-to-left shunts (RTLSs) are associated with ischaemic stroke, though not always with a clear causal association. Contrast-enhanced transoesophageal echocardiography (cTOE) is the diagnostic gold standard for detection of right-to-left intracardiac shunts. However, comparable diagnostic accuracy is achieved by contrast-enhanced TCD with bilateral monitoring of the MCA (15). The contrast agent is prepared by vigorously mixing 9 mL of saline with 1 mL of air and administered immediately intravenously. Air microbubbles are not able to cross the pulmonary capillary bed, and they enter the systemic circulation only in the presence of RTLSs. TCD detects microbubbles during their passage through the MCA as gaseous MES. The test is considered positive if at least one MES is detected

Box 9.2 Quantification of right-to-left shunt

- Test negative: no microbubble
- Low-grade shunt: 1–10 microbubbles
- Medium-grade shunt: ≥10 microbubbles but without 'curtain/shower effect'
- High-grade shunt: curtain/shower effect, seen when the microbubbles are numerous and no longer distinguishable separately.

within 40 seconds after terminating the air contrast injection. In case of little or no detection of MES, the examination should be repeated with a preferably 10-second long Valsalva manoeuvre starting 5 seconds after air contrast injection. Quantification of RTLSs should be reported as suggested in Box 9.2 (16). Contrast-enhanced TOE has the advantage of being able to determine the anatomical location of a cardiac RTLS and detect a possible concomitant atrial septal aneurysm. However, contrast-enhanced TOE is a semi-invasive technique requiring the patient's compliance and does not detect latent shunts or extracardiac shunts. Contrast-enhanced TCD should therefore be performed also in case of a normal contrast-enhanced TOE if a RTLS is suspected.

Assessment of cerebral vasoreactivity

Cerebral vasoreactivity (CVR) describes the response of intracranial arterioles to external vasomotor stimuli. Vasodilation of the intracranial arterioles may be induced by exogenous stimuli increasing extracellular partial pressure of carbon dioxide (pCO_2) (lowering pH) or decreasing mean blood pressure. Intracranial vasodilation leads to increased blood flow volume and blood flow velocity in the supplying large arteries which may be monitored by transcranial ultrasound. Breath-holding, inspiration of CO_2 through a mask, or intravenous acetazolamide (1 g or 0.15 mg/kg weight) are the most commonly used stimuli administered under continuous TCD monitoring to test CVR. An increase in blood flow velocity of more than 20% is normal (17). Impaired CVR (blood flow velocity increase ≤20%) may suggest a higher stroke risk. Hypertension, diabetes mellitus, and small vessel disease are associated with impaired CVR (18). CVR may be useful in risk stratification of patients with large artery disease, either asymptomatic or symptomatic. Impaired CVR indicates failure of collateral flow to adapt to the stenosis and may identify high-risk patients (19).

Monitoring of patients with sickle cell disease

Young patients with sickle cell disease are at high risk to suffer a stroke before the age of 20 years from steno-occlusive disease of the carotid siphon and the proximal MCA. Mean velocity higher than 200 cm/s in the carotid siphon or the proximal MCA, or both, indicates need for transfusion therapy (20). Serial transcranial ultrasonographic examinations are recommended for selection of patients requiring transfusion therapy. The ultrasonographic screening should start at the age of 2 years (21). Useful information may also be gained at the extracranial carotid level in case of poor transtemporal insonation.

Extracranial cerebrovascular ultrasound

Atherosclerosis

The three main risk factors for young patients with acute ischaemic stroke in Europe are modifiable hypertension, dyslipidaemia, and active smoking (22). These are also the most common risk factors for atherosclerosis. The Trial of Org 10172 in Acute Stroke Treatment (TOAST) classification from the early 1990s classifies atherosclerosis only as such when there is a stenosis of at least 50%. As CTA then was most available and as most stroke patients in the Western world have a mean age above 70 years, this was a reasonable decision. However, atherosclerosis develops gradually from slightly and increasing intima–media thickness (IMT) to stable and unstable plaques (23). IMT has since 1986 been described as reflexes between the arterial lumen and the intima and between the media and adventitia interfaces of the arterial wall (24). Plaques have since the first Mannheim consensus been defined as focal structures that encroach into the arterial lumen by at least 50% of the surrounding IMT value or at measurements of at least 1.5 mm (25). Improved technology has documented that most young patients frequently have subtle signs of atherosclerosis. Apart from young ischaemic patients with TOAST-classified atherosclerosis, also patients with small artery occlusion and unknown cause of stroke have more atherosclerosis than controls (26). Young stroke patients should therefore no longer be diagnosed by angiography alone. Ultrasound after acute ischaemic stroke at a young age may contribute to secure the cause of the stroke, even when angiography, regarded as the 'gold standard' is described as normal (Fig. 9.3).

Bedside monitoring

Bedside ultrasound monitoring after thrombolysis or interventional therapy, or both, may give early information about clinical development of either improvement by increasing recanalization and vascular and clinical stabilization, or

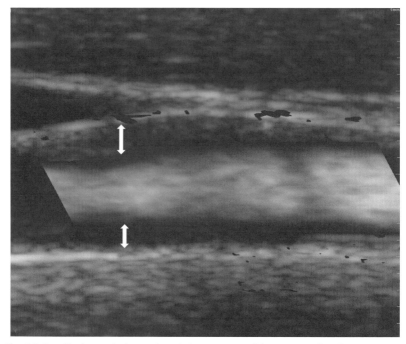

Fig. 9.3 Familiar hypercholesterolaemia in a 42-year-old woman with ischaemic stroke. The carotid bifurcation and proximal part of the internal carotid artery with thickened near and far walls due to familiar hypercholesterolaemia after angiography of the neck arteries with 'normal findings'.

worsening by increasing stenosis, occlusion, and deterioration of cerebral haemodynamics. Improvement or worsening may also depend on the patient's individual anatomy of the circle of Willis, hypoplasia or atresia of a vertebral artery, and actual collateral function monitoring. Dynamic changes of the collateral function from hour to hour or day to day may give valuable information for a necessary change of treatment (27). In case of dissection, occurring in about 20% of young ischaemic stroke patients, the role of ultrasound may be limited for anatomical reasons. Most dissections occur distally from a possible direct view on the artery by ultrasound, and special diagnostic series by magnetic resonance imaging/MRA are necessary to verify the diagnosis. But in case of dissection located in well-visible carotid or vertebral artery segments, ultrasound delivers versatile information, such as fresh vessel wall bleeding with maximum echolucency or visible flow in the false lumen, monitoring and counting of MES, monitoring of flow, flow direction, and pulsatility. Ultrasound allows control of dynamic changes during the first days and control of treatment effects as long as the patient is regarded as clinically unstable. Other changes, such as segmental fibromuscular dysplasia or general arterial wall changes in suspected familial hypercholesterolaemia or inflammatory disease, such as Takayasu disease, may provide valuable information for the cause of the stroke.

Staging of arteries

Staging of arteries may be an educational tool for better compliance and prophylaxis.

Pathological studies show that atherosclerosis is present at all ages, and is differently expressed at different sites of arteries (28). During recent years, several European long-term studies after ischaemic stroke up to the age of 50 years show high mortality rates. Cardiovascular mortality was most often caused by coronary disease, thereafter by recurrent stroke, and long-term survivors showed high rates of recurrent stroke and cognitive problems (29–31). These findings led to the idea that ischaemic stroke at a young age has aspects of a 'malign disease' of the brain. Oncologists have for decades performed staging of tumours for best treatment and prevention. Ultrasound can serve as a readily available, non-invasive tool to perform staging of arteries after acute ischaemic stroke. This was performed in the 5-year inclusion phase of the Norwegian Stroke in the Young Study (NOR-SYS) (32). IMT measurements at standardized sites of the arteries in a three-generation project contributed to broader understanding of arterial wall disease and served as an aid for defining best medical secondary prophylaxis (Fig. 9.4a–c).

To achieve this best prophylaxis and to prevent additional cardiovascular clinical events, patients do have to reach their treatment goals.

However, previous studies have shown that treatment goals are often not reached. Ultrasound pictures should therefore be used immediately after the examination as an educational tool demonstrating any arterial wall changes to the patient. This was done in the NOR-SYS in order to explain why continuous daily use of medication was regarded as necessary and to motivate the patient in addition for necessary lifestyle changes.

In conclusion, ultrasound can be quickly used on nearly any patient, and delivers a look into physiology, haemodynamics, and arterial disease. Knowledge about leading risk factors and high rates of death and cardiovascular events among young stroke patients, together with a rate of unknown cause of stroke about 40%, make ultrasound a very valuable diagnostic tool. Treating patients by acute ultrasound is still a research topic. Concerning diagnostics, however, the optimal use of ultrasound is to examine patients as soon as possible, consolidate findings from angiography, obtain supplementary information on the state of the arteries, gain information about extracranial and intracranial

(a)

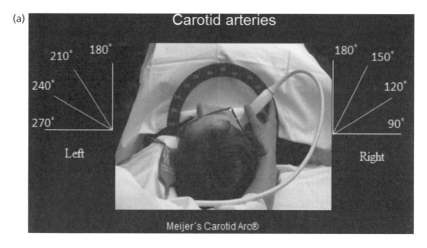

(b)

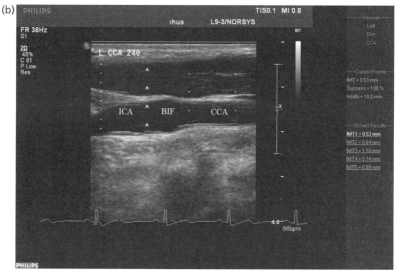

Fig. 9.4 Staging of carotid and femoral arteries. (a) The four-angle approach of measuring carotid arteries, used in the Norwegian Stroke in the Young Study. (b) Example of the mean intima–media thickness far-wall measurement of the left common carotid artery (CCA), at 240° in the end-diastolic phase. The ^-sign on the screen marks the location of the tip of the flow divider (TFD) and the pointed rows mark the standardized 1 cm segments. Carotid segments are standardized by defining the distal CCA as 2 cm distal from the TFD, the bifurcation (BIF) or carotid bulb as 1 cm distal from the TFD, and the carotid internal artery (ICA) as 1 cm proximal from the TFD. (c) Example of the mean intima–media thickness (IMT) far-wall measurement of the right superficial femoral artery (SFA). IMT and plaque measurements are performed at both sides for common femoral arteries (CFA) and SFA in the end-diastolic phase.

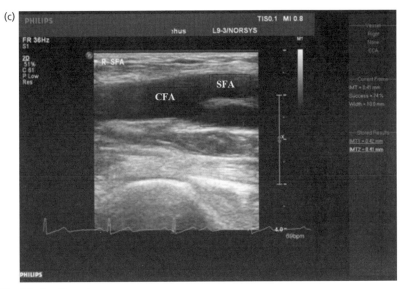

Fig. 9.4 Continued

haemodynamics, monitor MES, monitor unstable patients, and use ultrasound pictures with documented IMT changes and plaques to teach the patient why daily medication and lifestyle changes are necessary. Today, there is still a gap between acute treatment and lasting achievement of treatment goals.

Future challenges are to work for standardized models in each diagnostic field, and to train and certify young colleagues to use these models for future research.

References

1. **Aaslid R, Markwalder TM, Nornes H.** Noninvasive transcranial Doppler ultrasound recording of flow velocity in basal cerebral arteries. J Neurosurg. 1982;57(6):769–74.

2. **Toni D, Fiorelli M, Zanette EM, Sacchetti ML, Salerno A, Argentino C,** et al. Early spontaneous improvement and deterioration of ischemic stroke patients. A serial study with transcranial Doppler ultrasonography. Stroke. 1998;29(6):1144–48.

3. **Alexandrov AV, Black SE, Ehrlich LE, Caldwell CB, Norris JW.** Predictors of hemorrhagic transformation occurring spontaneously and on anticoagulants in patients with acute ischemic stroke. Stroke. 1997;28(6):1198–202.

4. **Logallo N, Lind J, Naess H, Idicula T, Brogger J, Waje-Andreassen U,** et al. Middle cerebral artery stenosis: transcranial color-coded sonography based on continuity equation versus CT-angiography. Ultraschall Med. 2012;33(7):E326–32.

5. **Guan J, Zhang S, Zhou Q, Li C, Lu Z.** Usefulness of transcranial Doppler ultrasound in evaluating cervical-cranial collateral circulations. Interv Neurol. 2013;2(1):8–18.

6. **Kaps M, Dorndorf W, Damian MS, Agnoli L.** Intracranial haemodynamics in patients with spontaneous carotid dissection. Transcranial Doppler ultrasound follow-up studies. Eur Arch Psychiatry Neurol Sci. 1990;239(4):246–56.

7. Saqqur M, Tsivgoulis G, Nicoli F, Skoloudik D, Sharma VK, Larrue V, et al. The role of sonolysis and sonothrombolysis in acute ischemic stroke: a systematic review and meta-analysis of randomized controlled trials and case-control studies. J Neuroimaging. 2014;**24**(3):209–20.

8. Schellinger PD, Alexandrov AV, Barreto AD, Demchuk AM, Tsivgoulis G, Kohrmann M, et al. Combined lysis of thrombus with ultrasound and systemic tissue plasminogen activator for emergent revascularization in acute ischemic stroke (CLOTBUST-ER): design and methodology of a multinational phase 3 trial. Int J Stroke. 2015;**10**(7):1141–48.

9. Schleicher N, Tomkins AJ, Kampschulte M, Hyvelin JM, Botteron C, Juenemann M, et al. Sonothrombolysis with BR38 microbubbles improves microvascular patency in a rat model of stroke. PLoS One. 2016;**11**(4):e0152898.

10. Nacu A, Kvistad CE, Logallo N, Naess H, Waje-Andreassen U, Aamodt AH, et al. A pragmatic approach to sonothrombolysis in acute ischaemic stroke: the Norwegian randomised controlled sonothrombolysis in acute stroke study (NOR-SASS). BMC Neurol. 2015;**15**:110.

11. Csiba L. Ultrasound in acute ischemic stroke. In: Brainin M, Heiss WD, Tabernig S, eds. Textbook of Stroke Medicine, 2nd ed. Cambridge: Cambridge University Press; 2014, 82–99.

12. Markus HS, Thomson ND, Brown MM. Asymptomatic cerebral embolic signals in symptomatic and asymptomatic carotid artery disease. Brain. 1995;**118**(Pt 4):1005–11.

13. Vicenzini E, Giannoni MF, Puccinelli F, Ricciardi MC, Altieri M, Di Piero V, et al. Detection of carotid adventitial vasa vasorum and plaque vascularization with ultrasound cadence contrast pulse sequencing technique and echo-contrast agent. Stroke. 2007;**38**(10):2841–43.

14. Keunen RWM, van Sonderen A, Hunfeld M, Remmers M, Tavy DL, de Bruijn SFTM, et al. Exploration of a zero-tolerance regime on cerebral embolism in symptomatic carotid artery disease. Perspect Med. 2012;**1**(1–12):218–23.

15. Horner S, Niederkorn K, Fazekas F. Patent foramen ovale. Perspect Med. 2012;**1**(1–12):228–31.

16. Jauss M, Zanette E. Detection of right-to-left shunt with ultrasound contrast agent and transcranial Doppler sonography. Cerebrovasc Dis. 2000;**10**(6):490–96.

17. Markus H, Cullinane M. Severely impaired cerebrovascular reactivity predicts stroke and TIA risk in patients with carotid artery stenosis and occlusion. Brain. 2001;**124**(Pt 3):457–67.

18. Settakis G, Molnar C, Kerenyi L, Kollar J, Legemate D, Csiba L, et al. Acetazolamide as a vasodilatory stimulus in cerebrovascular diseases and in conditions affecting the cerebral vasculature. Eur J Neurol. 2003;**10**(6):609–20.

19. Reinhard M, Schwarzer G, Briel M, Altamura C, Palazzo P, King A, et al. Cerebrovascular reactivity predicts stroke in high-grade carotid artery disease. Neurology. 2014;**83**(16):1424–31.

20. Lee MT, Piomelli S, Granger S, Miller ST, Harkness S, Brambilla DJ, et al. Stroke Prevention Trial in Sickle Cell Anemia (STOP): extended follow-up and final results. Blood. 2006;**108**(3):847–52.

21. Meschia JF, Bushnell C, Boden-Albala B, Braun LT, Bravata DM, Chaturvedi S, et al. Guidelines for the primary prevention of stroke: a statement for healthcare

professionals from the American Heart Association/American Stroke Association. Stroke. 2014;**45**(12):3754–832.

22. **Putaala J, Yesilot N, Waje-Andreassen U, Pitkaniemi J, Vassilopoulou S, Nardi K**, et al. Demographic and geographic vascular risk factor differences in European young adults with ischemic stroke: the 15 cities young stroke study. Stroke. 2012;**43**(10):2624–30.

23. **Ross R.** Atherosclerosis—an inflammatory disease. N Engl J Med. 1999;**340**(2):115–26.

24. **Pignoli P, Tremoli E, Poli A, Oreste P, Paoletti R.** Intimal plus medial thickness of the arterial wall: a direct measurement with ultrasound imaging. Circulation. 1986;**74**(6):1399–406.

25. **Touboul PJ, Hennerici MG, Meairs S, Adams H, Amarenco P, Desvarieux M**, et al. Mannheim intima-media thickness consensus. Cerebrovasc Dis. 2004;**18**(4):346–49.

26. **Fromm A, Haaland OA, Naess H, Thomassen L, Waje-Andreassen U.** Atherosclerosis in Trial of Org 10172 in Acute Stroke Treatment subtypes among young and middle-aged stroke patients: the Norwegian Stroke in the Young Study. J Stroke Cerebrovasc Dis. 2016;**25**(4):825–30.

27. **Vicenzini E, Toscano M, Maestrini I, Petolicchio B, Lenzi GL, Di Piero V.** Predictors and timing of recanalization in intracranial carotid artery and siphon dissection: an ultrasound follow-up study. Cerebrovasc Dis. 2013;**35**(5):476–82.

28. **Pasterkamp G, Schoneveld AH, Hillen B, Banga JD, Haudenschild CC, Borst C.** Is plaque formation in the common carotid artery representative for plaque formation and luminal stenosis in other atherosclerotic peripheral arteries? A post mortem study. Atherosclerosis. 1998;**137**(1):205–10.

29. **Waje-Andreassen U, Thomassen L, Jusufovic M, Power KN, Eide GE, Vedeler CA**, et al. Ischaemic stroke at a young age is a serious event—final results of a population-based long-term follow-up in Western Norway. Eur J Neurol. 2013;**20**(5):818–23.

30. **Aarnio K, Haapaniemi E, Melkas S, Kaste M, Tatlisumak T, Putaala J.** Long-term mortality after first-ever and recurrent stroke in young adults. Stroke. 2014;**45**(9):2670–76.

31. **Rutten-Jacobs LC, Arntz RM, Maaijwee NA, Schoonderwaldt HC, Dorresteijn LD, van Dijk EJ**, et al. Cardiovascular disease is the main cause of long-term excess mortality after ischemic stroke in young adults. Hypertension. 2015;**65**(3):670–75.

32. **Fromm A, Thomassen L, Naess H, Meijer R, Eide GE, Krakenes J**, et al. The Norwegian Stroke in the Young Study (NOR-SYS): rationale and design. BMC Neurol. 2013;**13**:89.

Chapter 10

Echocardiography

Sahrai Saeed and Eva Gerdts

Transthoracic echocardiography, transoesophageal echocardiography, or both

Echocardiography plays an essential role in the diagnosis of cardiac as well as aortic sources of embolism in ischaemic stroke and transient ischaemic attack patients (1). Criteria for the appropriate use of transthoracic echocardiography (TTE) and transoesophageal echocardiography (TOE) in the evaluation of cardiac sources of emboli are presented in the recent American Society of Echocardiography guidelines (2). However, the selection of echocardiographic methods and modalities should be based on individual evaluation of the ischaemic stroke patient and pretest probability of identifying a cardiac source of embolism. Generally, TTE is the method of choice for the assessment of structural heart changes, systolic and diastolic function, and detection of thrombus in the left ventricle (LV), while TOE is more useful when the region of interest is in the basis of heart (left atrium (LA), LA appendage (LAA), and atrial septum), and in patients with prosthetic heart valves, or when acoustic windows for TTE are limited. TOE is also mandatory in the evaluation of a patient for possible infective endocarditis. In such cases, the sensitivity of TOE for detection of vegetations is 87–100% compared to 30–63% by TTE (3). However, assessment of consequences of the vegetation for valve function and myocardial load will require combined TTE and TOE in most cases. Since TTE and TOE represent complementary echocardiographic methods, a good rule of thumb is to consider TTE as the primary echocardiographic method in ischaemic stroke patients and TOE as a supplement in selected cases.

Heart rhythm during echocardiography

During performance of echocardiography, three electrocardiographic (ECG) leads are placed on the patient and the heart rhythm is continuously displayed on the screen of the echocardiogram. However, this does not replace a standard 12-lead ECG recorded at a paper speed of 50 mm/s and with 1 mV/cm, which should be recorded in the supine position in all ischaemic stroke patients. The 12-lead ECG is an easy and inexpensive method for the detection of atrial fibrillation (AF), LA enlargement, cardiac overload in the form of left ventricular hypertrophy (LVH), prior myocardial infarction (Q-wave and/or persistent ST-segment elevation), actual myocardial ischaemia (ST segment depression, T-wave inversion), and conduction abnormalities, all of which may be associated with ischaemic stroke (4). AF, characterized by an irregular R–R interval and the absence of P waves on ECG, is associated with a fivefold increased risk of developing ischaemic stroke (4). Heart rhythm monitoring should be conducted routinely after an acute cerebrovascular event to screen for serious cardiac arrhythmias. For the detection of paroxysmal AF in ischaemic stroke patients, Holter monitoring is superior to the routine 12-lead ECG (5). A review found that new AF was detected by Holter ECG in approximately 5% of patients with recent ischaemic stroke or transient ischaemic attack, irrespective of findings on 12-lead ECG and clinical examination (6). In the Norwegian Stroke in the Young Study (NOR-SYS), the overall prevalence of AF defined by history of AF or detected by either resting 12-lead ECG at admission or 24-hour Holter monitoring was 5.6% (7). Holter monitoring beyond 24 hours may further improve the detection rates of AF (8). Other important indicators of cardiac abnormalities on ECG are findings indicating LA enlargement or LVH. LA enlargement can be detected using the duration of the P wave in any lead greater than 0.11 s, from the shape and axis of the P wave, area of negative P terminal forces in lead V1 greater than 0.04 s/mm, and positive P terminal force in lead aVL greater than 0.5 mm (9). LVH may be detected by ECG from a number of well-validated criteria. In particular, the Cornell voltage-duration product [(RaVL + SV3)× QRS duration in males; (RaVL + SV3 + 6 mm)× QRS duration in females] greater than 2440 mm × ms or the Sokolow–Lyon voltage criterion [SV1 + (RV5 or RV6)] greater than 38 mm are often used (10, 11).

AF and other arrhythmias present during echocardiography require that more cardiac cycles are stored for analysis, since measurements have to be averaged over several heart cycles to give accurate results, and analyses may not be performed on heart cycles involving supra- or ventricular ectopic beats. Still, validation of cardiac structure and function is possible in most patients with arrhythmias.

Standardized transthoracic echocardiography

A standardized two-dimensional (2D) TTE should be performed, including images from the parasternal, apical, and subcostal acoustic windows. The echocardiographic parameters, which should be included in a standard TTE, in particular in young stroke patients, are listed in Box 10.1.

B-mode images are used for assessment of cardiac structure and LV systolic function. From parasternal images, interventricular septum and posterior wall thickness, and LV internal diameter at end-diastole and end-systole may

---

Box 10.1 Echocardiographic parameters to be included in a standard TTE of ischaemic stroke patients

- Heart rhythm
- Aortic valve annulus diameter
- Aortic sinuses diameter
- Proximal ascending aorta diameter
- LA anterior–posterior diameter at end-systole
- LA volume indexed for body surface area
- LV internal diameter at end-diastole and end-systole
- Interventricular septum thickness at end-diastole and end-systole
- Posterior wall thickness at end-diastole and end-systole
- LV geometric pattern[*]
- LV systolic function (global and regional)
- LV ejection fraction
- LV diastolic function and filling pressure
- RV free wall thickness at end-diastole
- RV internal diameter at end-diastole
- RV systolic function
- Right atrium size
- Pulmonary artery systolic pressure
- Assessment of heart valves function
- Assessment of aortic valve anatomy and the extent of calcification
- Mitral annular calcification
- Pericardial effusion
- Intracardiac tumour, mass, thrombus, vegetation, excrescences.

[*] Based on left ventricular indexed mass and relative wall thickness.
LA, left atrium; LV, left ventricle; RV, right ventricle.

be measured and used for calculation of LV geometry, LV systolic function, and wall stress. From parasternal images, the anterior–posterior dimension of the aortic root may be measured at several levels (aortic valve annulus, aortic sinuses, sinotubular junction, and proximal ascending aorta). In addition, the anterior–posterior dimension of the LA in end systole may be measured in the parasternal long-axis projection. The measurement of LA dimensions from 2D anterior–posterior diameter, may lead to underestimation of the true LA size and volume when the LA is enlarged due to either AF, valvular heart disease, abnormal LV function, or any cause of increased LV filling pressure. In these circumstances, an asymmetric enlargement of LA will not be captured by a single plane measurement. LA enlargement is a cardiovascular risk marker, in particular for AF and stroke, and an index of the chronicity of diastolic dysfunction (12, 13). Therefore, LA end-diastolic and end-systolic volume calculated by the biplane Simpson's technique is the preferred technique. The apical four-chamber and two- or three-chamber images may also be used for a more accurate calculation of LV ejection fraction (LVEF) by the modified Simpson's biplane method.

The assessment of LV diastolic function and filling pressures should be an integral part of TTE. Diastolic function is assessed by measuring LV mitral inflow pattern in diastole using pulsed Doppler modality, by which typically the peak early (E) and late (A, atrial contribution) diastolic velocities and their ratio (E/A ratio) are recorded. Mitral inflow pattern measured by pulsed Doppler can be combined with the measurements of the early diastolic mitral annulus velocity by tissue Doppler (e′) to have an estimation of LV filling pressure (E/e′ ratio) (13, 14). The severity of LV diastolic dysfunction may be graded by combining these measures of LV mitral filling and diastolic mitral annulus velocity (13). The right atrium (RA), tricuspid valve, and right ventricle can be evaluated in apical four-chamber view and the pulmonary valve in parasternal short-axis view (14).

For assessment of heart valve function, pulsed wave and continuous wave Doppler may be used. Typically, continuous wave Doppler is used for measuring the maximal blood velocity through a stenotic or regurgitant valve, while pulsed wave Doppler is used to measure flow at a specific level or site. For regurgitant valve disease, colour Doppler is also used for semi-quantitative assessment of the severity of the regurgitation. In a standardized TTE examination, the functions of all four heart valves are routinely reported.

From the subcostal windows, the atrial septum may be visualized in most subjects by TTE. Colour Doppler mode in this position may diagnose an atrial septal defect, but detailed evaluation of the atrial septum and any patent foramen ovale (PFO) may be difficult by TTE alone. From the suprasternal acoustic window, the aortic arch and its branches may be visualized.

Transthoracic echocardiography in conditions associated with ischaemic stroke

Echocardiography can reveal a number of conditions that may predispose to cerebral embolism or be associated with ischaemic stroke. These conditions may be classified as major, minor, or uncertain risk sources of embolism (Table 10.1).

Left ventricular hypertrophy

Hypertension is a major risk factor for cardiovascular disease and stroke (15). One in three adults in the United States has hypertension (15). Similarly, in the Norwegian population, the prevalence of hypertension is estimated to be 30%, and more common among men than women in the population below 50 years of age. In the NOR-SYS population in western Norway, hypertension was found in 44% of patients (16). LVH may be found in 20–50% of subjects with mild uncomplicated hypertension. The prevalence of LVH increases with the severity of hypertension, and with the co-presence of other cardiovascular risk factors such as obesity, diabetes, and renal dysfunction. Moreover, LVH is associated with a threefold increased risk for subsequent clinical cardiovascular events including stroke and a five- to ninefold increased risk for sudden

Table 10.1 Potential cardioembolic sources of ischaemic stroke

Major risk factors	Minor or uncertain risk factors
Atrial fibrillation	Mitral valve prolapse
Recent myocardial infarction	Mitral annular calcification
Previous myocardial infarction	Calcified aortic stenosis
Left ventricular thrombus	Atrial septal aneurysm
Left atrial cavity thrombus	Patent foramen ovale
Left atrial appendage thrombus	Left ventricular aneurysm
Dilated cardiomyopathy (left ventricular ejection fraction <35%)	Spontaneous contrast on the echocardiogram
	Aortic aneurysm
Rheumatic valve disease	False tendon in the left ventricle
Intracardiac tumours	Moderate to severe left atrium enlargement
Valvular vegetation or mass	Left ventricular hypertrophy
Prosthetic valve disease	Concentric left ventricular geometry
Marantic or infective endocarditis	
Atheroma of the ascending aorta and aortic arch	

cardiac death. Echocardiographic signs of hypertensive heart disease, such as concentric remodelling and hypertrophy (concentric and eccentric), are markers of subclinical cardiovascular disease and strong predictors of higher risk for stroke in hypertensive patients (17, 18). Thus, when measuring the LV dimension and thickness, careful attention should be paid to the different LV geometric patterns as these patterns may add prognostic information in hypertensive patients beyond the assessment of LV mass alone (17) (Fig. 10.1).

Fabry disease is a rare, progressive, X-linked lysosomal storage disease due to deficient α-galactosidase A activity, resulting in accumulation of glycosphingolipids in internal organs including the heart (19). The disease is characterized by progressive clinical manifestations of early death from renal failure, stroke, and cardiac disease (20). Fabry disease is present in 4–5% of men with unexplained LVH or cryptogenic stroke. In Fabry cardiomyopathy, TTE typically demonstrates severe LVH, decreased myocardial function, LA enlargement, and valvular abnormalities (Fig. 10.2).

Echocardiographic findings in atrial fibrillation

TTE also plays a crucial role in the estimation of embolic risk, identification of aetiology and complications of AF, and in the indication for anticoagulant therapy based on CHA_2DS_2-VASc score. In this score, two components (congestive heart failure and hypertension-related structural changes in the LV geometry)

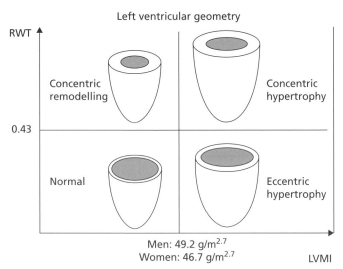

Men: 49.2 g/m^2.7
Women: 46.7 g/m^2.7

Fig. 10.1 Patterns of left ventricular (LV) geometry in women and men defined by partition values for LV mass indexed (LVMI) for height in the power of 2.7 and relative wall thickness (RWT).

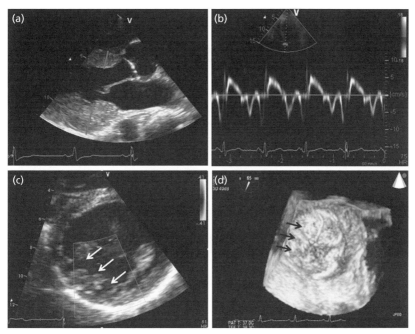

Fig. 10.2 Transthoracic echocardiography images. Typical findings in Fabry cardiomyopathy (a, b). Apical long-axis view illustrating a severe left ventricular hypertrophy (a). Tissue Doppler recording of the septal annular mitral velocities showing a significant decrease in early diastolic and systolic annular velocity (b). Parasternal short-axis view with colour Doppler in left ventricle non-compaction shows blood flow (arrows) in the interventricular recesses (c). Closure of patent foramen ovale with a Gore® Septal Occluder device (d, black arrows).

can be evaluated by TTE. In addition, typical abnormalities seen on TTE in AF patients are LA enlargement, LA thrombus, and spontaneous echo contrast (Fig. 10.3a) (8).

LA dilatation reflects the chronicity of AF and subsequent adverse remodelling. However, it is still a subject of debate whether LA dilatation is the cause or result of AF (21).

Acute ischaemic heart disease

Patients with acute myocardial infarction, in particular anterior wall infarction and LV dysfunction, are at particular risk of LV thrombus formation and embolization to the cerebral circulation (22). Global and regional wall motion abnormalities due to myocardial injury result in blood stasis and give rise to LV thrombus formation (2). Fresh, protruding, and mobile LV thrombi may be easily diagnosed with TTE and are particularly prone to embolize, while older

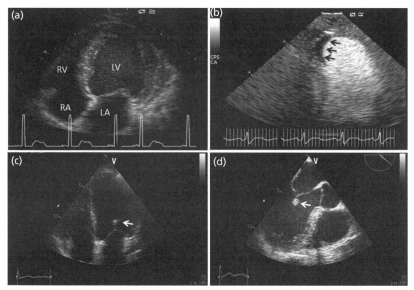

Fig. 10.3 Transthoracic echocardiographic images (a–c). (a) Apical four-chamber view demonstrates spontaneous contrast in LV; (b) contrast-enhanced image of apical four-chamber view shows an old thrombus in the LV apex (arrows); (c) apical four-chamber view shows papillary fibroelastoma attached to tip of anterior mitral leaflet (arrow); (d) transoesophageal echocardiography, long-axis image shows papillary fibroelastoma attached to tip of anterior mitral leaflet (arrow).

mural thrombi in the LV apex are more stable and may require use of ultra-sound contrast to be diagnosed (Fig. 10.3b) (1).

Non-ischaemic cardiomyopathies

Non-ischaemic LV dilation and dysfunction is also associated with an increased risk of LV thrombus and stroke (23). Typical findings are enlarged LV cavity, hypokinetic myocardium, reduced LVEF, and spontaneous contrast. Several rare cardiomyopathies such as LV non-compaction and others are associated with an increased risk of systemic thromboembolism. Non-compaction car-diomyopathy is caused by incomplete endomyocardial development of the LV in early fetal life, and the echocardiographic changes are typically seen in the apex, distal, and middle segments of the inferior and lateral walls (24). In non-compaction cardiomyopathy, these myocardial segments have a two-lay-ered contour with a normally organized epicardial layer, and an endocardial layer consisting of a prominent trabecular meshwork with deep intertrabecular recesses, where thrombus formation may occur (Fig. 10.2c) (24). Additional imaging with magnetic resonance imaging is recommended in non-compac-tion cardiomyopathy.

Valvular heart disease

TTE may be used for quantification and assessment of aetiology and functional consequences of valve calcification, in particular in mitral and aortic valves. Current joint European and American guidelines recommend TTE for the evaluation and monitoring of valvular heart disease (25, 26). Aortic valve calcification is increasingly recognized as a source of systemic embolism due to microthrombi or calcified emboli (27). In young subjects, aortic stenosis is mainly due to bicuspid aortic valve, found in 1 in 2000 newborns, which may lead to development of aortic stenosis, aortic regurgitation, or a combination of these. In aortic stenosis, peak jet velocity, mean aortic gradient, and efficient aortic valve opening area are reported in a standard TTE (25, 28).

Rheumatic fever is the most common cause of mitral stenosis in young immigrants from developing countries. Mitral stenosis is associated with a high risk of systemic embolization and stroke, and the risk further increases with age and in the presence of AF (26). In mitral stenosis, the doming appearance of the anterior mitral leaflet, restricted leaflet tips due to commissural fusion, and scarring are typically found by TTE. In addition, the measurement of pressure half-time for the calculation of mitral valve area, pulmonary artery pressure, and associated mitral or aortic regurgitation should be thoroughly reported. In patients with mitral stenosis and LA thrombi, long-term anticoagulant therapy has been shown to result in the resolution of LA thrombi (29).

Ischaemic stroke in patients with prosthetic valves typically requires combined TTE and TOE. Mitral annular calcification has been associated with an increased risk of ischaemic stroke in general populations as well as treated hypertensive patients with LVH, and is an independent predictor of incident ischaemic stroke (30).

Furthermore, in young patients, antiphospholipid syndrome is associated with a higher prevalence of valvular heart disease as well as an increased risk of cerebrovascular events (31). Patients with combined Libman–Sacks endocarditis and antiphospholipid syndrome are particularly exposed to a higher risk of thromboembolic events (32). Anticoagulation therapy should be considered as a key component of primary prophylactic treatment for these patients. TTE and TOE may reveal mitral valve leaflet thickening and vegetations consistent with Libman–Sacks endocarditis as well as mitral valve prolapse, which is commonly seen in adults.

Arterial stiffness

Arterial stiffness increases with age and higher systolic blood pressure, and is often elevated in ischaemic stroke patients. Based upon a two-element Windkessel model, arterial stiffness may be assessed by echocardiography as the ratio between pulse pressure and LV stroke volume (33). A more accurate measure of aortic stiffness can be made by carotid–femoral pulse wave velocity (PWV), which is considered the gold standard method (34, 35). In a Danish general population study, each one standard deviation increment in aortic stiffness (3.4 m/s) increased the cardiovascular disease risk by 16% to 20% (36). Aortic stiffness has also demonstrated an added predictive value for cardiovascular events, which goes beyond the cardiovascular risk stratification achieved by use of well-accepted risk scores (37–39). Aortic stiffness assessed by carotid–femoral PWV is an independent predictor of fatal stroke in patients with essential hypertension (40). High-for-age PWV is also common among younger ischaemic stroke patients, and is particularly associated with clustering of cardiovascular risk factors (41). Increased aortic stiffness can influence ischaemic stroke risk through several mechanisms. As the aorta becomes stiffer, systolic blood pressure rises and diastolic blood pressure decreases, leading to increased pulse pressure and increased cardiac load and LVH (42). The association between higher pulse pressure and the risk of ischaemic stroke has been described (43, 44). Higher pulse pressure may induce arterial remodelling, increased wall thickening, as well as plaque formation in both intra- and extracranial arteries (45). On the other hand, stiffer arteries may contribute to mechanical rupture and ulceration of atherosclerotic plaques (46, 47). Another proposed mechanism for the association of arterial stiffness with stroke, in particular small vessel disease in the brain, is the impedance matching between central and peripheral arteries which occurs in presence of aortic stiffness (48).

Standardized transoesophageal echocardiography

Currently, TOE is considered the standard modality for the identification of the cardiac or aortic source of embolism in particular when TTE, ECG, and Holter recording have not identified the ischaemic stroke aetiology (49). However, TOE is a semi-invasive test, and the individual indication should be decided after collaboration between the cardiologist and the attending neurologist. In a study of ischaemic stroke patients with an unknown aetiology, who all underwent both TTE and TOE, a potential embolic source was detected in 55% of patients, among them 17% were identified on both TTE and TOE, and 39% only on TOE (49). The diagnostic yield of TOE is highest in young ischaemic stroke patients without clinical evidence of cardiovascular disease (50).

A standardized TOE protocol includes adequate visualization of all cardiac chambers, the LAA, atrial septum, all four valves, all four pulmonary veins, and the ascending and descending aorta. In general, TOE is highly effective in diagnosing atrial septal abnormalities, left-sided cardiac valve disease, intrapulmonary shunt (delayed shunts), and in evaluating size, morphology, and function of the LA or LAA (Fig. 10.4a, b), which may all be associated with an increased risk of ischaemic stroke (51–53).

Transoesophageal echocardiography in conditions associated with ischaemic stroke

Atria, left atrial appendage, and atrial septum abnormalities

The LAA represents one of the most common sites of thrombus formation in patients with AF (54). A LAA thrombus is diagnosed by TOE as the presence of an echo-dense mass in the LAA (Fig. 10.4b). A LAA thrombus should be differentiated from the pectinate muscles of the LAA and the ligament of Marshall which separates the LAA from the left upper pulmonary vein (Fig. 10.4b). In a study of 932 patients with AF who were scheduled to undergo catheter ablation, cardiac computer tomography and magnetic resonance imaging of the

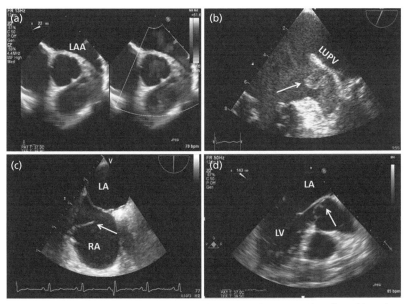

Fig. 10.4 Transoesophageal echocardiography images showing colour flow (a) and thrombus in LAA (b) in mid-oesophageal window, atrial septum and Eustachian valve (c, arrow), and Lambl's excrescence: a thin, linear, echo-dense, and free mobile structure on the non-coronary cusp of aortic valve in aortic long-axis view (d, arrow). LA, left atrium; LAA, left atrial appendage; LV, left ventricle; LUPV, left upper pulmonary vein; RA, right atrium.

LAA identified four different morphologies of the LAA morphology: 'cactus', 'chicken wing', 'windsock', and 'cauliflower' (55). Patients with 'chicken wing' LAA morphology were less likely to have an embolic event.

Flow within the LAA should be assessed with colour Doppler and by pulsed wave Doppler placing the sample volume approximately 1 cm into the LAA. LAA slow-flow velocity is defined as a peak velocity of 20–30 cm/s or less. Lower LAA blood velocity is associated with the presence of spontaneous contrast and LAA thrombus, and with a history of stroke (53). In TOE, the LAA is seen best in the mid-oesophageal window. However, the complex shape, multilobed structure, and unusual orientation of the LAA in some patients may make it difficult to visualize it in conventional views. Similarly, a reverberation artefact originating from the ridge at the orifice of the left upper pulmonary vein (Coumadin ridge) may create the impression of a pseudo-mass within the LAA (56).

The atrial septum should be carefully assessed in several views for the presence of abnormalities such as PFO, characterized by a channel in the atrial septum (Fig. 10.5a–c), atrial septum defect, and atrial septum aneurysm (Fig. 10.5d).

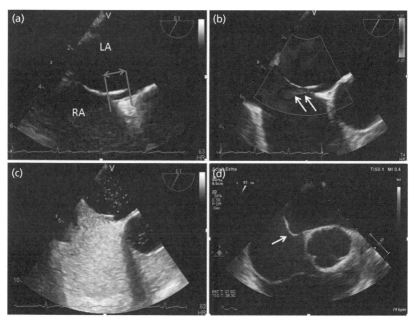

Fig. 10.5 Transoesophageal echocardiography images from basal short-axis windows show septal overlap and the length of PFO tunnel (a, arrow), colour Doppler flow across the PFO (b, arrow), passage of agitated saline bubbles to the LA across the PFO (c), and atrial septum aneurysm (d, arrow). LA, left atrium; PFO, patent foramen ovale; RA, right atrium.

On TOE, a PFO is assessed by 2D (Fig. 10.5a) or colour Doppler (Fig. 10.5b). If the atrial shunt could not be demonstrated by colour Doppler, intravenous injection of agitated saline contrast should be performed at baseline and after the Valsalva manoeuvre (Fig. 10.5c) (1). Prior to the TOE procedure, the patients should be given sufficient instructions to perform an optimal Valsalva manoeuvre. A Valsalva manoeuvre should be initiated when the contrast has arrived in the right atrium. If the agitated saline contrast is seen in the LA within three cardiac cycles, a PFO is assumed present. If the agitated saline contrast is seen in the LA more than five cardiac cycles after complete opacification of the RA, pulmonary arteriovenous malformations must be suspected (1). A loop of 15–20 cardiac cycles should be recorded for bubble studies. A moderate–severe shunt secondary to a PFO is defined as passage of a cloud of bubbles, or intense opacification of the LA (1, 2).

In the 15–45° basal TOE short-axis view, also called the procedural view, cross-sections of the aorta, atrial septum, LA, and RA can be demonstrated. In addition, a bi-caval 80–110° view may be needed for a detailed assessment of a PFO, in particular for the measurement of the diameter and oblique length of the PFO tunnel, also called septal overlap (Fig. 10.5a). A PFO provides a potential conduit for paradoxical embolism from the venous circulation or the right heart. The prevalence of PFO in the general population is estimated to 26% (57), and as high as 56% in patients with a cryptogenic stroke (58). However, the presence of a PFO in a population-based study did not increase the risk of a cryptogenic stroke or transient ischaemic attack compared with the risk among age-matched control subjects (57).

Atrial septum aneurysms are considered present if the protrusion during mobility is 10 mm or greater into the atrium (1). In addition, the extent, direction of bulging, severity (mild, moderate, and severe), and spontaneous oscillation should be evaluated properly (1). By the Olivares classification, atrial septum aneurysm is classified according to which atrium the aneurysm bulges into: type 1R if the bulging is only in the RA; type 2L if the bulging is only in the LA; type 3RL if the extent of bulging is greater towards the RA and the lesser towards the LA; type 4LR if the extent of bulging is greater towards the LA and lesser towards the RA; and type 5 if the atrial septal aneurysm movement is bidirectional (59).

The Eustachian valve should be looked for in the RA, although the clinical significance of this structure is not fully understood. A prominent Eustachian valve is defined as having a valve thickness of at least 1 mm with at least 10 mm protrusion within the RA as measured from the border of inferior vena cava (Fig. 10.4c) (60).

Spontaneous contrast, defined as a dynamic and slowly swirled smoke-like signal caused by aggregation of red blood cells secondary to slow flow, may be seen in any cardiac chamber and is associated with an increased risk of thromboembolic events (51, 61). The severity of the spontaneous contrast is classified from none to mild (minimal echogenicity only with optimal gain settings), moderate (a dense swirling pattern), or severe (intense echogenicity and very slow swirling patterns in the LA or LAA) (62).

Infective endocarditis

TOE is highly sensitive in the diagnosis of infective endocarditis in both native and prosthetic heart valves, perivalvular complications to endocarditis such as paravalvular blood flow (leakage) or abscess, as well as pacemaker lead infection (2). The modified Duke criteria are widely used for the diagnosis of infective endocarditis (63). Major echocardiographic criteria for the diagnosis of infective endocarditis are (a) oscillating intracardiac mass on valve or supporting structures, in the path of regurgitant jets, or on implanted material in the absence of an alternative anatomic explanation; (b) abscess; (c) new partial dehiscence of prosthetic valve; and (d) new valvular regurgitation (63).

Intracardiac tumours

The prevalence of primary cardiac tumours is 0.05%. Although most primary cardiac tumours are histologically benign, they may have fulminant clinical course due to risk for embolism (2). After myxoma and lipoma, papillary fibroelastoma is the third most common type of primary cardiac tumours on heart valves. Fibroelastoma is primarily located on the aortic valve, and rarely on the mitral valve (Fig. 10.3c, d). Usually, papillary fibroelastoma does not cause valvular dysfunction, and symptoms are generally caused by either mechanical effects of the tumour mass or due to systemic embolization (64, 65). Contrast-enhanced images after the intravenous administration of ultrasound contrast agent may help to differentiate a thrombus from an intracardiac tumour. A thrombus is avascular and does not have contrast uptake, while tumours are either poorly (myxoma) or highly vascularized (malignant tumours), and have contrast uptake (66). Lambl's excrescence is a thin, linear, echo-dense, and free mobile structure which is believed to be caused by valvular tear and wear and fibrin deposition (Fig. 10.4d) (67). Lambl's excrescence should not be confused with fibroelastoma or infective endocarditis. Therefore, cardiologists and cardiac sonographers should pay careful attention to the precise echocardiographic features and differentiation of vegetations, paravalvular complications, and calcified debris and excrescence.

Aortic arch and thoracic aorta

TOE may visualize dilatation, aneurysm, dissections, intramural haematoma and complex aortic atheroma, a marker of atherosclerosis and a direct substrate for thromboembolism in the thoracic aorta. This is an essential part of TOE in ischaemic stroke. However, computed tomography may offer an even more detailed examination. Aortic atherosclerosis is graded as 1: intimal thickening less than 4 mm; 2: a diffuse intimal thickening of 4 mm or greater; 3: atheromas less than 5 mm; 4: atheromas greater than 5 mm; and 5: any mobile atheroma. Grade 2 or higher is considered a causal factor in ischaemic stroke (1). The most important TOE views of the thoracic aorta are middle or lower oesophageal 0° for the short axis and 90° for the long axis, and 0° upper oesophageal view to image the aortic arch. The ascending aorta, aortic root, and aortic valve can be visualized from the long-axis 120–150° and short-axis 30–60° views (2).

Aortic dissection, intramural haematoma (in the absence of a dissection, intimal flap, and double lumen), and penetrating atherosclerotic ulcer are clinical emergencies. Alongside with computed tomography angiography, TOE is the most commonly used imaging modality for aortic dissections with a sensitivity of 90–100% and specificity of 94% (68). A careful search should also be performed for complications of aortic dissection such as acute aortic regurgitation, pericardial effusion, and LV dysfunction.

Three-dimensional echocardiography

Three-dimensional (3D) and multiplane imaging are advanced echocardiographic imaging for the assessment of cardiac structure and function. Although standard 2D imaging is still largely used in cardiac investigations, 3D and multiplane imaging can better visualize areas often missed or overlooked by 2D. Furthermore, in experienced hands, LV mass and LVEF are more accurately measured by 3D echocardiography. In some patients, 3D echocardiography may be useful in detection of a LAA thrombus and its differentiation from pectinate muscle, a ridge-like protrusion within the LAA wall (69). This differentiation can sometime be difficult even with conventional 2D TOE (69). Atrial myxoma, its localization and movement in LA, and its attachment to atrial septum may also be better visualized by 3D imaging (2). 3D imaging is also increasingly used in the follow-up of young patients after catheter-based PFO/atrial septal defect closure (Fig. 10.2d).

Speckle tracking echocardiography

Subclinical impairment of the LV systolic function despite normal conventional LVEF has been demonstrated by speckle tracking echocardiography (STE) in a wide range of diseases including LVH (70, 71), hypertension (72), aortic stenosis (70), and Fabry disease (73), all associated with an increased risk of ischaemic stroke. STE imaging is a relatively new and angle-independent strain method, which enables evaluation of global and regional myocardial deformation by tracking movement of speckles in the myocardium through the cardiac cycle. Routine grey-scale digital images of the myocardium contains pattern of bright and dark pixels, termed speckles. In STE, a user-defined region of interest is placed on the myocardial wall and speckles within these regions are tracked from frame to frame.

Conclusion

In conclusion, complete TTE should be routinely performed in all ischaemic stroke and transient ischaemic attack patients to identify cardiac and proximal aortic sources of emboli and as part of a general cardiovascular risk assessment. TOE should be used in selected patients, in particular if LA abnormality, LA appendix thrombus, or infective endocarditis is suspected, and in patients with prosthetic heart valves or limited acoustic windows for TTE.

References

1. **Pepi M, Evangelista A, Nihoyannopoulos P, Flachskampf FA, Athanassopoulos G, Colonna P**, et al. Recommendations for echocardiography use in the diagnosis and management of cardiac sources of embolism: European Association of Echocardiography (EAE) (a registered branch of the ESC). Eur J Echocardiogr. 2010;**11**:461–76.

2. **Saric M, Armour AC, Arnaout MS, Chaudhry FA, Grimm RA, Kronzon I**, et al. Guidelines for the use of echocardiography in the evaluation of a cardiac source of embolism. J Am Soc Echocardiogr. 2016;**29**:1–42.

3. **Jacob S, Tong AT.** Role of echocardiography in the diagnosis and management of infective endocarditis. Curr Opin Cardiol. 2002;**17**:478–85.

4. **Camm AJ, Kirchhof P, Lip GY, Schotten U, Savelieva I, Ernst S**, et al. Guidelines for the management of atrial fibrillation: the Task Force for the Management of Atrial Fibrillation of the European Society of Cardiology (ESC). Eur Heart J. 2010;**31**:2369–429.

5. **Gunalp M, Atalar E, Coskun F, Yilmaz A, Aksoyek S, Aksu NM**, et al. Holter monitoring for 24 hours in patients with thromboembolic stroke and sinus rhythm diagnosed in the emergency department. Adv Ther. 2006;**23**:854–60.

6. **Liao J, Khalid Z, Scallan C, Morillo C, O'Donnell M.** Noninvasive cardiac monitoring for detecting paroxysmal atrial fibrillation or flutter after acute ischemic stroke: a systematic review. Stroke. 2007;**38**:2935–40.

7. **Saeed S, Waje-Andreassen U, Fromm A, Øygarden H, Naess H, Gerdts E.** Prevalence and covariates of masked hypertension in ischemic stroke survivors: the Norwegian Stroke in the Young Study. Blood Press Monit. 2016;**21**:244–50.

8. **Jabaudon D, Sztajzel J, Sievert K, Landis T, Sztajzel R.** Usefulness of ambulatory 7-day ECG monitoring for the detection of atrial fibrillation and flutter after acute stroke and transient ischemic attack. Stroke. 2004;**35**:1647–51.

9. Tsao CW, Josephson ME, Hauser TH, O'Halloran TD, Agarwal A, et al. Accuracy of electrocardiographic criteria for atrial enlargement: validation with cardiovascular magnetic resonance. J Cardiovasc Magn Reson. 2008;**10**:1–7.

10. Okin PM, Roman MJ, Devereux RB, Kligfield P. Electrocardiographic identification of increased left ventricular mass by simple voltage—duration products. J Am Coll Cardiol. 1995;**25**:417–23.

11. Sokolow M, Lyon TP. The ventricular complex in left ventricular hypertrophy as obtained by unipolar precordial and limb leads. Am Heart J. 1949;**37**:16–86.

12. Gerdts E, Wachtell K, Omvik P, Otterstad JE, Oikarinen L, Boman K, et al. Left atrial size and risk of major cardiovascular events during antihypertensive treatment: losartan intervention for endpoint reduction in hypertension trial. Hypertension. 2007;**49**:311–16.

13. Nagueh SF, Smiseth OA, Appleton CP, Byrd BF, Dokainish H, Edvardsen T, et al. Recommendations for the evaluation of left ventricular diastolic function by echocardiography: an update from the American Society of Echocardiography and the European Association of Cardiovascular Imaging. J Am Soc Echocardiogr. 2016;**29**:277–314.

14. Lang RM, Badano LP, Mor-Avi V, Afilalo J, Armstrong A, Ernande L, et al. Recommendations for cardiac chamber quantification by echocardiography in adults: an update from the American Society of Echocardiography and the European Association of cardiovascular imaging. J Am Soc Echocardiogr. 2015;**28**:1–39.

15. Go AS, Mozaffarian D, Roger VL, Benjamin EJ, Berrry DJ, Blaha MJ, et al. On behalf of the American Heart Association Statistics Committee and Stroke Statistics Subcommittee. Heart Disease and Stroke Statistics—2014 Update A Report From the American Heart Association. Circulation. 2014;**129**:399–410.

16. Saeed S, Waje-Andreassen U, Lønnebakken MT, Fromm A, Øygarden H, Naess H, et al. Covariates of non-dipping and elevated night-time blood pressure in ischemic stroke patients: the Norwegian Stroke in the Young Study. Blood Press. 2015;**23**:1–7.

17. Gerdts E, Cramariuc D, de Simone G, Wachtell K, Dahlöf B, Devereux RB. Impact of left ventricular geometry on prognosis in hypertensive patients with left ventricular hypertrophy (the LIFE study). Eur J Echocardiogr. 2008;**9**:809–15.

18. Verdecchia P, Porcellati C, Reboldi G, Gattobigio R, Borgioni C, Pearson TA, et al. Left ventricular hypertrophy as an independent predictor of acute cerebrovascular events in essential hypertension. Circulation. 2001;**104**:2039–44.

19. Linhart A, Elliott PM. The heart in Anderson-Fabry disease and other lysosomal storage disorders. Heart. 2007;**93**:528–35.

20. Mehta A, Ricci R, Widmer U, Dehout F, Garcia de Lorenzo A, Kampmann C, et al. Fabry disease defined: baseline clinical manifestations of 366 patients in the Fabry Outcome Survey. Eur J Clin Invest. 2004;**34**:236–42.

21. Casaclang-Verzosa G, Gersh BJ, Tsang TS. Structural and functional remodeling of the left atrium: clinical and therapeutic implications for atrial fibrillation. J Am Coll Cardiol. 2008;**51**:1–11.

22. Meurin P, Brandao Carreira V, Dumaine R, Shqueir A, Milleron O, Safar B, et al. Incidence, diagnostic methods, and evolution of left ventricular thrombus in patients with anterior myocardial infarction and low left ventricular ejection fraction: a prospective multicenter study. Am Heart J. 2015;**170**:256–62.

23. **Koniaris LS, Goldhaber SZ.** Anticoagulation in dilated cardiomyopathy. J Am Coll Cardiol. 1998;**31**:745–48.

24. **Saeed S, Vegsundvåg J, Lode I.** Noncompaction of the left ventricular myocardium. Tidsskr Nor Laegeforen. 2009;**129**:1104–107.

25. **Vahanian A, Alfieri O, Andreotti F, Antunes MJ, Barón-Esquivias G, Baumgartner H,** et al. Guidelines on the management of valvular heart disease (version 2012): the Joint Task Force on the Management of Valvular Heart Disease of the European Society of Cardiology (ESC) and the European Association for Cardio-Thoracic Surgery (EACTS). Eur Heart J. 2012;**33**:2451–96.

26. **Nishimura RA, Otto CM, Bonow RO, Carabello BA, Erwin JP, 3rd, Guyton RA,** et al. 2014 AHA/ACC guideline for the management of patients with valvular heart disease: a report of the American College of Cardiology/American Heart Association Task Force on Practice Guidelines. Circulation. 2014;**129**:521–643.

27. **Stein P, Sabbath H, Apitha J.** Continuing disease process of calcific aortic stenosis. Am J Cardiol. 1977;**39**:159–63.

28. **Baumgartner H, Hung J, Bermejo J, Chambers JB, Evangelista A, Griffin BP,** et al. Echocardiographic assessment of valve stenosis: American Society of Echocardiography/European Association of Echocardiography recommendations for clinical practice. J Am Soc Echocardiogr. 2009;**22**:1–23.

29. **Silaruks S, Thinkhamrop B, Tantikosum W, Wongvipaporn C, Tatsanavivat P, Klungboonkrong V.** A prognostic model for predicting the disappearance of left atrial thrombi among candidates for percutaneous transvenous mitral commissurotomy. J Am Coll Cardiol. 2002;**39**:886–91.

30. **De Marco M, Gerdts E, Casalnuovo G, Migliore T, Wachtell K, Boman K,** et al. Mitral annular calcification and incident ischemic stroke in treated hypertensive patients: the LIFE study. Am J Hypertens. 2013;**26**:567–73.

31. **Levine JS, Branch DW, Rauch J.** The antiphospholipid syndrome. N Engl J Med. 2002;**346**:752–63.

32. **Lønnebakken MT, Gerdts E.** Libman-Sacks endocarditis and cerebral embolization in antiphospholipid syndrome. Eur J Echocardiogr. 2008;**9**:192–93.

33. **de Simone G, Roman MJ, Koren MJ, Mensah GA, Ganau A, Devereux RB.** Stroke volume/pulse pressure ratio and cardiovascular risk in arterial hypertension. Hypertension. 1999;**33**:800–805.

34. **Laurent S, Cockcroft J, Van Bortel L, Boutouyrie P, Giannattasio C, Hayoz D,** et al. Expert consensus document on arterial stiffness: methodological issues and clinical applications. Eur Heart J. 2006;**27**:2588–605.

35. **Nilsson PM, Khalili P, Franklin SS.** Blood pressure and pulse wave velocity as metrics for evaluating pathologic ageing of the cardiovascular system. Blood Press. 2013;**23**:17–30.

36. **Willum-Hansen T, Staessen JA, Torp-Pedersen C, Rasmussen S, Thijs L, Ibsen H,** et al. Prognostic value of aortic pulse wave velocity as index of arterial stiffness in the general population. Circulation. 2006;**113**:664–70.

37. **Mitchell GF, Hwang SJ, Vasan RS, Larson MG, Pencina MJ, Hamburg NM,** et al. Arterial stiffness and cardiovascular events: the Framingham Heart Study. Circulation. 2010;**121**:505–11.

38. **Muiesan ML, Salvetti M, Paini A, Monteduro C, Rosei CA, Aqqiusti C**, et al. Pulse wave velocity and cardiovascular risk stratification in a general population: the Vobarno study. J Hypertens. 2010;**28**:1935–43.

39. **Sehestedt T, Jeppesen J, Hansen TW, Wachtell K, Ibsen H, Torp-Pedersen C**, et. al. Risk prediction is improved by adding markers of subclinical organ damage to SCORE. Eur Heart J. 2010;**31**:883–91.

40. **Laurent S, Katsahian S, Fassot C, Tropeano AI, Gautier I, Laloux B, Boutouyrie P.** Aortic stiffness is an independent predictor of fatal stroke in essential hypertension. Stroke. 2003;**34**: 1203–206.

41. **Saeed S, Waje-Andreassen U, Lønnebakken MT, Fromm A, Øygarden H, Naess H**, et al. Early vascular aging in young and middle-aged ischemic stroke patients: the Norwegian Stroke in the Young Study. PLoS One. 2014;**9**:e112814.

42. **London GM, Guerin AP.** Influence of arterial pulse and reflected waves on blood pressure and cardiac function. Am Heart J. 1999;**138**:220–24.

43. **Mattace-Raso FU, van der Cammen TJ, van Popele NM, van der Kuip DA, Schalekamp MA, Hofman A**, et al. Blood pressure components and cardiovascular events in older adults: the Rotterdam study. J Am Geriatr Soc. 2004;**52**:1538–42.

44. **Domanski MJ, Davis BR, Pfeffer MA, Kastantin M, Mitchell GF.** Isolated systolic hypertension: prognostic information provided by pulse pressure. Hypertension. 1999;**34**:375–80.

45. **Witteman JC, Grobbee DE, Valkenburg HA, van Hemert AM, Stijnen T, Burger H**, et al. J-shaped relation between change in diastolic blood pressure and progression of aortic atherosclerosis. Lancet. 1994;**343**:504–507.

46. **Laurent S, Boutouyrie P, Asmar R, Gautier I, Laloux B, Guize L**, et al. Aortic stiffness is an independent predictor of all-cause and cardiovascular mortality in hypertensive patients. Hypertension. 2001;**37**:1236–41.

47. **Cheng GC, Loree HM, Kamm RD, Fishbein MC, Lee RT.** Distribution of circumferential stress in ruptured and stable atherosclerotic lesions: a structural analysis with histopathological correlation. Circulation. 1993;**87**:1179–87.

48. **O'Rourke MF, Safar ME.** Relationship between aortic stiffening and microvascular disease in brain and kidney. Cause and logic of therapy. Hypertension. 2005;**46**:200–204.

49. **De Bruijn SF, Agema WR, Lammers GJ, van der Wall EE, Wolterbeek R, Holman ER**, et al. Transesophageal echocardiography is superior to transthoracic echocardiography in management of patients of any age with transient ischemic attack or stroke. Stroke. 2006;**37**:2531–34.

50. **Kizer JR, Devereux RB.** Clinical practice: patent foramen ovale in young adults with unexplained stroke. N Engl J Med. 2005;**353**:2361–72.

51. **Bernhardt P, Schmidt H, Hammerstingl C, Lüderitz B, Omran H.** Patients with atrial fibrillation and dense spontaneous echo contrast at high risk a prospective and serial follow-up over 12 months with transesophageal echocardiography and cerebral magnetic resonance imaging. J Am Coll Cardiol. 2005;**45**:1807–12.

52. **Goldman ME, Pearce LA, Hart RG, Zabalgoitia M, Asinger RW, Safford R**, et al. Pathophysiologic correlates of thromboembolism in nonvalvular atrial fibrillation: I. Reduced flow velocity in the left atrial appendage. J Am Soc Echocardiogr. 1999;**12**:1080–87.

53. Uretsky S, Shah A, Bangalore S, Rosenberg L, Sarji R, Cantales DR, et al. Assessment of left atrial appendage function with transthoracic tissue Doppler echocardiography. Eur J Echocardiogr. 2009;10:363–71.

54. Hart RG, Halperin JL. Atrial fibrillation and stroke: concepts and controversies. Stroke. 2001;32:803–808.

55. Di Biase L, Santangeli P, Anselmino M, Mohanty P, Salvetti I, Gili S, et al. Does the left atrial appendage morphology correlate with the risk of stroke in patients with atrial fibrillation? Results from a multicenter study. J Am Coll Cardiol. 2012;60:531–38.

56. Patti G, Pengo V, Marcucci R, Cirillo P, Renda G, Santilli F, et al. Working Group of Thrombosis of the Italian Society of Cardiology. The left atrial appendage: from embryology to prevention of thromboembolism. Eur Heart J. 2017;38(12):877–87.

57. Meissner I, Khandheria BK, Heit JA, Petty JW, Sheps SG, Schwartz GL, et al. Patent foramen ovale: innocent or guilty? Evidence from a prospective population-based study. J Am Coll Cardiol. 2006;47:440–45.

58. Furlan AJ, Reisman M, Massaro J, Mauri L, Adams H, Albers GW, et al. Closure or medical therapy for cryptogenic stroke with patent foramen ovale. N Engl J Med. 2012;366:991–99.

59. Olivares-Reyes A, Chan S, Lazar EJ, Bandlamudi K, Narla V, Ong K. Atrial septal aneurysm: a new classification in two hundred five adults. J Am Soc Echocardiogr. 1997;10:644–56.

60. Rigatelli G, Dell'Avvocata F, Cardaioli P, Giordan M, Braggion G, Aggio S, et al. Permanent right-to-left shunt is the key factor in managing patent foramen ovale. J Am Coll Cardiol. 2011;58:2257–61.

61. Leung DY, Black IW, Cranney GB, Hopkins AP, Walsh WF. Prognostic implications of left atrial spontaneous echo contrast in nonvalvular atrial fibrillation. J Am Coll Cardiol. 1994;24:755–62.

62. Vincelj J, Sokol I, Jaksić O. Prevalence and clinical significance of left atrial spontaneous echo contrast detected by transesophageal echocardiography. Echocardiography. 2002;19:319–24.

63. Baddour LM, Wilson WR, Bayer AS, Fowler VG Jr, Tleyjeh IM, Rybak MJ, et al. Infective endocarditis in adults: diagnosis, antimicrobial therapy, and management of complications: a scientific statement for healthcare professionals from the American Heart Association. Circulation. 2015;132:1435–86.

64. Mezilis NE, Dardas PS, Tsikaderis DD, Zaraboukas T, Hantas A, Makrygiannakis K, et al. Papillary fibroelastoma of the cardiac valves: a rare cause of embolic stroke. Hellenic J Cardiol. 2005;46:310–13.

65. Liebeskind DS, Buljubasic N, Saver JL. Cardioembolic stroke due to papillary fibroelastoma. J Stroke Cerebrovasc Dis. 2001;10:94–95.

66. Porter TR, Abdelmoneim S, Belcik JT, McCulloch ML, Mulvagh SL, Olson JJ, et al. Guidelines for the cardiac sonographer in the performance of contrast echocardiography: a focused update from the American Society of Echocardiography. J Am Soc Echocardiogr. 2014;27:797–810.

67. Voros S, Nanda NC, Thakur AC, Winokur TS, Samal AK. Lambl's excrescences (valvular strands). Echocardiography. 1999;16:399–414.

68. Moore AG, Eagle KA, Bruckman D, Moon BS, Malouf JF, Fattori R, et al. Choice of computed tomography, transesophageal echocardiography, magnetic resonance

imaging, and aortography in acute aortic dissection: International Registry of Acute Aortic Dissection (IRAD). Am J Cardiol. 2002;**89**:1235–38.

69. **Karakus G, Kodali V, Inamdar V, Nanda NC, Suwanjutah T, Pothineni KR.** Comparative assessment of left atrial appendage by transesophageal and combined two- and three-dimensional transthoracic echocardiography. Echocardiography. 2008;**25**:918–24.

70. **Cramariuc D, Gerdts E, Davidsen ES, Segadal L, Matre K.** Myocardial deformation in aortic valve stenosis: relation to left ventricular geometry. Heart. 2010;**96**:106–12.

71. **Edvardsen T, Helle-Valle T, Smiseth OA.** Systolic dysfunction in heart failure with normal ejection: speckle-tracking ehcocardiography. Prog Cardiovasc Dis. 2006;**49**:207–14.

72. **Rosen BD, Saad MF, Shea S, Nasir K, Edvardsen T, Burke G,** et al. Hypertension and smoking are associated with reduced regional left ventricular function in asymptomatic: individuals the Multi-Ethnic Study of Atherosclerosis. J Am Coll Cardiol. 2006;**47**:1150–58.

73. **Morris DA, Blaschke D, Canaan-Kühl S, Krebs A, Knobloch G, Walter TC,** et al. Global cardiac alterations detected by speckle-tracking echocardiography in Fabry disease: left ventricular, right ventricular, and left atrial dysfunction are common and linked to worse symptomatic status. Int J Cardiovasc Imaging. 2015;**31**:301–13.

Chapter 11

Genetics

Alessandro Pezzini

Genetic contribution to ischaemic stroke

Ischaemic stroke (IS) is a complex and multifactorial disease caused by the combination of vascular risk factors, environment, and genetic factors. A genetic predisposition to IS has been largely documented in animal models (1). By using different experimental approaches such as spontaneously hypertensive stroke-prone rats, and genetic engineering to generate transgenic mice, several genes directly or indirectly implicated in the mechanisms leading to IS have been proposed. Most of them are involved in thrombosis, inflammation, and lipid metabolism (2). A large body of evidence clearly indicates that this genetic contribution is also operant in humans. First, studies conducted in twins and families support the assumption of a genetic contribution to IS, although the extent of this genetic predisposition is uncertain. In twins, concordance rates for the disease were reported to be about 65% greater in monozygotic than in dizygotic twins, but most twin studies have been relatively small (3). In case–control studies, a family history of stroke was shown to increase the risk of IS, which is in line with the data from studies in twins, but a precise estimate is difficult to ascertain. Flossmann et al. (4) summarized the evidence for a genetic contribution to IS across nine cohort studies, 27 case–control studies, and three twin studies and reported that having a positive family history of stroke was associated with an approximately 30–76% increase in stroke risk (odds ratio (OR)=1.3–1.76). In the Framingham Study, a parental history of IS by 65 years of age was associated with a 2.22-fold increase in IS risk in offspring ($P <0.05$) after adjusting for stroke risk factors (5). The biggest limitation lies in the interpretation of the familial aggregation itself because it is not only an indicator for shared genes between family relatives but also shared environments. More recent approaches using population samples and genetic polymorphisms across the entire genome can circumvent this limitation (6, 7). This genotype-based heritability method estimates the similarity among individuals based on their actual genotypes at markers throughout the genome (i.e. genetic relatedness).

Heritability is then defined as the proportion of phenotype variation (e.g. in stroke liability) explained by the genotypes across the chromosome. Two recent studies using this approach estimated the heritability of IS to be 37–38% (estimate statistically different than zero at $P <0.001$), indicating a significant genetic contribution to IS (8, 9). This appears higher for young-onset IS (10).

Second, conventional vascular risk factors for IS, including hypertension, diabetes, and hyperlipidaemia, may be also influenced by genetics, as well as environmental factors. The American Heart Association Council on Epidemiology and Prevention, the Stroke Council, and the Functional Genomics and Translational Biology Interdisciplinary Working Group recently stated that 'Identification of important intermediate phenotypes (i.e. phenotypes that mediate disease as opposed to phenotypes that represent the ultimate manifestation of a disease or endophenotypes) may prove to be more amenable to genetic analysis' (11). Given the complexity of most common forms of IS, the intermediate phenotypes as markers of subclinical disease may be more helpful in identifying genes related to the disease. Studies on these stroke intermediate phenotypes support this view. Carotid intima–media thickness (cIMT) and carotid plaque, as well as cerebral white matter lesions (also known as leucoaraiosis), are among the most frequently investigated endophenotypes for IS. Heritability estimates for cIMT, a surrogate measure for subclinical atherosclerosis, range from about 30% to 60%, while estimates for cerebral white matter lesions, a surrogate marker for cerebral small vessel disease, range from 55% to 70% (12).

Finally, modifiable risk factors account for about 60% of the attributable risk for stroke, leading to the assumption that a significant proportion of stroke risk might be explained by other conditions, including genetic factors.

Genetic influences could act at various levels: by predisposing to conventional risk factors, by modulating the effects of such risk factors on the end organs, or, alternatively, by a direct independent effect on stroke risk, infarct size, and outcome. Similarly, interactions between genes and the environmental factors could occur at various levels. In addition, to make it more complex, genetic predisposition could differ depending on age and stroke subtype. Both twin and family-history studies found a stronger genetic component in younger stroke patients than in older individuals, and stronger in large vessel and small vessel stroke than in cryptogenic stroke or in cardioembolic stroke (12).

Monogenic ischaemic stroke versus polygenic ischaemic stroke

Genetic determinants of IS are traditionally divided into single-gene disorders (mainly Mendelian conditions, characterized by classic autosomal dominant, autosomal recessive, or X-linked patterns of inheritance) and polygenic disorders (where multiple genes act together to result in a certain phenotype). The monogenic diseases following Mendelian inheritance patterns tend to be caused by highly penetrant and rare mutations, whereas more common variants or polymorphisms (presenting with at least 1–5% frequency in the general population) may contribute to the great majority of IS cases which are sporadic and genetically complex. This distinction, however, is over-simplistic, as additional genetic and environmental risk factors often play a modifying role in the final disease phenotype even in Mendelian conditions. This has been conceptualized as a spectrum of the effect of genetic variation.

Single-gene disorders

Although monogenic disorders are an important cause of IS, they comprise less than 1% of all cases. To what extent these specific heritable disorders contribute to the population of patients with cerebral ischaemia at young age is currently unknown. However, indirect data indicate that the frequency of single-gene conditions in this age category is probably higher because they often remain undiagnosed, reflecting the substantial variability in their phenotypic expression. Monogenic disorders are typically associated with stroke in childhood or young adulthood, with certain stroke types and subtypes, with the absence of other stroke risk factors, and with specific phenotypes of the associated diseases (13). In order to recognize Mendelian stroke syndromes it is essential to perform a systematic family inquiry and to search for neurological and non-neurological signs and symptoms in index cases and relatives. Family history also may be negative because the disease can be caused by new mutations. Within recent years, considerable progress has been made in defining the underlying genetic basis of many Mendelian and mitochondrial diseases which can cause IS and most of the major genes have been mapped. This has provided new insights into the mechanisms underlying these disorders and the more common sporadic stroke. At present, there is no uniform classification for Mendelian stroke syndromes. Criteria that may be useful include underlying mechanisms, mode of inheritance, and the presence or absence of associated symptoms. Table 11.1 lists the single-gene disorders which more frequently cause IS in young adults and summarizes their molecular defects and clinical features.

The following paragraphs focus on some of the representative forms with different patterns of Mendelian inheritance and report on the molecular mechanisms underlying the pathogenesis of these paradigmatic diseases. The reader is referred to websites such as OMIM (14), the Genetic Testing Registry (15), and Orphanet (16) for specific details of these uncommon diseases.

Table 11.1 Single-gene disorders causing ischaemic stroke

Syndrome	Acronym	Chromosome	Gene region	Clinical features
Cerebral autosomal dominant subcortical infarcts and leucoencephalopathy	CADASIL	19p13.2–p13.1	NOTCH3	Migraine, cognitive problems, depression, seizures, stroke
Cerebral autosomal recessive arteriopathy with subcortical infarcts and leucoencephalopathy	CARASIL	10q26.3	HTRA1	Spasticity, stroke, cognitive problems, scalp hair loss, back pain
Fabry disease		X	GLA	Episodes of pain in hands and feet, angiokeratomas, corneal opacity, renal affection, heart affection, stroke
Sickle cell disease		11p15.5	HBB	Anaemia, pain episodes, infections, affection of lungs including pulmonary hypertension, kidneys, spleen, and brain including stroke
Hereditary endotheliopathy with retinopathy, nephropathy and stroke	HERNS	3p21.31	TREX1	Visual loss, cognitive problems, stroke-like episodes, renal dysfunction
Marfan syndrome		15q21.1	FBN1	Lens dislocation, cataract, myopia, aortic aneurysm, aortic dissection, cerebral aneurysms, cerebral haemorrhage, arthritis, tall habitus, pectus excavatum, dural ectasia
Ehlers–Danlos syndrome type IV		2q31	COL3A1	Joint hypermobility, cerebral aneurysm, arterial dissection, short stature, thin skin that easily bruises, intestinal and uterine fragility, joint subluxation and pain
Pseudoxanthoma elasticum		16p13.1	ABCC6	Papules in flexor areas of skin, visual loss, hypertension, arterial dissection

Table 11.1 Continued

Syndrome	Acronym	Chromosome	Gene region	Clinical features
Homocystinuria		21q22.3, 1p36.3, and other	*CBS, MTHFR,* and other	Varies, e.g. cognitive problems, myopia, lens dislocation, osteoporosis, thromboembolic events
Neurofibromatosis type 1 (von Recklinghausen's disease)		17q11.2	*NF1*	Café au lait skin spots, neurofibromas, optic glioma, cerebral ischaemia, intracranial aneurysm
von Hippel–Lindau syndrome		3p25.3	*VHL*	Haemangioblastoma in brain, spinal cord, retina. Intracerebral haemorrhage, phaeochromocytoma, hearing loss
COL4A1-related brain small vessel disease		13q34	*COL4A1*	Haemorrhagic stroke, white matter changes, seizures, migraine
Hereditary haemorrhagic telangiectasia (Osler–Weber–Rendu disease)		Several	Several	Telangiectasia, arteriovenous malformations in lungs, brain, liver, intestines. Intracerebral haemorrhage. Ischaemic stroke
Mitochondrial encephalopathy lactic acidosis and stroke-like episodes	MELAS	Mitochondrial DNA	Several	Muscle weakness, headache episodes, seizures, stroke-like episodes

Cerebral autosomal dominant arteriopathy with subcortical infarcts and leucoencephalopathy (CADASIL)

CADASIL is an autosomal dominant small vessel disease caused by mutations in the *NOTCH3* gene (17, 18). Although the disorder is one of the most common inherited neurological conditions, the frequency is probably underestimated and the prevalence of *NOTCH3* gene mutations has been estimated from 1.98 to more than 4 per 100,000 adults (17, 19). The onset of symptoms occurs around the age of 20–30 years, with subsequent cerebral vascular accidents, mainly recurrent subcortical IS, progressive cognitive impairment, psychiatric dysfunction, depressive syndrome and mood disturbances, and migraine most commonly with aura (17, 20, 21). *NOTCH3*, mapped on chromosome 19p13.1, consists of 33 exons encoding a transmembrane receptor of 2321 amino acids involved in signal transduction and cell differentiation (18). The extracellular domain contains 34 EGF-like repeats (with six cysteine residues in each). NOTCH3 is mainly expressed in vascular smooth muscle cells and pericytes and plays an important role in the control of different processes of vascular development and vascular smooth muscle cell differentiation. Pathogenic mutations, consisting of loss or gain of cysteine residues of extracellular domains lead to the deposition of NOTCH3 fragments in the vascular basal membrane (22, 23).

Cerebral autosomal recessive arteriopathy with subcortical infarcts and leucoencephalopathy (CARASIL)

CARASIL is a non-hypertensive cerebral small vessel arteriopathy transmitted in an autosomal recessive manner first identified in the Japanese population under the name of Maeda syndrome (24). The disease is characterized by a mean age of onset of 32 years, and common clinical features are atherosclerotic leucoencephalopathy, alopecia, lumbago, spondylosis deformans, and psychiatric disorders. A study conducted by Hara et al. on five families with CARASIL indicated an association of this disease with mutations affecting *HTRA1* (25). This gene is localized on chromosome 10q and is expressed in the blood vessels, skin, and bone in relationship with the baldness, cerebrovascular, and back symptoms. It encodes a serine protease that represses signalling by TGF-beta family members.

Fabry disease

Fabry disease (FD) is an X-linked recessive lysosomal storage disorder. In males, the classical form of the disease occurs usually during childhood. Manifestations of FD have also been reported in heterozygote females, ranging from asymptomatic or with mild manifestations to rare cases showing severe disease as in affected males (26). Major clinical features of this pathology include renal failure, cardiomyopathy, multiple strokes, and neuropathic pain. This multisystemic involvement derives from mutations affecting the alpha-galactosidase A gene at Xq22 (27). Reported mutations include all types of genetic defects and are distributed over the entire gene. To date, more than 600 mutations have been identified and are listed in the online FD database (http://fabry-database.org/) (28). The enzyme deficiency results in uncleaved glycosphingolipids (particularly globotriaosylceramide, Gb3), which accumulates in lysosomes within the intima and media of blood vessels in different organs and tissues (vascular smooth muscle and endothelial cells, carotid, heart, brain, peripheral nerves, and kidney) leading to cell dysfunction, organ failure, and development of tissue ischaemia and infarction. Although ISs and transient ischaemic attacks are the most prevalent types of overt cerebrovascular events in FD, cases of intracerebral haemorrhages, subarachnoid haemorrhage, microbleeds, cerebral venous thrombosis, and cervical carotid dissection have also been reported (29).

Retrospective studies in small cohorts of FD patients have reported a wide range of stroke incidence (24–48%) (30). An analysis of a large cohort of 2446 patients in the Fabry Registry (https://www.registrynxt.com/) reported that stroke occurs in 6.9% of men and 4.3% of women over 66 months. Of these, 87% of first strokes were found to be ischaemic, with haemorrhagic stroke reported in 13% of cases. The incidence of stroke among patients with FD is markedly higher than that observed in the general US population across all age categories (31). For example, in men aged 35–45 years, the relative risk of stroke is 12.2 times higher in FD patients when compared with healthy subjects. In the Fabry Registry cohort, a majority of FD patients experienced a first stroke between the age of 20 and 50 years, with 22% of patients having a first stroke at less than 30 years of age (10). Data from the Fabry Registry reported that women with FD were more likely to experience a stroke than men with FD although female patients were likely to be older at first stroke (29).

Previous hypotheses about FD prevalence in the cryptogenic (undetermined) young stroke cohort (32) could not be supported by several subsequent studies. Therefore, a regular FD screening tool remains out of reach. Three screening studies did not identify any patients with FD, but others have reported FD in 0.5–3.9% of the stroke population (29). This variation in reported prevalence may be because of differences in the studied stroke populations (age and sex ratios), the stroke types studied, and the diagnosis of FD.

Mitochondrial encephalomyopathy, lactic acidosis and stroke episodes (MELAS)

MELAS is a maternally inherited multisystem disorder caused by mutations affecting mitochondrial DNA (mtDNA). Onset of symptoms is typically during childhood with mitochondrial encephalopathy initially characterized by tonic– clonic seizures, migrainous headaches, anorexia, and vomiting. The heteroplasmy, a variable distribution of mutant and wild-type mtDNA among different tissues, explains the phenotypic diversity of this disorder (3). The multisystemic involvement leads to progressive developmental delay and cognitive decline, sensorineural hearing loss, and short stature, but in some cases monosymptomatic stroke episodes have been described. The stroke-like episodes in MELAS differ from typical ischaemic infarcts involving not only the vascular territories but also the brain parenchyma leading to tissue ischaemia, since the underlying cause is likely an energetic imbalance instead of vascular occlusion. The most frequent mutation of MELAS, reported in approximately 80% of patients with typical clinical findings, is an A to G transition at nucleotide 3243 on the *MT-TL1* mitochondrial gene, which encodes tRNALeu (UUR). Another transition of T to C at nucleotide position 3271 is found in approximately 10% of cases (33). MtDNA mutations can lead to dysfunctional mitochondrial oxidative phosphorylation with impairment of cellular respiratory capacity and ATP synthesis (3). Recently, a systematic mtDNA testing for MELAS was performed in a relatively young phenotype-selected IS subpopulation from the Stroke in Young Fabry Patients (sifap1) registry, which disclosed a considerable number of previously unrecognized m.3243A>G mutations in the *MT-TL1* gene of mitochondrial DNA, although it remains uncertain whether mitochondrial disease was the cause of IS in these cases (34).

Common multifactorial ischaemic stroke

The genetic contribution to common multifactorial stroke seems to be polygenic, with many alleles involved having individual small effect sizes (relative risk <1.5). However, because of their wide distribution, on a population basis the impact on stroke is large. It is increasingly recognized that the effects of some alleles are limited to one or a few stroke subtypes and that effect sizes may vary depending on sex and ethnic origin (2, 3). A strategy successfully used to identify genetic determinants of other common complex diseases has been to focus on early-onset disease which may be enriched for high-penetrance variants. Variants that are highly penetrant or highly predictive of diseases may be easier to detect and also produce useful insights about disease pathways, even if the same variants play a lesser role in late-onset disease.

Candidate gene studies

Most previous studies investigating genetic risk factors for human stroke have taken a candidate gene approach using case–control methodologies. One of the great limitations of candidate gene studies is that any given genetic variant has a low pre-test probability of being truly associated with a phenotype. Candidate gene studies also presuppose more understanding about pathophysiology than is usually the case. This might explain why, although large numbers of candidate genes have been investigated, few associations have been consistently replicated. In individuals of European descent, non-stratified by age, associations have been observed for common variants in the genes for coagulation factor V, prothrombin, methylenetetrahydrofolate reductase (*MTHFR*), and angiotensin-converting enzyme and replicated in individuals of non-European descent (mainly Chinese, Japanese, and Korean) (35). A meta-analysis of studies conducted on patients with early-onset, adult IS (aged 18–50 years) found associations with modest effect for common variants in the genes for *MTHFR* and apolipoprotein E (*APOE*) (36). Though non-independently associated to an increased risk of premature stroke, factor V Leiden (FVG1691A mutation) and prothrombin mutation (PTG20210A mutation) might predispose to brain ischaemia in specific subgroups of young individuals, such as those who carry cardiac interatrial abnormalities, such as patent foramen ovale (37), and those taking oral contraceptives (38). However, to be reliably detected, small relative risks require large sample sizes, probably in the order of 1000 patients or more. Few studies have achieved such numbers and none have included only juvenile stroke cases. This difficulty, together with differences in sample characteristics and study design, could explain much of the inconsistency between studies. The modest success of candidate-gene studies provides support to alternative systematic hypothesis-free approaches, such as genome-wide linkage and genome-wide association studies (GWASs) (see Table 11.2).

Genome-wide studies

Genome-wide *linkage* studies utilize family structure and large numbers of tagging single-nucleotide polymorphisms (SNPs) to track the inheritance of stroke risk with the transmission of the SNP alleles. Although genome-wide linkage

Table 11.2 Results of the candidate gene studies targeting early-onset ischaemic stroke

Age	Ethnicity	Genetic variant	Risk variant (frequency)	No. of ischaemic stroke cases/ controls	Effect of the risk allele (genetic model)
18–50 years	Mixed	F5 G1691A	A (0–0.008)	1543/5267	OR=1.17, P=0.28 (dominant)
		F2 G20210A	A (0.016–0.022)	1279/5036	OR=1.40, P=0.06 (dominant)
		MTHFR C677T	T (0.11–0.51)	1093/1757	OR=1.44, P=0.002 (recessive)
		ITGB3 PLA1/ A2	A2 (0.01–0.16)	488/837	OR=1.27, P=0.49 (dominant)
		ITGA2 C807T	T (0.27–0.49)	308/614	OR=1.50, P=0.01 (dominant)
		APOE ε2/ ε3/ε4	e4 (0.07–0.08)	326/338	OR=2.53, P<0.001 (dominant)
		NOS3 4ab	4b (0.09–0.26)	365/419	OR=1.37, P=0.61 (recessive)

studies have the ability to detect single risk loci with relatively large effect, success has been limited. Early findings of a linkage between stroke and SNPs in *PDE4D* (encoding cAMP-specific 3′,5′-cyclic phosphodiesterase 4D) (39) and *ALOX5AP* (encoding arachidonate 5-lipoxygenase-activating protein) (40) were not replicated consistently. This could be due, in part, to a limited number and low frequency in the population of genes of large effect for stroke, as well as difficulty in procuring stroke family materials that would be required for replication of the previous findings. More recently, a whole-genome linkage scan of 109 families from a genetically homogeneous region of Northern Sweden failed to identify any new major loci for IS (41).

Genome-wide *association* studies (GWASs) analyse subsets of the 3 million or so DNA polymorphisms that make us individuals. By testing 1 million or so SNPs in a single test of an individual's DNA, the pattern seen in patients with a common disease such as IS can be compared to normal controls, and patterns of polymorphisms associated with the disease state. The polymorphisms associated with the disease are often not pathogenic, but just mark a region of the chromosome where a certain variant of that region likely predisposes to disease. However, in some cases the SNPs can be directly pathogenic. GWASs can identify novel genetic loci, do not require a pre-specified hypothesis implicating a particular candidate pathway, and allow the application of the association testing in a genome-wide manner. GWASs appear to be much more powerful than genome-wide linkage studies for the identification of genetic variants underlying multifactorial diseases. So far, GWASs have identified SNPs implicating hundreds of robustly replicated loci for common traits, revealing the unexpected involvement of certain functional and mechanistic pathways in a variety of disease processes, thus, opening doors to potential novel therapeutic targets. Although numerous analyses have been conducted to investigate complex diseases, relatively few GWASs have been performed in the context of IS, especially targeting patients with early-onset disease.

The first GWAS in stroke was reported from the Ischemic Stroke Genetics Study (ISGS) in 2007 (42) and found no genetic locus specifically and robustly associated with the disease. After that, the same group investigated the potential association between IS and variants in the chromosome 9p21 region, which was previously found to be associated with coronary atherosclerotic heart disease. Although the pooled analysis demonstrated that six SNPs were independently associated with atherosclerotic stroke, it is notable that only a small subgroup of young stroke patients was included (43). A separate analysis of over 400 patients with premature IS did not confirm the association in young adults (44). None of the other loci or genes of interest (45), initially shown to be potentially associated with IS based on GWASs, has been consistently replicated or has been tested in large cohorts of young stroke patients yet (see Table 11.3).

Table 11.3 Significant findings from genome-wide association studies
for ischaemic stroke

Chromosome	Gene/locus	Risk allele frequency	Odds ratio (95% confidence intervals)	P-values
7p21.1	HDAC9	0.09	1.39 (1.27–1.53)	2.03×10^{-12}
4q25	PITX2	0.19	1.36 (1.27–1.47)	2.8×10^{-16}
9q21.3	CDKN2A/B	0.51	1.17 (1.09–1.25)	2.93×10^{-5}
12p13.33	NINJ2	0.23	1.41 (1.27–1.56)	2.3×10^{-10}
16q22.3	ZFHX3	0.17	1.25 (1.15–1.35)	2.28×10^{-8}
11q12	AGTRL1		1.3 (1.14–1.47)	6.66×10^{-5}
	CELSR1		1.85 (1.29–2.61)	1×10^{-4}
5q12	PDE4D	0.16		1.5×10^{-6}
13q12–13	ALOX5AP	0.15	1.67	9.5×10^{-5}
	PRKCH		1.4	5.1×10^{-7}
6q21.1	rs556621		1.21	4.7×10^{-8}

In this regard, the results of two GWASs targeting juvenile IS have been recently reported. The first GWAS targeting 1393 patients with cervical artery dissection (CeAD), the most frequent cause of IS at young age, and 14,416 controls was conducted in the setting of the Cervical Artery Dissection and IS Patients (CADISP) study (http://www.cadisp.org) (46). The study identified one previously unreported genome-wide significant risk locus for CeAD at *PHACTR1* and some additional highly suggestive loci. In particular, the rs9349379(G) allele at *PHACTR1* was associated with lower CeAD risk, with confirmation in independent follow-up samples (659 CeAD cases and 2648 controls). Interestingly, the rs9349379(G) allele was previously shown to be associated with lower risk of migraine, a putative risk factor for CeAD, and increased risk of myocardial infarction.

In the largest GWAS of early-onset IS reported to date, including a total of 4505 early-onset cases and 21,968 controls from three ethnic groups, Cheng and co-workers identified a novel locus at 10q25 associated with all IS in a young adult population. This locus is located near *HABP2*, which encodes an extracellular serine protease involved in coagulation, fibrinolysis, and even inflammatory pathways, suggesting a plausible biological mechanism leading to increased risk of stroke. This locus did not appear to have a significant effect in older cases, indicating this may be a genetic susceptibility locus for early-onset stroke (47). Although findings from these studies are promising, further replication and additional studies investigating the potential age of onset effect are needed. Similarly, it will be also relevant to explore whether genes supposed to influence major stroke risk factors based on the results of GWASs have any impact on juvenile stroke.

Mitochondrial studies

Common variants in the mitochondrial genome are supposed to influence the occurrence of sporadic IS, based on the observation that so-called metabolic strokes and rarely even cardioembolic strokes are part of the clinical spectrum of the MELAS syndrome. This hypothesis has been tested in sparse case–control analyses, including a recent multicentre GWAS (13). This multicentre mitochondrial GWAS of IS characterized 144 SNPs that were either directly genotyped or imputed (48). A genetic risk score incorporating information from all the SNPs showed a statistically significant association with IS with minimal heterogeneity across study cohorts. However, no individual variant reached statistical significance. The study, which involved 2284 IS cases, did not confirm a previously reported association with haplogroups H1 and K. Again, none of these analyses specifically targeted young stroke patients.

Clinical implications

Recognition of individuals—and families—carrying rare mutations that cause Mendelian diseases with stroke as a phenotypic manifestation remains an important consideration for clinicians. Because of its characteristics of treatable disorder, FD represents a relevant example. In general, Mendelian disorders can be recognized by their familial aggregation, relatively young age of onset, more severe clinical course, and higher recurrence rates compared with sporadic diseases. Identification of people carrying mutations is important to provide appropriate genetic counselling. Moreover, accurate genetic diagnosis might improve clinical care, because specific preventive measures can be implemented on the basis of known natural evolution of some disorders. For the majority of sporadic IS cases, however, the main challenge for stroke genetics (as for genetics of any complex trait) is to transform findings into actionable clinical methods. One promising translational application is the improvement of prediction models. Unfortunately, risk prediction based on common genetic variation has proven disappointing so far, and findings of several studies indicate that improvements in prediction ability are either low or, if considerable, no different than those obtained from a thorough assessment of family history (49, 50). Genetic research is likely to modify the clinical care of stroke patients in coming years through contributions to personalized medicine. This notion encompasses not only the possibility of estimating an individual's risk of disease but also the ability to tailor all procedures implicated in clinical care, including preventive, diagnostic, prognostic, therapeutic, and rehabilitation strategies. In stroke and other cardiovascular diseases, however, risk stratification on the basis of multiple genetic variants is unfeasible because of the poor predictive ability, especially at young age (51).

Future directions

A number of new methodologies and technologies have been recently developed, including gene expression profiling, proteomics, and metabolomics, aimed at detecting functional changes induced by genetic variations as well as by coexistent non-genetic factors. These offer the potential for identifying blood biomarkers that can be useful in clinical practice in assessing the magnitude of risk associated with specific mutations. Similarly, pharmacogenomics, the study of how genetic variants can influence drug response, offers the opportunity to personalize treatments and reduce side effects. Finally, the next-generation whole-sequencing technologies will be able to explore the unassayed genome, to obtain the entire coding sequence in a short time, and to make comparisons between genomes due to advances in computational methods and processing power. Since this approach might enable the identification of rare variants with intermediate to large effects (as opposed to GWASs, which have so far targeted mainly common variants), it might be of particular interest for stroke of unexplained aetiology occurring in the very young. So far, these techniques have been rarely applied to IS. As to the specific subgroup of younger patients, the challenge will be to set up larger and well-phenotyped samples in order to detect more reliable age-specific risk variants and, eventually, individualized treatment protocols.

References

1. **Herrera VL, Ruiz-Opazo N.** Genetic studies in rat models: insights into cardiovascular disease. Curr Opin Lipidol. 2005;**16**:179–91.
2. **Guo JM, Liu AJ, Su DF.** Genetics of stroke. Acta Pharmacol Sin. 2010;**31**:1055–64.
3. **Dichgans M.** Genetic of ischemic stroke. Lancet Neurol. 2007;**6**:149–61.
4. **Flossmann E, Schulz UG, Rothwell PM.** Systematic review of methods and results of studies of the genetic epidemiology of ischemic stroke. Stroke. 2004;**35**:212–27.
5. **Seshadri S, Beiser A, Pikula A, Himali JJ, Kelly-Hayes M, Debette S,** et al. Parental occurrence of stroke and risk of stroke in their children: the Framingham study. Circulation. 2010;**121**:1304–12.
6. **Yang J, Lee SH, Goddard ME, Visscher PM.** GCTA: a tool for genomewide complex trait analysis. Am J Hum Genet. 2011;**88**:76–82.

7. Lee SH, Wray NR, Goddard ME, Visscher PM. Estimating missing heritability for disease from genome-wide association studies. Am J Hum Genet. 2011;**88**:294–305.

8. Bevan S, Traylor M, Adib-Samii P, Malik R, Paul NL, Jackson C, et al. Genetic heritability of ischemic stroke and the contribution of previously reported candidate gene and genome-wide associations. Stroke. 2012;**43**:3161–67.

9. Holliday EG, Maguire JM, Evans TJ, Koblar SA, Jannes J, Sturm JW, et al. Common variants at 6p21.1 are associated with large artery atherosclerotic stroke. Nat Genet. 2012;**44**:1147–51.

10. Bluher A, Devan WJ, Holliday EG, Nalls M, Parolo S, Bione S, et al. Heritability of young- and old-onset ischaemic stroke. Eur J Neurol. 2015;**22**:1488–91.

11. Arnett DK, Baird AE, Barkley RA Basson CT, Boerwinkle E, Ganesh SK, et al. Relevance of genetics and genomics for prevention and treatment of cardiovascular disease: a scientific statement from the American Heart Association Council on Epidemiology and Prevention, the Stroke Council, and the Functional Genomics and Translational Biology Interdisciplinary Working Group. Circulation. 2007;**115**:2878–901.

12. Ferro JM, Massaro AR, Mas JL. Aetiological diagnosis of ischaemic stroke in young adults. Lancet Neurol. 2010;**9**:1085–96.

13. Meschia JF, Worral BB, Rich SS. Genetic susceptibility to ischemic stroke. Nat Rev Neurol. 2011;**7**:369–78.

14. Online Mendelian Inheritance in Man (OMIM). An Online Catalog of Human Genes and Genetic Disorders. http://omim.org

15. Genetic Testing Registry. https://www.ncbi.nlm.nih.gov/gtr/

16. Orphanet. The portal for rare diseases and orphan drugs. http://www.orpha.net/consor/cgi-bin/Disease.php?lng=EN

17. Andre C. CADASIL: pathogenesis, clinical and radiological findings and treatment. Arq Neuropsiquiatr. 2010;**68**:287–99.

18. Joutel A, Corpechot C, Ducros A, Vahedi K, Chabriat H, Mouton P, et al. Notch3 mutations in CADASIL, a hereditary adult-onset condition causing stroke and dementia. Nature. 1996;**383**:707–10.

19. Razvi SS, Davidson R, Bone I, Muir KW. The prevalence of cerebral autosomal dominant arteriopathy with subcortical infarcts and leucoencephalopathy (CADASIL) in the west of Scotland. J Neurol Neurosurg Psychiatry. 2005;**76**:739–41.

20. Francis J, Raghunathan S, Khanna P. The role of genetics in stroke. Postgrad Med J. 2007;**83**:590–95.

21. Baird AE. Genetics and genomics of stroke: novel approaches. J Am Coll Cardiol. 2010;**56**:245–53.

22. Caplan LR, Arenillas J, Cramer SC, Joutel A, Lo EH, Meschia J, Savitz S, Tournier-Lasserve E. Stroke-related translational research. Arch Neurol. 2011;**68**:1110–23.

23. Mawet J, Vahedi K, Aout M, Vicaut E, Duering M, Touboul PJ, et al. Carotid atherosclerotic markers in CADASIL. Cerebrovasc Dis. 2011;**31**:246–52.

24. Fukutake T, Hirayama K. Familial young-adult-onset arteriosclerotic leukoencephalopathy with alopecia and lumbago without arterial hypertension. Eur Neurol. 1995;**35**:69–79.

25. Hara K, Shiga A, Fukutake T, Nozaki H, Miyashita A, Yokoseki A, et al. Association of HTRA1 mutations and familial ischemic cerebral small-vessel disease. N Engl J Med. 2009;**360**:1729–39.

26. **Deegan PB, Baehner AF, Barba Romero MA, Hughes DA, Kampmann C, Beck M; European FOS Investigators**. Natural history of Fabry disease in females in the Fabry Outcome Survey. J Med Genet. 2006;**43**:347–52.

27. **Brady RO.** Enzymatic abnormalities in diseases of sphingolipid metabolism. Clin Chem. 1967;**13**:565–77.

28. **Saito S, Ohno K, Sakuraba H.** Comparative study of structural changes caused by different substitutions at the same residue on α-galactosidase A. PLoS One. 2013;**8**:e84267.

29. **Kolodny E, Fellgiebel A, Hilz MJ, Sims K, Caruso P, Phan TG**, et al. Cerebrovascular involvement in Fabry disease. Current status of knowledge. Stroke. 2015;**46**:302–13.

30. **Buechner S, Moretti M, Burlina AP, Cei G, Manara R, Ricci R**, et al. Central nervous system involvement in Anderson-Fabry disease: a clinical and MRI retrospective study. J Neurol Neurosurg Psychiatry. 2008;**79**:1249–54.

31. **Sims K, Politei J, Banikazemi M, Lee P.** Stroke in Fabry disease frequently occurs before diagnosis and in the absence of other clinical events: natural history data from the Fabry Registry. Stroke. 2009;**40**:788–94.

32. **Rolfs A, Böttcher T, Zschiesche M, Morris P, Winchester B, Bauer P**, et al. Prevalence of Fabry disease in patients with cryptogenic stroke: a prospective study. Lancet. 2005;**366**:1794–96.

33. **El-Hattab AW, Adesina AM, Jones J, Scaglia F.** MELAS syndrome: clinical manifestations, pathogenesis, and treatment options. Mol Genet Metab. 2015;**116**:4–12.

34. **Tatlisumak T, Putaala J, Innilä M, Enzinger C, Metso TM, Curtze S**, et al. Frequency of MELAS main mutation in a phenotype-targeted young ischemic stroke patient population. J Neurol. 2016;**263**:257–62.

35. **Cheng YC, Cole JW, Kittner SJ, Mitchell BD.** Genetics of ischemic stroke in young adults. Circ Cardiovasc Genet. 2014;**7**:383–92.

36. **Xin XY, Song YY, Ma JF, Fan CN, Ding JQ, Yang GY**, et al. Gene polymorphisms and risk of adult early-onset ischemic stroke: a meta-analysis. Thromb Res 2009;**124**:619–24.

37. **Pezzini A, Grassi M, Del Zotto E, Giossi A, Volonghi I, Costa P**, et al. Do common prothrombotic mutations influence the risk of cerebral ischaemia in patients with patent foramen ovale? Systematic review and meta-analysis. Thromb Haemost. 2009;**101**:813–17.

38. **Pezzini A, Grassi M, Iacoviello L, Del Zotto E, Archetti S, Giossi A**, et al. Inherited thrombophilia and stratification of ischemic stroke risk among users of oral contraceptives. J Neurol Neurosurg Psychiatry 2007;**78**:271–76.

39. **Gretarsdottir S, Thorleifsson G, Reynisdottir ST, Manolescu A, Jonsdottir S, Jonsdottir T**, et al. The gene encoding phosphodiesterase 4D confers risk of ischemic stroke. Nat Genet. 2003;**35**:131–38.

40. **Helgadottir A, Manolescu A, Thorleifsson G, Gretarsdottir S, Jonsdottir H, Thorsteinsdottir U**, et al. The gene encoding 5-lipoxigenase activating protein confers risk of myocardial infarction and stroke. Nat Genet. 2004;**36**:233–39.

41. **Nilsson-Ardnor S, Janunger T, Wiklund PG, Lackovic K, Nilsson AK, Lindgren P**, et al. Genomewide linkage scan of common stroke in families from northern Sweden. Stroke. 2007;**38**:34–40.

42. **Matarín M, Brown WM, Scholz S, Simón-Sánchez J, Fung HC, Hernandez D**, et al. A genome-wide genotyping study in patients with ischaemic stroke: initial analysis and data release. Lancet Neurol. 2007;**6**:414–20.

43. **Gschwendtner A, Bevan S, Cole JW, Plourde A, Matarin M, Ross-Adams H**, et al. Sequence variants on chromosome 9p21.3 confer risk for atherosclerotic stroke. Ann Neurol. 2009;**65**:531–39.

44. **Di Castelnuovo A, Pezzini A, Latella MC, Lichy C, Iacoviello L.** Polymorphisms in chromosome 9 and risk of ischemic stroke in two European white populations, and a meta-analysis. J Thromb Haemost. 2009;**7**:365–67.

45. **Sharma P, Yadav S, Meschia JF.** Genetics of ischaemic stroke. J Neurol Neurosurg Psychiatry. 2013;**84**:1302–308.

46. **Debette S, Kamatani Y, Metso TM, Kloss M, Chauhan G, Engelter ST**, et al. Common variation in PHACTR1 is associated with susceptibility to cervical artery dissection. Nat Genet. 2015;**47**:78–83.

47. **Cheng YC, Stanne TM, Giese AK, Ho WK, Traylor M, Amouyel P**, et al. Genome-wide association analysis of young-onset stroke identifies a locus on chromosome 10q25 near HABP2. Stroke. 2016;**47**:307–16.

48. **Anderson CD, Biffi A, Rahman R, Ross OA, Jagiella JM, Kissela B**, et al. Common mitochondrial sequence variants in ischemic stroke. Ann Neurol. 2010;**69**:471–80.

49. **Ripatti S, Tikkanen E, Orho-Melander M, Havulinna AS, Silander K, Sharma A**, et al. A multilocus genetic risk score for coronary heart disease: case-control and prospective cohort analyses. Lancet. 2010;**376**:1393–400.

50. **Van't Hof FN, Ruigrok YM, Baas AF, Kiemeney LA, Vermeulen SH, Uitterlinden AG**, et al. Impact of inherited genetic variants associated with lipid profile, hypertension, and coronary artery disease on the risk of intracranial and abdominal aortic aneurysms. Circ Cardiovasc Genet. 2013;**6**:264–70.

51. **Markus HS.** Stroke genetics: prospects for personalized medicine. BMC Med. 2012;**10**:113.

Chapter 12

Stroke in women

Kirsi Rantanen and Karoliina Aarnio

Risk factors more prevalent in women

The underlying aetiology, causes, and burden of stroke are different for men and women, as is shown in Fig. 12.1 (1). Endogenous oestrogen might protect from cardiovascular events, but exogenous hormones seem to lack this beneficial effect. As the ageing population increases substantially in the next few decades, the prevalence of stroke survivors is increasing particularly among elderly women (2). Possibly, cardiovascular risk factors go unrecognized and therefore untreated in middle-aged women, who have been traditionally seen as having a very low risk for cardiovascular diseases. The prevalence of hypertension is higher in women after the age of 65 years and lower before 45 years, making it important to focus on preventing hypertension in women who are approaching middle age (3). Hypertensive women are also significantly more likely to be treated than men, but less likely to have achieved blood pressure control. Migraine with aura has been identified as an independent stroke risk factor and is more common in women (1). The pooled adjusted odds ratio (OR) of having ischaemic stroke was 2.3 for migraineurs compared with non-migraineurs (4). Limited evidence suggests a two- to fourfold increased risk of stroke among women with migraine who use combined oral contraceptives (COCs) compared with non-users (5). Premenopausal women are increasingly likely to have abdominal obesity, which used to be a male problem in the past (6). The prevalence of atrial fibrillation is growing and it will be a challenge in the ageing female population in the coming decades. Women with atrial fibrillation are at higher risk of stroke than men (7). The female gender as a stroke risk factor was incorporated in the stroke stratification risk model CHA_2DS_2-VASc in 2009 and this has improved stroke prevention in women with atrial fibrillation, who actually achieve greater risk reduction with full anticoagulation compared with men (8).

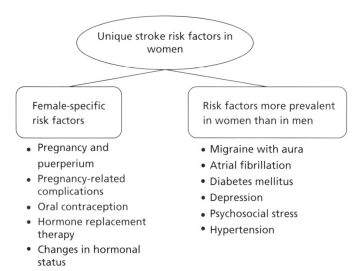

Fig. 12.1 Unique or more prevalent stroke risk factors in women.

How does combined oral contraceptive use affect the risk of ischaemic stroke?

The concern on the safety of COCs has persisted ever since they were first introduced in the 1960s (9). The first report of a woman who had a stroke while receiving COC treatment was published in 1961 and a few case–control studies followed (10–12). The first reported patient was using Enovid, the first-ever commercially available COC that contained 150 micrograms of mestranol and 9.85 milligrams of norethynodrel and was approved by the US Food and Drug Administration in 1959 for use as a birth control method (13).

A systematic review of 16 studies conducted in the United States and Europe between 1960 and 1999 analysed whether COC use is associated with an increased risk of stroke. These cohort and case–control studies showed that the current use of COC was associated with an increased risk of ischaemic stroke (relative risk (RR) 2.75; 95% confidence interval (CI) 2.24–3.38). Small oestrogen doses were associated with a lower risk, but the risk was significantly increased for all doses. The elevated risk of ischaemic stroke fell from a RR of 4.53 with more than 50 micrograms of oestrogen to a RR of 2.08 with less than 50 micrograms. A RR of 1.93 (95% CI 1.35–2.74) was recorded for low-oestrogen preparations in population-based studies that controlled for smoking and hypertension. Based on these figures, there are an additional 4.1 ischaemic strokes for 100,000 normotensive women using low-oestrogen COCs, or one additional ischaemic stroke annually for 24,000 women.

Altogether, 425 strokes per year would be attributed to COC use in the United States. Analysis of progesterone type suggested a non-significant decreasing risk with the newer formulations, with an RR of 3.2 (95% CI 2.16–4.77) in first-generation preparations and an RR of 2.11 (95% CI 0.96–4.64) in third-generation preparations (14). A later meta-analysis identified 20 studies from 1970 to June 2000 and included four additional studies compared with the earlier study by Gillum et al. (14, 19). These include three cohort studies with 119,061, 15,000, and 935,000 subjects, and 93, 1, and 9 cases of stroke respectively, as well as one case–control study with 896 controls and 323 stroke cases (15–19). In this meta-analysis, the overall pooled OR for the risk of stroke in women exposed to COCs was 1.79 (95% CI 1.62–1.97). The OR for ischaemic stroke associated with COC exposure was 2.74 (95% CI 2.24–3.35). The ORs were significant both for women taking COCs containing less than 50 micrograms of ethinyl oestradiol and for women taking the higher dose of greater than 50 microgram of ethinyl oestradiol. Women aged over 35 years seemed to have a greater risk of stroke associated with COC use than younger women, and smokers an increased risk of stroke combined with COC use. The association was strongest for hypertensive (OR 9.82; 95% CI 6.97–13.84) compared with normotensive individuals (OR 2.06; 95% CI 1.46–2.92). In a following meta-analysis by Baillargeon et al., the literature search was limited to 1980–2002, excluding the very early studies with first-generation COCs (20). Fourteen independent studies reported in 12 articles compared current versus non-current use of COC, except for one study that compared current versus never use. The OR for myocardial infarction was 1.84 (95% CI 1.38–2.44) and for ischaemic stroke 2.12 (95% CI 1.56–2.86). The second-generation COCs were associated with a significantly increased risk of both myocardial infarction (OR 1.85, 95% CI 1.03–3.32) and ischaemic stroke (OR 2.54; 95% CI 1.96–3.28). Third-generation COCs were associated with an increased risk of ischaemic stroke (OR 2.03; 95% CI 1.15–3.57), but not of myocardial infarction. The studies that controlled for cardiovascular risk factors were analysed separately and these women still had a two- to threefold increased risk for cardiovascular disease. Other meta-analyses yielded similar results, confirming the findings that in current COC users the risk of MI is increased, but the risk of past users is similar to non-users (21, 22).

A Swedish cohort study included 49,259 women from the Women's Lifestyle and Health Cohort, aged 30–49 years at baseline in 1991 to 1992. There were 285 cases of stroke during follow-up, 193 of which were ischaemic, 72 haemorrhagic, and 20 of unknown type. In this cohort study, no association was found between either ischaemic or haemorrhagic stroke and COC use, not even in hypertensive and smoking women (23).

A large historical cohort study from Denmark included 1,626,158 women followed up for 15 years. During the study period, 3311 thrombotic strokes were identified translating to 21.4 strokes per 100,000 person-years and 1725 myocardial infarctions translating to 10.1 myocardial infarctions per 100,000 person-years. The overall risk of ischaemic stroke and myocardial infarction associated with hormonal contraception was low, but existed even with the lowest dose of 20 micrograms of ethinyl oestradiol with which it was increased by a factor of 0.9–1.7. With the dose of ethinyl oestradiol of 30–40 micrograms, similarly the risk was increased by a factor of 1.3–2.3. The risk of stroke was also increased in users of transdermal patches (RR 3.2; 95% CI 0.8–12.6) and vaginal rings (RR 2.5; 95% CI 1.4–4.4) (24).

COC use doubles the risk of ischaemic stroke in the general population in the presence of hypertension, cigarette smoking, migraine with aura, obesity, and thrombophilia as well as with increasing age. For example, in women who smoke, the risk of stroke varies from two- to eightfold in COC users versus non-users (25). Women who use COCs and have migraine with aura are eight times more likely to have ischaemic stroke than those who only have migraine with aura or those who use COCs but do not have migraine with aura, and 16 times more likely to have ischaemic stroke than those who lacked either of these risk factors (26). In a Finnish Young Stroke Registry Study, female stroke victims were preponderant among those under 30 years of age (27), which may have associations with female-specific risk factors such as COC use.

The Cochrane collaboration published a review of COCs and the risk of myocardial infarction and ischaemic stroke in August 2015. Women younger than 50 years were included and 28 articles identified. The Cochrane review showed that the risk of ischaemic stroke was increased by 1.7-fold in women using COCs compared with non-users. The risk seemed to be doubled in women using higher doses of oestrogen and the risk did not vary clearly according to progestogen type. The overall quality of evidence was moderate (28).

Progesterone-only contraceptives and the risk of stroke

A meta-analysis of epidemiological studies was carried out in 2009 (29). The authors identified six case–control studies conducted mainly in the 1990s in Denmark, France, United States, and worldwide by the World Health Organization, but no randomized controlled trials. This meta-analysis is the first one assessing stroke risk in progesterone-only contraceptive (POC) users. They found no association between POC use and stroke risk with an overall OR of 0.96 (95% CI 0.70–1.31). The small sample sizes resulted in lack of statistical power and the definition of stroke cases was rather heterogeneous. POCs are often prescribed to women who are older, who have cardiovascular risk factors, and have a family history of stroke, as well as in developing countries due to their relatively low cost. There are also no studies addressing the risk of POC use in stroke survivors.

Cerebral venous thrombosis and combined oral contraceptive

The annual overall incidence of cerebral venous thrombosis (CVT) has been historically underestimated being three to four cases per million, mainly due to poor imaging techniques in the past (30). A Dutch series reported an incidence of 13.2 per million person-years in 2008–2010 (31). There is a marked gender preference for this disease, and the median age of first thrombosis may occur as early as in the fourth decade of life (32). In the largest ever ISCVT study, gender-specific risk factors were present in 65% of women, and 46% of women were taking COCs. In a pooled analysis of 17 case–control studies and 263 women with CVT, the OR for the association of COC use was 5.59 (95% CI 3.95–7.91) (33). Though every CVT case in a young otherwise healthy woman is a tragic event (as is shown in Fig. 12.2), it seems that CVTs associated with COC use are not larger than CVTs with other aetiologies, and death and dependency are rarer outcomes in patients with COC use-associated CVTs compared with other types (34). However, in a single-centre study, 25% of the CVT patients remained unemployed and 16% became retired due to CVT-borne disabilities during long-term follow-up (35).

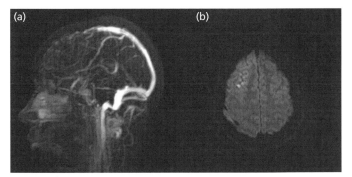

Fig. 12.2 Brain magnetic resonance imaging of a young woman who smoked, used combined oral contraceptives, and had a factor V Leiden mutation presenting with (a) thrombosis in the superior sagittal sinus (b) and a right frontal venous infarction.

Pregnancy, puerperium, and the risk of ischaemic stroke

Thromboembolism was the leading cause of maternal death in the report from the Confidential Enquiries into Maternal Deaths in the UK (36). Despite its relative rareness, stroke contributes to 12% of all maternal deaths. Maternal deaths have slumped in the high-income countries during the last decades, but remain a serious problem globally. There were 342,900 maternal deaths in 2008 worldwide, down from 526,300 in 1980 (37). The physiological changes during pregnancy are substantial, including hypercoagulable state, venous stasis, and blood pressure variation. Normal pregnancy in a previously healthy mother is associated with a 50% increase in blood volume and a corresponding increase in cardiac output (38).

The incidence of pregnancy-related stroke varies substantially in different studies, most of which were completed before 2000, were retrospective, and hospital based (Table 12.1). The incidence of ischaemic stroke in non-pregnant women aged 15–44 years has been reported to be 5.1 per 100,000 women-years (39). In a large retrospective analysis from Canada, 34 pregnant or puerperal patients with stroke diagnosis were identified among 50,700 admissions during the years 1980–1997. The analysis included a postpartum period of 6 weeks. There were 21 infarctions and 13 haemorrhages, of the infarctions eight were venous and 13 arterial. Most venous occlusions occurred postpartum and nine of 13 arterial infarctions in the third trimester or puerperium (40). In a population-based study from the US Nationwide Inpatient Sample, data from 1000 hospitals were used and altogether 2850 pregnancy-related strokes were identified translating into the rate of 34.2 per 100,000 deliveries, which would mean a threefold risk of a stroke event compared with non-pregnant women (41). The majority of pregnancy-related strokes, 48%, occurred in the postpartum period (as is the case in Fig. 12.3), 41% at delivery, and 11% during pregnancy. Risk factors for pregnancy-related stroke include age over 35 years, black ethnicity, hypertension, smoking, heart disease, diabetes, systemic lupus erythematosus, migraine headaches, sickle cell disease, alcohol and other substance use, caesarean delivery, thrombophilia, multiple gestation, greater parity, postpartum infection, pre-eclampsia, eclampsia, and disorders of fluid, electrolytes, and acid–base balance.

The incidence of pregnancy-related intracerebral haemorrhage (ICH) was studied in a large sample derived from the US Nationwide Inpatient Sample, which identified 423 patients with pregnancy-related ICH from 1993 to 2002. This corresponds to 6.1 pregnancy-related ICHs per 100,000 deliveries. The in-hospital mortality rate was almost 20% and the risk was greatest with advanced age, hypertensive disease, African American race, coagulopathy, and substance abuse. In addition, 18% of patients were discharged to a skilled nursing or other treatment facility, and only 44% of ICH patients returned home (42).

Table 12.1 Incidence of ischaemic stroke during pregnancy and the postpartum period

Study	Methods	Study period	Incidence of ischaemic stroke	
			Pregnancy	**Postpartum**
Scott et al. (43)	Prospective, population based	2007–2010	0.9 per 100,000 deliveries	
Hovsepian et al. (44)	Retrospective, registry based	2005–2011		3.6 per 100,000 deliveries[a]
Kamel et al. (45)	Retrospective, registry based	2005–2010		7.1 per 100,000 deliveries[a]
James et al. (41)	Retrospective, registry based	2000–2001	9.2 per 100,000 deliveries	
Liang et al. (46)	Retrospective, hospital based	1992–2004	13.5 per 100,000 deliveries[a]	
Skidmore et al. (47)	Retrospective, hospital based	1992(1994)–1999	35.9 per 100,000 deliveries[b]	
Sharshar et al. (48)	Retro-and prospective, population based	1989–1992	4.3 per 100,000 deliveries[c]	
Bashiri et al. (49)	Retrospective, hospital based	1988–2004	5.2 per 100,000 deliveries	
Kittner et al. (50)	Retrospective, population based	1988–1991	11.0 per 100,000 deliveries[a]	
Ros et al. (51)	Retrospective, population based	1987–1995	4.0 per 100,000 deliveries[a]	
Jaigobin et al. (40)	Retrospective, hospital based	1980–1997	25.6 per 100,000 deliveries[a,d]	
Witlin et al. (52)	Retrospective, single centre	1978–1998		4.6 per 100,000 deliveries
Cross et al. (53)	Hospital based	1956–1965	5.0 per 100,000 births	

[a] Until 6 weeks postpartum; [b] until 12 weeks postpartum; [c] until 2 weeks postpartum; [d] including patients referred from outside the city of Toronto.

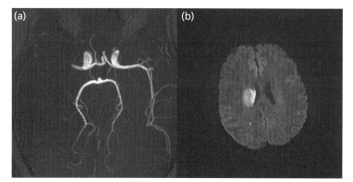

Fig. 12.3 Brain magnetic resonance imaging and magnetic resonance angiography of a young woman with an acute cerebral infarction 10 days after emergency caesarean section due to impending fetal asphyxia with (a) right M1 occlusion on hospital arrival, and (b) acute cerebral infarction of the right hemisphere in diffusion-weighted imaging 24 hours after intravenous thrombolysis and thrombectomy.

Pre-eclampsia

Pre-eclampsia is defined as a new onset of raised blood pressure after 20 weeks of gestation together with proteinuria. It evolves into eclampsia, if seizures occur. Pre-eclampsia affects 2–10% of all pregnancies. An increased risk of both haemorrhagic and ischaemic stroke is associated with eclampsia (48). As much as 25% of ischaemic strokes during pregnancy were caused by eclampsia (50). The Nationwide Inpatient Sample analysis from 1993 to 2002 showed that pre-eclampsia and gestational hypertension were associated with a tenfold risk of pregnancy-related ICH (42). It has been reported that women with pre-eclampsia onset before 34 gestational weeks have elevated carotid intima–media thickness as a measure of sub-clinical atherosclerosis, compared with nulliparous women and women with normal pregnancies (54). A portion of patients with pre-eclampsia also present with haemolysis, elevated liver enzyme levels, and low platelet levels (HELLP syndrome). Stroke is the most common cause of death in a mother with HELLP syndrome (55). As concluded by Bushnell, it is important to recognize that pre-eclampsia is a risk factor for vasculopathy or stroke during delivery and postpartum, and it poses a risk for stroke later in life as a result of endothelial dysfunction, hypertension, and an increase in cardiovascular risk factors (56).

Antithrombotic agents during and after pregnancy-related stroke

Earlier studies have indicated that aspirin may have a teratogenic effect during the first 12 weeks of pregnancy, but this has not been confirmed in prospective studies. In the CLASP study, aspirin was used after the first 12 weeks without any evidence of harm to either the fetus or the mother (57). In patients with ischaemic stroke, it is advisable to use aspirin as secondary prevention during pregnancy after the first trimester and while breastfeeding, after balancing the benefits and hazards. The use of no medication or unfractionated heparin (UFH), or low-molecular-weight heparin (LMWH) during the first trimester should be evaluated individually (58). During the second and third trimesters, low-dose aspirin is the drug of choice as an antiplatelet therapy (59). There is no data on the use of clopidogrel, dipyridamole, or novel oral anticoagulants during pregnancy.

If anticoagulation is indicated, it is best to use adjusted-dose LMWH or UFH compared with warfarin during the first trimester. Warfarin crosses the placenta while heparins do not. Warfarin is potentially teratogenic in the first trimester and increases the risk of fetal cerebral microhaemorrhages and haemorrhage at delivery. Adjusted-dose LMWH or UFH can be used throughout the pregnancy. Alternatively, UFH or LMWH could be replaced by warfarin after the 13th week and then resumed close to delivery. Both warfarin and heparin are safe during breastfeeding. Compared to UFH, LMWHs have a more stable coagulant response and a lower incidence of thrombocytopenia and osteoporosis. LMWHs have been shown to be safe during pregnancy in a large systematic review in patients with underlying thrombophilic disorders and prophylactic doses are not associated with risk of severe bleeding. Higher treatment doses are indicated in patients with prosthetic heart valves, carotid or vertebral dissections, sinus thrombosis, or with some thrombophilic conditions, and this might increase the risk of maternal postpartum haemorrhage (59, 60). Fig. 12.4 provides a schematic overview of the primary aetiological and risk factor profile workup in general, as well as secondary preventive treatment suggestions during pregnancy, although this field lacks strong evidence in the form of clinical trials (1, 58, 59).

Pregnancy, pregnancy complications, and late vascular disease

Higher parity is associated with the risk of ischaemic heart disease and incident stroke (61, 62). It also accelerates preclinical atherosclerosis (63). This is partly due to the lifestyle changes associated with child-rearing, but also the persistent risk factor profile, which includes the increased prevalence of overweight and obesity (64). Even when controlled for lifestyle changes and cardiovascular risk factors, the association between parity and cardiovascular disease remains. Pregnancy might give a rapid progression to atherosclerosis. Skilton

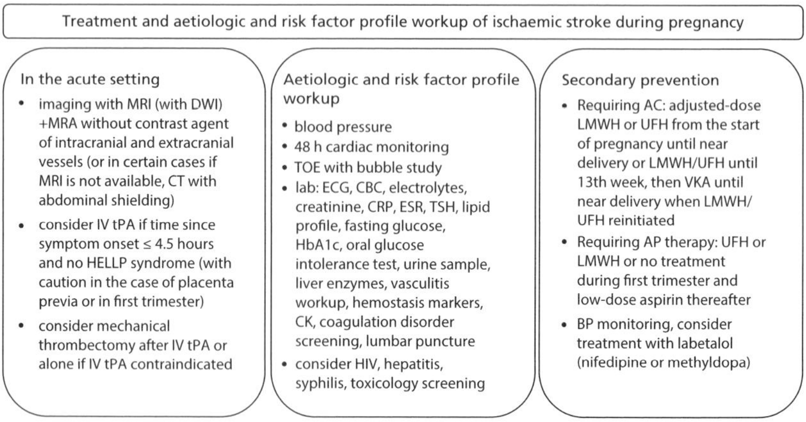

Treatment and aetiologic and risk factor profile workup of ischaemic stroke during pregnancy

In the acute setting
- imaging with MRI (with DWI) +MRA without contrast agent of intracranial and extracranial vessels (or in certain cases if MRI is not available, CT with abdominal shielding)
- consider IV tPA if time since symptom onset ≤ 4.5 hours and no HELLP syndrome (with caution in the case of placenta previa or in first trimester)
- consider mechanical thrombectomy after IV tPA or alone if IV tPA contraindicated

Aetiologic and risk factor profile workup
- blood pressure
- 48 h cardiac monitoring
- TOE with bubble study
- lab: ECG, CBC, electrolytes, creatinine, CRP, ESR, TSH, lipid profile, fasting glucose, HbA1c, oral glucose intolerance test, urine sample, liver enzymes, vasculitis workup, hemostasis markers, CK, coagulation disorder screening, lumbar puncture
- consider HIV, hepatitis, syphilis, toxicology screening

Secondary prevention
- Requiring AC: adjusted-dose LMWH or UFH from the start of pregnancy until near delivery or LMWH/UFH until 13th week, then VKA until near delivery when LMWH/UFH reinitiated
- Requiring AP therapy: UFH or LMWH or no treatment during first trimester and low-dose aspirin thereafter
- BP monitoring, consider treatment with labetalol (nifedipine or methyldopa)

Fig. 12.4 Treatment and aetiological and risk factor profile workup of ischaemic stroke during pregnancy. AC, anticoagulation; AP, antiplatelet; BP, blood pressure; CBC, complete blood count; CK, creatinine kinase; CRP, c-reactive protein; CT, computed tomography; DWI, diffusion-weighted imaging; ECG, electrocardiography; ESR, erythrocyte sedimentation rate; HbA1c, glycated haemoglobin; HELLP, haemolysis, elevated liver enzyme levels, and low platelet levels; HIV, human immunodeficiency virus; IV, intravenous; LMWH, low-molecular-weight heparin; MRI, magnetic resonance imaging; TOE, transoesophageal echocardiography; tPA, tissue type plasminogen activator; TSH, thyroid stimulating hormone; UFH, unfractionated heparin; VKA, vitamin K antagonist.

et al. studied a relationship between parity and carotid atherosclerosis during a 6-year follow-up in a Finnish sample of Cardiovascular Risk in Young Finns Study. They included 1786 subjects, 1005 females and 781 male controls. They found that the progression of carotid atherosclerosis over the studied period was indeed increased in females who gave birth during that period, independent of traditional vascular risk factors (65).

Hypertension affects up to 8% of pregnancies and can be due to pre-eclampsia, eclampsia, superimposed on chronic hypertension, or gestational hypertension (66). Two meta-analyses reported all the available data in this area around 2005, but many of the studies had short-comings such as a lack of control for age and traditional risk factors, were retrospective, and registry-based (67, 68). In the US Family Blood Pressure Program Study, the women with a history of hypertension during pregnancy had an increased risk of all outcomes (50% hypertensive at the age of 53 vs 60, coronary heart disease 14% estimated event rate vs 11%, and stroke 12% estimated event rate vs 5%). After controlling for traditional risk factors, the increased risk for stroke remained statistically significant (hazard ratio 2.10; 95% CI 1.19–3.71) (69). In a cross-sectional study, 81,983,216 pregnancy hospitalizations were gathered from the 1994–2011

Nationwide Inpatient Sample. It showed that between 1994–1995 and 2010–2011 the nationwide rate of stroke with hypertensive disorders of pregnancy increased from 0.8 to 1.6 per 10,000 pregnancy hospitalizations. Women with hypertensive disorders of pregnancy were 5.2 times more likely to have a stroke than those without (70). History of pre-eclampsia symptoms in young women seems to be an independent risk factor of future stoke according to data from the Stroke Prevention in Young Women study, which is a population-based case–control study of risk factors for ischaemic stroke in women aged 15–44 years. A patient with a history of pre-eclampsia could have an up to 60% increased risk (OR 1.63; 95% CI 1.02–2.62) of suffering an ischaemic stroke after pregnancy (71).

Stroke recurrence and pregnancy outcomes in future pregnancies after stroke

There is very little evidence to guide the decision-making of future family planning for patients who have suffered an ischaemic stroke. In a French study published 17 years ago, 489 young women with first-ever ischaemic stroke or CVT were identified. Information on stroke recurrence and reproductive history were obtained by written questionnaire or telephone contact. The risk of stroke recurrence was higher with a definite cause of stroke, with 11 strokes occurring outside of pregnancy and two during a subsequent pregnancy. The outcome of 187 pregnancies in these women was similar to that expected in the general population. The numbers in the study are low, 34% of the women did not have subsequent pregnancies and were unhappy with this for multiple reasons. The women who did have subsequent pregnancies had milder deficits and were younger. The reasons for not having more children were most commonly concern of stroke recurrence, medical advice against a new pregnancy, and residual deficit (72). One retrospective study from Spain identified 32 new pregnancies in 192 women, who had suffered a transient ischaemic attack, stroke, or CVT in 1996–2011. There were no recurrent strokes, but many women refrained from becoming pregnant based on medical advice or fear of recurrent stroke (73).

Conclusion

COC doubles the risk of stroke and is extremely widely used in the Western world. It would be important to educate young women of the risk as well and not only the family planning benefits and evaluate the risk factor profile including hypertension, obesity, migraine with aura, smoking, and family history especially for venous thrombosis prior to start of medication. Stroke in pregnancy is luckily not very common, but as it often affects young, healthy individuals at the height of their career and family life, it is probably not exaggerating to say that stroke in these women is a particularly disabling disease in multiple dimensions. There are also a growing number of middle-aged pregnant females, who already may have a variety of traditional vascular risk factors. Pre-menopause would be an ideal period in a woman's life to try to prevent or treat vascular risk factors.

Concerning stroke research and stroke in women, the lack of good quality studies or comprehensive registry data is striking. However, the publication of the first-ever American Heart Association/American Stroke Association guideline for Stroke Prevention in Women has marked a new era in this field and the recognition of female-specific factors in stroke research. Future research should specifically concentrate on randomizing more women to clinical trials, on selecting the most appropriate secondary prevention for patients with ischaemic stroke during and after pregnancy and puerperium, on determining the safety and efficacy of acute treatments such as thrombolysis and mechanical thrombectomy also for pregnant patients, and determining the long-term outcome for patients with pregnancy-related stroke. It is also vitally important to identify stroke risk factors that are either unique to females or more prevalent in women and aggressively treat them early on in order to prevent cardiovascular and cerebrovascular events later in life.

References

1. **Bushnell C, McCullough LD, Awas IA, Chireau MV, Fedder WN, Furie KL**, et al. Guidelines for the prevention of stroke in women. Stroke. 2014;**45**:1545–88.
2. **Reeves MJ, Bushnell CD, Howard G, Gargano JW, Duncan PW, Lynch G**, et al. Sex differences in stroke: epidemiology, clinical presentation, medical care, and outcomes. Lancet Neurol. 2008;**7**:915–26.
3. **Go AS, Mozaffarian D, Roger VL, Benjamin EJ, Berry JD, Blaha MJ**, et al. Heart disease and stroke statistics-2014 update: a report from the American Heart Association. Circulation. 2014;**129**:e28–e292.
4. **Spector JT, Kahn SR, Jones MR, Jayakumar M, Dalai D, Nazarian S.** Migraine headache and ischemic stroke risk: an update and meta-analysis. Am J Med. 2010;**123**:612–24.
5. **Tepper NK, Whiteman MK, Zapata LB, Marchbanks PA, Curtis KM.** Safety of hormonal contraceptives among women with migraine: a systematic review. Contraception. 2016;**94**:630–40.
6. **Towfighi A, Zheng L, Ovbiagele B.** Weight of the obesity epidemic: rising stroke rates among middle age women in the Unites States. Stroke. 2010;**41**:1371–75.
7. **Wagstaff AJ, Overvad TF, Lip GY, Lane AD.** Is female sex a risk factor for stroke and thromboembolism in patients with atrial fibrillation? A systematic review and meta-analysis. QJM. 2014;**107**:955–67.
8. **Cheng EY, Kong MH.** Gender differences of thromboembolic events in atrial fibrillation. Am J Cardiol. 2016;**117**:1021–27.

9. **Lewis MA.** The epidemiology of oral contraceptives use: a critical review of the studies on oral contraceptives and the health of young women. Am J Obstet Gynecol. 1998;**179**:1086–97.

10. **Lorentz IT.** Parietal lesion and Enovid (letter). BMJ. 1962; **2**:1191.

11. **Inman WHW, Vessey MP.** Investigation of death from pulmonary, coronary, and cerebral thrombosis and embolism in women of childbearing age. BMJ. 1968;**2**:193–99.

12. **Vessey MP, Doll R.** Investigation of the relation between use of oral contraceptives and thromboembolic disease. BMJ. 1968;**2**:199–205.

13. **Diczfalusy E.** Gregory Pincus and steroidal contraception: a new departure in the history of mankind. J Steroid Biochem. 1979;**11**(1A):3–11.

14. **Gillum LA, Mamidipudi SK, Johnston SC.** Ischaemic stroke risk with oral contraceptives. A meta-analysis. JAMA. 2000, **284**:72–78.

15. **Stampfer MJ, Willett WC, Colditz GA, Speizer FE, Hennekens CH.** A prospective study of past use of oral contraceptive agents and risk of cardiovascular diseases. N Engl J Med. 1988;**319**:1313–17.

16. **Porter JB, Hunter JR, Jick H, Stergachis A.** Oral contraceptives and nonfatal vascular disease. Obstet Gynecol. 1985;**66**:1–4.

17. **Hirvonen E, Idänpään-Heikkilä J.** Cardiovascular death among women under 40 years of age using low-oestrogen oral contraceptives and intrauterine devices in Finland from 1975 to 1984. Am J Obstet Gynecol. 1990;**163**:281–84.

18. **Chang KK, Chow LP, Rider RV.** Oral contraceptives and stroke: a preliminary report on an epidemiologic study in Taiwan, China. Int J Gynecol Obstet. 1986;**24**:421–30.

19. **Chan WS, Ray J, Wai EK, Ginsburg S, Hannah ME, Corey PN,** et al. Risk of stroke in women exposed to low-dose oral contraceptives. A critical evaluation of the evidence. Arch Intern Med. 2004;**164**:741–47.

20. **Baillargeon J-P, McClish DK, Essah PA, Nestler JE.** Association between the current use of low-dose oral contraceptives and cardiovascular arterial disease: a meta-analysis. J Clin Endocrinol Metab. 2005;**90**:3863–70.

21. **Spitzer WO, Faith JM, MacRae KD.** Myocardial infarction and third generation oral contraceptives: aggregation of recent studies. Hum Reprod. 2002;**17**:2307–14.

22. **Khader YS, Rice J, John L, Abueita O.** Oral contraceptives use and the risk of myocardial infarction: a meta-analysis. Contraception. 2003; **68**:11–17.

23. **Yang L, Kuper H, Sandin S, Margolis KL, Chen Z, Adami HL,** et al. Reproductive history, oral contraceptive use, and the risk of ischaemic and haemorrhagic stroke in a cohort study of middle-aged Swedish women. Stroke. 2009;**40**:1050–58.

24. **Lidegaard Q, Lokkegaard E, Jensen A, Skovlund CW, Keiding N.** Thrombotic stroke and myocardial infarction with hormonal contraception. N Engl J Med. 2012;**366**:2257–66.

25. **Siritho S, Thrift AG, McNeil JJ, You RX, Davis SM, Donnan GA,** et al. Risk of ischaemic stroke among users of the oral contraceptive pill. The Melbourne Risk Factor Study (MERFS) Group. Stroke. 2003; **34**:1575–80.

26. **Chang C, Donaghy M, Poulter N.** Migraine and stroke in young women: a case-control study. BMJ. 1999;**318**:13–18.

27. **Putaala J, Metso AJ, Metso TN, Konkola N, Kraemer Y, Haapaniemi E,** et al. Analysis of 1008 consecutive patients aged 15 to 49 with first-ever ischaemic stroke. Stroke. 2009; **40**:1195–203.

28. **Roach RE, Helmerhorst FM, Lijfering WM, Stijnen T, Algra A, Dekkers OM.** Combined oral contraceptives: the risk of myocardial stroke and ischaemic stroke. Cochrane Database Syst Rev. 2015;**8**:CD011054.

29. **Chakhtoura Z, Canonico M, Gompel A, Thalabard J-C, Scarabin P-Y, Plu-Bureau.** Progestogen-only contraceptives and the risk of stroke. A meta-analysis. Stroke. 2009;**40**:1059–62.

30. **Stam J.** Thrombosis of the cerebral veins and sinuses. N Engl J Med. 2005;**352**:1791–98.

31. **Coutinho JM, Zuurbier SM, Armideh M, Stam J.** The incidence of cerebral venous thrombosis: a cross-sectional study. Stroke. 2012;**43**:3375–77.

32. **Ferro JM, Canhao P, Stam J, Bousser MG, Barinagarrementeria F.** Prognosis of cerebral vein and dural sinus thrombosis: results of the International Study on Cerebral Vein and Dural Sinus Thrombosis (ISCVT). Stroke. 2004; **35**:664–70.

33. **Dentali F, Crowther M, Ageno W.** Thrombophilic abnormalities, oral contraceptives, and risk of cerebral vein thrombosis: a meta-analysis. Blood. 2006; **107**:2766–73.

34. **Coutinho JM, Ferro JM, Canhao P, Barinagarrementeria F, Cantu C, Bousser MG,** et al. Cerebral venous and sinus thrombosis in women. Stroke. 2009; **40**:2356–61.

35. **Hiltunen S, Putaala J, Haapaniemi E, Tatlisumak T.** Long-term outcome after cerebral venous thrombosis: analysis of functional and vocational outcome, residual symptoms, and adverse events in 161 patients. J Neurol. 2016;**263**:477–84.

36. **Department of Health, Scottish Executive Health Department, and Department of Health, Social Services and Public Safety, Northern Ireland**. Why Mothers Die. Sixth Report of Confidential Enquiries into Maternal Deaths in the United Kingdom, 2000–2002. London: RCOG Press, 2004.

37. **Hogan MC, Foreman KJ, Naghavi M, Ahn SY, Wang M, Makela SM,** et al. Maternal mortality for 181 countries, 1980-2008: a systematic analysis of progress towards Millennium Development Goal 5. Lancet. 2010;**375**:1609–23.

38. **van Oppen ACC, van der Tweel L, Alsbach GBJ, Heethaar RM, Bruinse HW.** A longitudinal study of maternal hemodynamics during normal pregnancy. Obstet. Gynecol. 1996; **88**:40–46.

39. **Petitti DB, Sidney S, Quesenberry CP, Bernstein A.** Incidence of stroke and myocardial infarction in women of reproductive age. Stroke. 1997; **28**:280–83.

40. **Jaigobin C, Silver FL.** Stroke and pregnancy. Stroke. 2000;**31**:2948–51.

41. **James AH, Bushnell CD, Jamison MG, Myers ER.** Incidence and risk factors for stroke in pregnancy and the puerperium. Obstet Gynecol. 2005;**106**:509–16.

42. **Bateman BT, Schumacher HC, Bushnell CD, Pile-Spellman J, Simpson LL, Sacco RL,** et al. Intracerebral haemorrhage in pregnancy. Neurology. 2006; **67**:424–29.

43. **Scott CA, Bewley S, Rudd A, Spark P, Kurinczuk JJ, Brocklehurst P,** et al. Incidence, risk factors, management, and outcomes of stroke in pregnancy. Obstet Gynecol. 2012;**120**(2 Pt 1):318–24.

44. **Hovsepian DA, Sriram N, Kamel H, Fink ME, Navi BB.** Acute cerebrovascular disease occurring after hospital discharge for labor and delivery. Stroke. 2014;**45**:1947–50.

45. **Kamel H, Navi BB, Sriram N, Hovsepian DA, Devereux RB, Elkind MS.** Risk of a thrombotic event after the 6-week postpartum period. N Engl J Med. 2014;**370**:1307–15.

46. **Liang CC, Chang SD, Lai SL, Hsieh CC, Chueh HY, Lee TH.** Stroke complicating pregnancy and the puerperium. Eur J Neurol. 2006;**13**:1256–60.

47. **Skidmore FM, Williams LS, Fradkin KD, Alonso RJ, Biller J.** Presentation, aetiology, and outcome of stroke in pregnancy and puerperium. J Stroke Cerebrovasc Dis. 2001;**10**:1–10.

48. **Sharshar T, Lamy C, Mas JL.** Incidence and causes of strokes associated with pregnancy and puerperium. A study in public hospitals of Ile de France. Stroke in Pregnancy Study Group. Stroke. 1995;**26**:930–36.

49. **Bashiri A, Lazer T, Burstein E, Smolin A, Lazer S, Perry ZH,** et al. Maternal and neonatal outcome following cerebrovascular accidents during pregnancy. J Matern Fetal Neonatal Med. 2007;**20**(3):241–47.

50. **Kittner SJ, Stern BJ, Feeser BJ, Hebel R, Nagey DA, Buchholz DB,** et al. Pregnancy and the risk of stroke. N Engl J Med. 1996;**335**:768–74.

51. **Ros H, Lichtenstein P, Bellocco R, Petersson G, Cnattingius S.** Increased risks of circulatory diseases in late pregnancy and puerperium. Epidemiology. 2001; **12**:456–60.

52. **Witlin AG, Mattar F, Sibai BM.** Postpartum stroke: a twenty-year experience. Am J Obstet Gynecol. 2000; **183**:83–88.

53. **Cross JN, Castro PO, Jennett WB.** Cerebral strokes associated with pregnancy and the puerperium. Br Med J. 1968;**3**:214–18.

54. **Blaauw J, van Pampus M, van Doormaal J.** Increased intima-media thickness after early-onset preeclampsia. Obstet Gynecol. 2006; **107**:1345–51.

55. **Isler CM, Rinehart BK, Terrone DA, Martin RW, Mugann EF, Martin JN Jr,** et al. Maternal mortality associated with HELLP. Am J Obstet Gynecol. 1999;**181**:924–28.

56. **Bushnell CD.** Stroke in Women: risk and prevention throughout the lifespan. Neurol Clin. 2008;**26**:1161–70.

57. **CLASP: a randomized trial of low-dose aspirin for prevention and treatment of pre-eclampsia among 9364 pregnant women.** CLASP (Collaborative Low-Dose Aspirin Study in Pregnancy) Collaborative Group. Lancet. 1994;**343**:619–29.

58. **Kernan WN, Ovbiagele B, Black HR, Bravata DM, Chimowitz MI, Ezekowitz MI.** Guidelines for the prevention of stroke in patients with stroke and transient ischaemic attack. A guideline for Healthcare professionals from the American Heart Association/American Stroke Association. Stroke. 2014;**45**:2160–236.

59. **Bates SM, Greer IA, Middeldorp S, Veenstra DI, Prabulos AM, Vandvik PO.** VTE, thrombophilia, antithrombotic therapy, and pregnancy: Antithrombotic therapy and prevention of thrombosis, 9th ed: American College of Chest Physician Evidence-Based Clinical Practice Guidelines. Chest. 2012;**141**(suppl):e691S-736S.

60. **Greer IA, Nelson-Pierce C.** Low-molecular weight heparins for thromboprophylaxis and treatment of venous thromboembolism in pregnancy: a systematic review of safety and efficacy. Blood. 2005;**106**:401–407.

61. **Lawlor DA, Emberson JR, Ebrahim S, Whincup PH, Wannamethee SG, Walker M,** et al. Is the association between parity and coronary heart disease due to biological effects of pregnancy or adverse lifestyle risk factors associated with child-rearing? Findings from the British Women's Heart and Health Study and the British Regional Heart Study. Circulation. 2003;**107**:1260–64.

62. **Zhang X, Shuh XO, Gao Y-T, Yang G, Li H, Zheng W.** Pregnancy, childrearing, and risk of stroke in Chinese women. Stroke. 2009;**40**:2680–84.

63. **Wolff B, Volzke H, Robinson D, Schwahn C, Ludemann J, Kessler C,** et al. Relation of parity with common carotid intima-media thickness among women of the study of health in Pomerania. Stroke. 2005;**36**:938–43.

64. **Skilton MR, Serusclat A, Begg L-M, Moulin P, Bonnet F.** Parity and carotid atherosclerosis in men and women: insights into the roles of childbearing and child-rearing. Stroke. 2009;**40**:1151–57.

65. **Skilton MR, Bonnet F, Begg LM, Juonala M, Kähönen M, Lehtimäki T,** et al. Childbearing, child-rearing, cardiovascular risk factors, and progression of carotid intima-media thickness. Stroke. 2010;**41**:1332–37.

66. Report of the National Blood Pressure Education Program Working Group on High Blood Pressure in Pregnancy. Am J Obstet Gynecol. 2000;**183**:S1–S22.

67. **Craici I, Wagner S, Garovic VD.** Preeclampsia and future cardiovascular risk: formal risk factor or failed stress test? Ther Adv Cardiovasc Dis. 2008;**2**:249–59.

68. **Bellamy L, Casas J-P, Hingorani AD, Williams DJ.** Preeclampsia and risk of cardiovascular disease and cancer in later life: systematic review and meta-analysis. BMJ. 2007;**335**:974.

69. **Garovic VD, Bailey GR, Boerwinkle E, Hunt SC, Weder AB, Curb D, Mosley TH,** et al. Hypertension in pregnancy as a risk factor for cardiovascular disease later in life. Hypertension. 2010;**28**:826–33.

70. **Leffert LR, Clancy CR, Bateman BT, Bryant AS, Kuklina EV.** Hypertensive disorders and pregnancy-related stroke: frequency, trends, risk factors, and outcomes. Obstet Gynecol. 2015; **125**:124–31.

71. **Brown DW, Dueker N, Jamieson DJ, Cole JW, Wozniak MA, Stern BJ.** Pre-eclampsia and the risk of ischaemic stroke among young women: results from the Stroke Prevention in Young Women Study. Stroke. 2006;**37**:1055–56.

72. **Lamy C, Hamon JB, Coste J, Mas JL** for the **French Study Group on Stroke in Pregnancy.** Ischaemic stroke in young women: risk of recurrence during subsequent pregnancies. Neurology. 2000;**55**:269–74.

73. **Cruz-Herrantz A, Ilan-Gala I, Martinez-Sanchez P, Fuentes B, Diez-Tejedor E.** Recurrence of stroke among women of reproductive age: impact of and on subsequent pregnancies. Eur J Neurol. 2015;**22**:681–87.

Chapter 13

Stroke in children

Bettina Henzi and Maja Steinlin

Introduction

This chapter will give an overview on the large spectrum of childhood arterial ischaemic stroke, a changing continuum from infancy through adolescence towards stroke in young adults. There are many similarities but also specific differences and this chapter will emphasize these particularities of stroke in children.

Epidemiology

Incidence of paediatric stroke ranges from 3 to 5 per 100,000 children per year and is similar to that of brain tumours in children. Stroke ranges among the top ten leading causes of death in children (1). Haemorrhagic stroke shows with 29% (2) the highest overall mortality followed by cerebral sinus venous thrombosis (11–17%) (3) and arterial ischaemic stroke (6–8%) (1, 4, 5). Within arterial ischaemic stroke, the incidence in neonates is high and rises up to 13 per 100,000 live births, compared to 2 per 100,000 children/year in childhood stroke. Predominantly preschool children suffer from stroke, but it can occur at any age. Boys are affected more frequently than girls (2:1) (6). Despite comparatively small numbers, the socioeconomic burden of stroke is tremendous. Costs for childhood arterial ischaemic stroke are $81,870 during acute hospitalization followed by $135,160 in the following 5 years as outpatients (7). As care for the majority of these children is ongoing at least until fulfilled social and professional integration in adult life, these costs will add up significantly.

Difficulty in diagnosis and the problem of stroke mimics

Nowadays, 28% of adults with stroke arrive in the emergency department within 1 hour of symptom onset (8). However, in children it takes about 6 hours for one-third of them to arrive at a hospital (9, 10). An important factor for this delay is the lack of algorithms to get children as fast as possible to adequate hospital care. Even in tertiary paediatric emergency departments, only 24–38% of strokes are managed on an adequate fast track (9).

Variable clinical stroke recognition tools have been developed to improve recognition of stroke symptoms in adults. The ROSIER scale and FAST score have been shown to be a reasonable starting point also for children. But differences in manifestation of stroke in children compared to adults ask for adjustments to improve the yield (11). One exemplary cause is that children with stroke more often present with a seizure than adult patients do, though in the ROSIER score a seizure does not account for high stroke risk (12).

In addition, the fact that many children present with fast improving symptoms or a stuttering onset of symptoms might have an influence on a delayed approach to adequate investigations. Moreover, children frequently do not complain about their symptoms, and/or have difficulty in verbalizing them due to their language development or to the higher incidence of speech problems compared to adults.

Diagnosis of childhood stroke is further hampered by the many mimics that exist. In adults, 73% of patients with acute focal neurological signs suffer from stroke, whereas in children only 7% do (13). The most important differential diagnoses are summarized in Table 13.1.

Manifestation/symptoms

Similarly to adults, 70–80% of children with ischaemic stroke present with hemiparesis with or without facial palsy at stroke onset. Compared to adults, children more frequently have strokes in the posterior circulation, and symptoms such as ataxia and ocular motor problems are therefore important to recognize. However, in children, ataxia is not limited to cerebellar lesions (14) (Table 13.2).

Aphasia is significantly more frequent in children than in adults. Due to the immature lateralization of language and yet broader network, aphasia is not only caused by a stroke of the dominant side and may also be prominent in thalamic lesions. Around 20% of children present with seizures, which are rarely the first manifestation but occur within the first hours or days after stroke onset (6, 11).

Some children show non-focal symptoms such as headache, vomiting, or changes in level of consciousness. Cephalalgia is present in 30% of children, before, with, or shortly after the onset of symptoms.

The age of the child suffering a stroke influences possible symptoms. Children under 1 year of age present more likely with seizures and altered level

Table 13.1 Important differential diagnoses of acute focal neurological deficit in children

Migraine accompagnée	28%
Febrile or afebrile seizure	15%
Bell's palsy	10%
Cerebrovascular disease	7%
Conversion disorder	6%
Syncope	5%
Headache	4%
Other encephalopathy	3%
Cerebellitis	3%
CNS demyelination	2%
Peripheral nerve	1.6%
CNS infection	1.3%
Drug intoxication	1.3%
CNS tumours	1%
Cord demyelination	0.7%
Other neurologic	6%
Other non-neurologic	6%

CNS, central nervous system.

Adapted from Neurology, 82(16), Mackay, M.T., et al., Stroke and nonstroke brain attacks in children, pp. 1434–40, Copyright (2014), with permission from Wolters Kluwer Health, Inc.

of consciousness. Older children are more likely to present with focal neurological deficits (15).

Risk factors

Current knowledge suggests that a stroke in childhood is the result of multiple risk factors. The understanding of the relationship between the different risk factors is still limited and evidence-based optimal treatment is missing (19). It has been shown that the aetiological profile of childhood stroke differs significantly from that in adult patients.

In contrast to adult stroke patients, non-arteriosclerotic arteriopathies are the most frequent risk factor and can be detected in about half of the patients. One-third of these arteriopathies consist of transient focal vasculopathies—a condition affecting typically the middle cerebral artery. Its aetiology is not entirely

Table 13.2 Comparison of symptoms at manifestation

	Adults, in % (16)	CH children, in % (4)	AU children, in % (11)	GB children, in % (17)
Headache	22	28	46	24
Vertigo	3	3	–	–
Seizures	3	26	17	29
Aphasia/dysarthria	26	41	46	46
Hemiparesis	87	79	57–63	72
Facial palsy	58	40	46	41
Visual problems*	17	14	19	5
Ataxia	–	13	10	–
Sensory problems	44	16	25	–

Adults from the Atherosclerosis Risk in Community Study (USA).

CH: all children from the Swiss Neuropaediatric Stroke Registry, population based.

AU: all children from the stroke registry of Royal Children's Hospital Melbourne.

GB: all children from the Southern England Stroke Registry, population based.

* Visual problems such as hemianopsia, diplopia.

Reproduced from Curr Treat Options Neurol, 17(5), Steinlin, M. and M.T. Mackay, Emergency management of ischemic stroke in children, pp. 349, Copyright (2015), with permission from Springer.

clear but an association with a parainfectious reaction is assumed. This reaction leads to a stenosis of the vessel through thickening of the intimal layer. The most frequently named pathogens associated with transient focal arteriopathy are varicella zoster, *Mycoplasma, Borrelia*, and entero- as well as parvovirus infections (Figs. 13.1 and 13.2).

Other causes of a cerebral arteriopathy are moyamoya disease and syndrome (22%), dissections (22%), fibromuscular dysplasia, and vasculitis of small cerebral vessels (20) (Fig. 13.3).

During the last decade, the importance of genetically determined vasculopathy is increasingly recognized. The list continuously expands and gene mutations of *COL4A1, ACTA2, ADA2,* and *JAG1* are only a few that could be mentioned (21).

Suspicion of a genetic vasculopathy has to be high when the family history is suggestive, when haemorrhagic and ischaemic stroke occur within the same family or if in a single patient multiple organs (e.g. the kidney and the brain) are affected by vascular abnormalities.

Cardiac disease is the second most common cause of stroke in children and represents a major risk factor. Complex congenital heart disease with

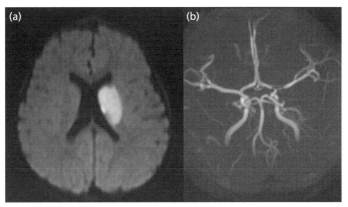

Fig. 13.1 Acute infarction of the left striatum in a 9-year-old boy pictured as a diffusion restriction in the diffusion-weighted sequence (a) and stenosis of the distal end of the carotid artery, the proximal anterior cerebral artery and middle cerebral artery on the left shown in arterial time of flight sequence (b).

right-to-left shunt is particularly prone to cause a stroke. Also, acquired cardiac disorders such as myocarditis or endocarditis may cause a stroke due to low ejection fraction and formation of thrombi.

Haematological disorders as hereditary coagulopathies are identified in 20–50% of children presenting with stroke (22, 23), but it is believed that those haematological risk factors mostly work in combination with other mechanisms, instead of being a causative factor on their own. In contrast, children

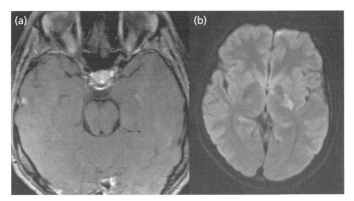

Fig. 13.2 Occlusion of the left distal internal carotid artery in a 14-year-old girl due to inflammation of the vessel with enlargement of the vessel wall with local wall enhancement pictured in T1 dark-blood sequence after application of contrast media (a) with the corresponding ischaemia in the left choroidal anterior vascular territory in the diffusion-weighted sequence (b).

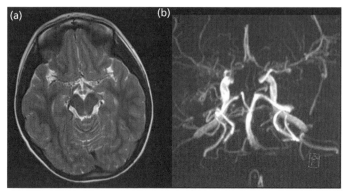

Fig. 13.3 Moyamoya disease in a 5-year-old boy. Obvious collaterals due to filiform internal carotid artery and middle cerebral artery bilaterally pictured in the T2-weighted sequence (a) and the arterial time of flight sequence (b), which gives it a foggy aspect.

with sickle cell disease represent an important group of patients with a high risk of stroke justified by the lone presence of their haematological burden.

Although rare, metabolic infarctions are important for the paediatric population. These lesions typically do not occur in a specific vascular territory since pathogenic mechanisms differ between the different entities. In mitochondrial disease, energy depletion leads to ischaemic damage of cells and in urea cycle disorders, toxic deposits destroy cerebral tissues. Fabry disease provokes a focal arteriopathy (24). Additionally, multisystemic metabolic disorders can form additional risk factors such as, for example, cardiomyopathy, which in turn can cause embolic stroke. Any systemic infectious disease, such as bacterial sepsis and meningitis, is a risk factor for paediatric stroke (25).

Diagnostic investigations

Magnetic resonance imaging, as the first choice in stroke diagnostics, has not only diagnostic purposes, but also aetiological evaluation and gives some information on prognosis concerning recovery. It reveals ischaemic lesions within minutes and can give accurate information about the lesion's extension (13, 26, 27). The importance of adequate neuroimaging is underlined by the long list of differential diagnoses of a child with suspected stroke. A broader investigation concerning aetiology of the stroke can be made by including magnetic resonance angiography to determine dissection, and dark blood sequences to look for vasculopathy.

The fact that brain computed tomography is positive in only 66% of children with ischaemic stroke, and the presence of the many mimics in the differential diagnosis, support magnetic resonance as the first choice in imaging. Moreover, computed tomography includes a relevant radiation exposure and has to be avoided in childhood whenever possible (28, 29). Magnetic resonance imaging is certainly the gold standard in paediatric patients. However, the younger the child, the more difficult it is to access this examination within a short time (30).

Once a paediatric ischaemic stroke has been confirmed, a thorough workup for risk factors has to be conducted, including cardiological and haematological investigations. The importance of neurovascular ultrasound is subsidiary and is more important for follow-up investigations than diagnostic investigations. As childhood stroke is a multiple risk problem in two-thirds of the children, laboratory investigations should always include a search for underlying infectious, immunological, haematological-haemostasiological, and metabolic problems. The add-on value of a lumbar puncture gains increasing importance, especially in suspected infectious-inflammatory risk profiles (31). Table 13.3 summarizes a suggested primary workup.

Therapy

Over the past three decades, acute treatment of adult patients with stroke developed rapidly. Defined algorithms for fast transportation to specialized stroke units and primary diagnosis decreased 'time to needle' significantly (32). Unfortunately, children did not yet benefit from this progress due to still missing awareness, lack of algorithms, and also lack of evidence-based treatment guidelines. Recommendations in published guidelines for paediatric stroke treatment are mostly based on expert consensus opinion or adaptation of adult guidelines.

The supportive measures to be taken in children with stroke are undisputed and they have their origin in the ABC algorithms from advanced life support guidelines. Careful respiratory monitoring and saturation of greater than 92% has to be maintained. As in adults, additional oxygen via facemask is not supported if saturation is stable (33). Arterial blood pressure is important to monitor. About two-thirds of children with stroke are hypertensive in the first 24 hours after stroke onset, but normalize their blood pressure within a short time spontaneously (34). This may be caused by cerebral autoregulation to maintain cerebral perfusion or if persistent, might be the first sign of increased intracranial pressure. As chronic hypertension in children, without a history or without signs of chronic vasculopathies, is rare, persistent arterial hypertension has to be evaluated carefully. When adequate cerebral perfusion is ensured, and elevated intracranial pressure is excluded, arterial hypertension has to be lowered cautiously in line with adult recommendations.

Table 13.3 Suggested laboratory investigations for paediatric ischaemic stroke

	At admittance	At diagnosis	Within follow-up
Blood	BC, ESR, CRP, electrolytes, glucose, liver and renal functions, coagulation, lactate	Viral serology (e.g. varicella/herpes simplex/*Borrelia* maybe: *Mycoplasma*/enterovirus etc.), vasculitis screen (e.g. ACLA, ANA, LA, ANCA) Amino acids*	Lipid profile, homocysteine, prothrombotic studies (factor V Leiden, prothrombin and *MTHFR* mutation, lipoprotein A, protein C and S)
Urine		Organic acids*	
Cerebrospinal fluid		Opening pressure, cell count, protein, glucose, lactate, PCR or antibodies of varicella and herpes, if needed other PCR/antibodies	

ACLA, anticardiolipin antibody; ANA, antinuclear antibody; ANCA, antineutrophil cytoplasmic antibody; BC, blood count; CRP, C-reactive protein; ESR, erythrocyte sedimentation rate; PCR, polymerase chain reaction.

* If suspecting metabolic origin of stroke.

Reproduced from Curr Treat Options Neurol, 17(5), Steinlin, M. and M.T. Mackay, Emergency management of ischemic stroke in children, pp. 349, Copyright (2015), with permission from Springer.

Glucose problems in children with no underlying metabolic disorder are rare, but should be excluded. As in adults, it is suggested to maintain a body temperature between 36.5°C and 37.0°C. This is of special importance for pre-schoolers, who are at risk for symptomatic seizure. If necessary, an antiepileptic treatment needs to be installed (18).

Children with large volume ischaemic lesions or lesions in the posterior fossa are especially at high risk for brain oedema. Malignant middle cerebral infarction or large ischaemic lesions in the posterior fossa are associated with a bad outcome and similar to what is described in adults, neurosurgical intervention may be beneficial (35). Decompressive hemicraniectomy has to be considered with a low threshold.

In view of lacking evidence, therapy decisions in children have to be made cautiously, considering the individual situation and also the underlying aetiology or risk profile of the individual, or both (6, 36, 37).

Antithrombotic therapy is recommended after exclusion of haemorrhagic stroke and should be started as soon as possible. Concerning the specific indications of antithrombotic therapy and use of different pharmaceutical agents, controversies prevail. Guidelines differ about the use of unfractionated heparin, low-molecular-weight heparin, and aspirin. An analysis of current practice showed a trend for aspirin in Europe and one towards anticoagulation in North America (38). Most experts accept prophylactic use of aspirin in a dosage of 3–5 mg/kg body weight in the acute phase, after exclusion of cardioembolic aetiology or dissections.

There is a tendency towards the use of anticoagulant therapy in children with stroke due to cardioembolism. However, a single randomized controlled trial of children with cardiac disease showed that heparin was equal to aspirin in preventing thrombotic events after palliative surgery (36), but did not search for silent infarctions by imaging. Stence et al. showed that it is justifiable to anticoagulate children with extracranial dissection, if there is no elevated risk of bleeding (39). However, new studies in adults do not show a benefit of anticoagulation over aspirin in dissections (40). These studies will likely also influence current practice in children.

Another aspect of stroke treatment in paediatric patients are steroids and immunosuppressive agents. Infection and inflammation play an important role in paediatric stroke. In recent studies (41–44), changes in inflammatory biomarker profiles have been detected. Therefore the additive therapy with steroids to antithrombotic agents might be beneficial in certain underlying pathologies such as transient focal arteriopathies (18, 45). In view of the association with varicella virus, but also the detection or reactivated herpes infection in children (46) with vasculopathy, accompanying aciclovir has to be considered. The add-on value of cerebrospinal fluid investigations for polymerase chain reaction or serologies for varicella or herpes virus, or both, to assist a decision on treatment with steroids plus or minus aciclovir has to be shown in the future. In cases of primary central nervous system vasculitis, the use of other immunosuppressive agents, such as mycophenolate, azathioprine, and cyclophosphamide has to be taken into consideration besides steroids.

Thrombolysis or thrombectomy in children

In adults, the target of acute treatment is the ischaemic penumbra, since recanalization and collaterals have been shown to be the most important factor to influence outcome (27). Endovascular thrombectomy has been shown to be the most successful treatment approach (47). In children, effects of recanalization and collaterals with thrombolysis and thrombectomy are not sufficiently investigated and present guidelines recommend these procedures only within (as yet non-existent) research protocols.

A review of patients of the International Stroke Registry detected that 2% of 687 children with stroke between 2003 and 2007 received tissue plasminogen activator (tPA) (48). The application of the thrombolytic agent was frequently outside the therapeutic windows defined for adults, which might be the explanation for the increased rate of intracranial haemorrhage (26%) compared to adults (7%). A study of our own data combined with a literature review summarizes thrombolysis and thrombectomy in 34 children (49). Partial or complete recanalization was achieved in 63% of the children. One-third of the children had periprocedural complications, in none of them with clinical worsening. Complications were more frequent in thrombolysed patients than in patients undergoing thrombectomy. The role of mechanical thrombectomy in children should be investigated in more depth. In a prospective population-based study (Swiss Neuropediatric Stroke Registry), 6.4% (n=16) of the children received thrombectomy or thrombolysis, or both. Only one child had clinically significant complications caused by bleeding, but with almost complete recovery after decompressive hemicraniectomy. Outcome was favourable in all 16 patients with median Paediatric Stroke Outcome Measure (PSOM) of 1.5 (range 0–7) (50).

The appropriate dose of tPA in children is not defined. It is assumed that due to developmental differences in the coagulation cascade, higher doses of tPA are needed for clot lysis (51, 52). In many case reports and series, the use of tPA in children in similar dosages as in adults has been shown to be safe.

There are increasing reports of cases and case series, where thrombolysis or thrombectomy, or both, have been used successfully in children. There is probably a subgroup of children with stroke who may 'benefit' from acute therapies. In any case, children have to be thoroughly evaluated for dispatch to the appropriate treatment. Furthermore, performance of these treatments should be centred in primary stroke units experienced in acute management of adults *and* children with stroke.

Prognostics

For decades there was the belief that acute brain damage in infancy or childhood would be less devastating than later in life. There are several studies indicating that damage to the developing brain in infancy and early childhood is prognostically less favourable than in later life. This has also been shown in childhood stroke (53). Mortality in children ranges between 6% and 8% (4, 5). More than half of the patients show persisting neurological symptoms (mostly hemiparesis) and even more children suffer from neurocognitive and behavioural problems as a lifelong handicap.

Knowledge on prognostic factors is limited. Known negative prognostic factors include the presence of seizures and altered consciousness at initial manifestation (38). Neuroimaging may direct clinicians during the first step: lesion location in basal ganglia or thalamus (or both) is a negative prognostic factor concerning neurological and cognitive outcome (54). Beside the fact that residual hemiparesis significantly influences the future quality of life (55), neurocognitive and behavioural problems have a great impact as they influence schooling, professional training, as well as social and family life.

The risk of stroke recurrence is particularly high in children with vasculopathies (56), which might indicate the necessity for prolonged aspirin treatment in these children. In addition, hereditary coagulopathies, as protein C deficiency and elevated lipoprotein A, might also have a negative influence (22). Risk of recurrent stroke in children must be evaluated thoroughly and treated respectively.

Summary

Stroke in childhood is rare and has an incidence similar to brain tumours in childhood. Symptoms are comparable to those in adults, but there is a significant delay in diagnosis of stroke in children. It is vital to raise awareness of childhood stroke in the public and in medical personnel, as treatment options are likely to be time dependent as in adults. Algorithms for diagnosis and treatment have to be supported by multicentre prospective trials to improve the outcome for children with arterial ischaemic stroke.

Acknowledgement

The authors would like to thank Christian Weisstanner, MD, for his help with the figures.

References

1. **Mallick AA, O'Callaghan FJ.** The epidemiology of childhood stroke. Eur J Paediatr Neurol. 2010;**14**(3):197–205.

2. **Jordan LC, Hillis AE.** Hemorrhagic stroke in children. Pediatr Neurol. 2007;**36**(2):73–80.

3. **Grunt S, Wingeier K, Wehrli E, Boltshauser E, Capone A, Fluss J**, et al. Cerebral sinus venous thrombosis in Swiss children. Dev Med Child Neurol. 2010;**52**(12):1145–50.

4. **Steinlin M, Pfister I, Pavlovic J, Everts R, Boltshauser E, Capone Mori A**, et al. The first three years of the Swiss Neuropaediatric Stroke Registry (SNPSR): a population-based study of incidence, symptoms and risk factors. Neuropediatrics. 2005;**36**(2):90–97.

5. **Christerson S, Stromberg B.** Stroke in Swedish children II: long-term outcome. Acta Paediatr. 2010;**99**(11):1650–56.

6. **Steinlin M.** A clinical approach to arterial ischemic childhood stroke: increasing knowledge over the last decade. Neuropediatrics. 2012;**43**(1):1–9.

7. **Gardner MA, Hills NK, Sidney S, Johnston SC, Fullerton HJ.** The 5-year direct medical cost of neonatal and childhood stroke in a population-based cohort. Neurology. 2010;**74**(5):372–78.

8. Saver JL, Smith EE, Fonarow GC, Reeves MJ, Zhao X, Olson DM, et al. The "golden hour" and acute brain ischemia: presenting features and lytic therapy in >30,000 patients arriving within 60 minutes of stroke onset. Stroke. 2010;**41**(7):1431–39.

9. Martin C, von Elm E, El-Koussy M, Boltshauser E, Steinlin M; Swiss Neuropediatric Stroke Registry study group. Delayed diagnosis of acute ischemic stroke in children—a registry-based study in Switzerland. Swiss Med Wkly. 2011;**141**:w13281.

10. Srinivasan J, Miller SP, Phan TG, Mackay MT. Delayed recognition of initial stroke in children: need for increased awareness. Pediatrics. 2009;**124**(2):e227–34.

11. Yock-Corrales A, Mackay MT, Mosley I, Maixner W, Babl FE. Acute childhood arterial ischemic and hemorrhagic stroke in the emergency department. Ann Emerg Med. 2011;**58**(2):156–63.

12. Yock-Corrales A, Babl FE, Mosley IT, Mackay MT. Can the FAST and ROSIER adult stroke recognition tools be applied to confirmed childhood arterial ischemic stroke? BMC Pediatr. 2011;**11**:93.

13. Mackay MT, Chua ZK, Lee M, Yock-Corrales A, Churilov L, Monagle P, et al. Stroke and nonstroke brain attacks in children. Neurology. 2014;**82**(16):1434–40.

14. Bigi S, Fischer U, Wehrli E, Mattle HP, Boltshauser E, Bürki S, et al. Acute ischemic stroke in children versus young adults. Ann Neurol. 2011;**70**(2):245–54.

15. Zimmer JA, Garg BP, Williams LS, Golomb MR. Age-related variation in presenting signs of childhood arterial ischemic stroke. Pediatr Neurol. 2007;**37**(3):171–75.

16. Rathore SS, Hinn AR, Cooper LS, Tyroler HA, Rosamond WD. Characterization of incident stroke signs and symptoms: findings from the atherosclerosis risk in communities study. Stroke. 2002;**33**(11):2718–21.

17. Mallick AA, Ganesan V, Kirkham FJ, Fallon P, Hedderly T, McShane T, et al. Childhood arterial ischaemic stroke incidence, presenting features and risk factors: a prospective population-based study. Lancet Neurol. 2014;**13**(1):35–43.

18. Steinlin M, Mackay MT. Emergency management of ischemic stroke in children. Curr Treat Options Neurol. 2015;**17**(5):349.

19. Bernard TJ, Goldenberg NA, Armstrong-Wells J, Amlie-Lefond C, Fullerton HJ. Treatment of childhood arterial ischemic stroke. Ann Neurol. 2008;**63**(6):679–96.

20. Amlie-Lefond C, Bernard TJ, Sébire G, Friedman NR, Heyer GL, Lerner NB, et al. Predictors of cerebral arteriopathy in children with arterial ischemic stroke: results of the International Pediatric Stroke Study. Circulation. 2009;**119**(10):1417–23.

21. Munot P, Crow YJ, Ganesan V. Paediatric stroke: genetic insights into disease mechanisms and treatment targets. Lancet Neurol. 2011. **10**(3):264–74.

22. Barnes C, Deveber G. Prothrombotic abnormalities in childhood ischaemic stroke. Thromb Res. 2006;**118**(1):67–74.

23. Barnes C, Newall F, Harvey AS, Monagle P. Thrombophilia interpretation in childhood stroke: a cautionary tale. J Child Neurol. 2004;**19**(3):218–19.

24. Sestito S, Ceravolo F, Concolino D. Anderson-Fabry disease in children. Curr Pharm Des. 2013;**19**(33):6037–45.

25. Fullerton HJ, Hills NK, Elkind MS, Dowling MM, Wintermark M, Glaser CA, et al. Infection, vaccination, and childhood arterial ischemic stroke: results of the VIPS study. Neurology. 2015;**85**(17):1459–66.

26. Husson B, Lasjaunias P. Radiological approach to disorders of arterial brain vessels associated with childhood arterial stroke-a comparison between MRA and contrast angiography. Pediatr Radiol. 2004;**34**(1):10–15.

27. **Jung S, Gilgen M, Slotboom J, El-Koussy M, Zubler C, Kiefer C**, et al. Factors that determine penumbral tissue loss in acute ischaemic stroke. Brain. 2013;**136**(Pt 12):3554–60.

28. **Miglioretti DL, Johnson E, Williams A, Greenlee RT, Weinmann S, Solberg LI**, et al. The use of computed tomography in pediatrics and the associated radiation exposure and estimated cancer risk. JAMA Pediatr. 2013;**167**(8):700–707.

29. **Mathews JD, Forsythe AV, Brady Z, Butler MW, Goergen SK, Byrnes GB, Giles GG**, et al. Cancer risk in 680,000 people exposed to computed tomography scans in childhood or adolescence: data linkage study of 11 million Australians. BMJ. 2013;**346**:f2360.

30. **Mallick AA, Ganesan V, Kirkham FJ, Fallon P, Hedderly T, McShane T**, et al. Diagnostic delays in paediatric stroke. J Neurol Neurosurg Psychiatry. 2015;**86**(8):917–21.

31. **Riou EM, Amlie-Lefond C, Echenne B, Farmer M, Sébire G.** Cerebrospinal fluid analysis in the diagnosis and treatment of arterial ischemic stroke. Pediatr Neurol. 2008;**38**(1):1–9.

32. **Jauch EC, Saver JL, Adams HP Jr, Bruno A, Connors JJ, Demaerschalk BM, Khatri P**, et al. Guidelines for the early management of patients with acute ischemic stroke: a guideline for healthcare professionals from the American Heart Association/American Stroke Association. Stroke. 2013;**44**(3):870–947.

33. **Ronning OM, Guldvog B.** Should stroke victims routinely receive supplemental oxygen? A quasi-randomized controlled trial. Stroke. 1999;**30**(10):2033–37.

34. **Brush LN, Monagle PT, Mackay MT, Gordon AL.** Hypertension at time of diagnosis and long-term outcome after childhood ischemic stroke. Neurology. 2013;**80**(13):1225–30.

35. **Shah S, Murthy SB, Whitehead WE, Jea A, Nassif LM.** Decompressive hemicraniectomy in pediatric patients with malignant middle cerebral artery infarction: case series and review of the literature. World Neurosurg. 2013;**80**(1–2):126–33.

36. **Monagle P, Cochrane A, Roberts R, Manlhiot C, Weintraub R, Szechtman B**, et al. A multicenter, randomized trial comparing heparin/warfarin and acetylsalicylic acid as primary thromboprophylaxis for 2 years after the Fontan procedure in children. J Am Coll Cardiol. 2011;**58**(6):645–51.

37. **Roach ES, Golomb MR, Adams R, Biller J, Daniels S, Deveber G**, et al. Management of stroke in infants and children: a scientific statement from a Special Writing Group of the American Heart Association Stroke Council and the Council on Cardiovascular Disease in the Young. Stroke. 2008;**39**(9):2644–91.

38. **Goldenberg NA, Bernard TJ, Fullerton HJ, Gordon A, deVeber G; International Pediatric Stroke Study Group**. Antithrombotic treatments, outcomes, and prognostic factors in acute childhood-onset arterial ischaemic stroke: a multicentre, observational, cohort study. Lancet Neurol. 2009;**8**(12):1120–7.

39. **Stence NV, Fenton LZ, Goldenberg NA, Armstrong-Wells J, Bernard TJ.** Craniocervical arterial dissection in children: diagnosis and treatment. Curr Treat Options Neurol. 2011;**13**(6):636–48.

40. **Markus HS, Hayter E, Levi C, Feldman A, Venables G, Norris J**, et al. Antiplatelet treatment compared with anticoagulation treatment for cervical artery dissection (CADISS): a randomised trial. Lancet Neurol. 2015;**14**(4):361–67.

41. **Bernard TJ, Fenton LZ, Apkon SD, Boada R, Wilkening GN, Wilkinson CC**, et al. Biomarkers of hypercoagulability and inflammation in childhood-onset arterial ischemic stroke. J Pediatr. 2010;**156**(4):651–56.

42. **Eleftheriou D, Ganesan V, Hong Y, Klein NJ, Brogan PA**. Endothelial injury in childhood stroke with cerebral arteriopathy: a cross-sectional study. Neurology. 2012;**79**(21):2089–96.

43. **Buerki SE, Grandgirard D, Datta AN, Hackenberg A, Martin F, Schmitt-Mechelke T**, et al. Inflammatory markers in pediatric stroke: An attempt to better understanding the pathophysiology. Eur J Paediatr Neurol. 2016;**20**(2):252–60.

44. **Mineyko A, Narendran A, Fritzler ML, Wei XC, Schmeling H, Kirton A**. Inflammatory biomarkers of pediatric focal cerebral arteriopathy. Neurology. 2012;**79**(13):1406–8.

45. **Cantez S, Benseler SM**. Childhood CNS vasculitis: a treatable cause of new neurological deficit in children. Nat Clin Pract Rheumatol. 2008;**4**(9):460–61.

46. **Elkind MS, Hills NK, Glaser CA, Lo WD, Amlie-Lefond C, Dlamini N**, et al. Herpesvirus Infections and Childhood Arterial Ischemic Stroke: results of the VIPS Study. Circulation. 2016;**133**(8):732–41.

47. **Rodrigues FB, Neves JB, Caldeira D, Ferro JM, Ferreira JJ, Costa J**. Endovascular treatment versus medical care alone for ischaemic stroke: systematic review and meta-analysis. BMJ. 2016;**353**:i1754.

48. **Amlie-Lefond C, deVeber G, Chan AK, Benedict S, Bernard T, Carpenter J**, et al. Use of alteplase in childhood arterial ischaemic stroke: a multicentre, observational, cohort study. Lancet Neurol. 2009;**8**(6):530–36.

49. **Ellis MJ, Amlie-Lefond C, Orbach DB**. Endovascular therapy in children with acute ischemic stroke: review and recommendations. Neurology. 2012;**79**(13 Suppl 1):S158–64.

50. **Dulcey-Husi A, Datta A, Fluss J, Hackenberg A, Meier O, Poloni C**, et al. Thrombolysis and thrombectomy in children with acute ischemic stroke. Neuropediatrics. 2016;**47**:FV02-08.

51. **Andrew M, Vegh P, Johnston M, Bowker J, Ofosu F, Mitchell L**. Maturation of the hemostatic system during childhood. Blood. 1992;**80**(8):1998–2005.

52. **Monagle P, Barnes C, Ignjatovic V, Furmedge J, Newall F, Chan A**, et al. Developmental haemostasis. Impact for clinical haemostasis laboratories. Thromb Haemost. 2006;**95**(2):362–72.

53. **Studer M, Boltshauser E, Capone Mori A, Datta A, Fluss J, Mercati D, Hackenberg A**, et al. Factors affecting cognitive outcome in early pediatric stroke. Neurology. 2014;**82**(9):784–92.

54. **Ganesan V, Ng V, Chong WK, Kirkham FJ, Connelly A**. Lesion volume, lesion location, and outcome after middle cerebral artery territory stroke. Arch Dis Child. 1999;**81**(4):295–300.

55. **Kornfeld S, Delgado Rodríguez JA, Everts R, Kaelin-Lang A, Wiest R, Weisstanner C**, et al. Cortical reorganisation of cerebral networks after childhood stroke: impact on outcome. BMC Neurol. 2015;**15**:90.

56. **Fullerton HJ, Wintermark M, Hills NK, Dowling MM, Tan M, Rafay MF**, et al. Risk of Recurrent Arterial Ischemic Stroke in Childhood: a prospective international study. Stroke. 2016;**47**(1):53–59.

Chapter 14

Acute treatment

Svetlana Lorenzano and Danilo Toni

Causes of stroke in the young are heterogeneous, ranging from easily identifiable causes related to traditional vascular risk factors to more uncommon and atypical causes (1). Advances in stroke diagnostic workups, particularly neuroimaging, and screening for cardiac disease, coagulation defects, and novel risk factors may have a significant impact on the profile of stroke in young adults. However, there may still be uncertainties in the diagnostic evaluation, even considering the higher chance of stroke mimics in younger patients compared to older ones, in the cause-specific management, and on whether uncommon aetiologies may benefit from specific acute treatments (1–3). This may have an impact on a timely delivery of treatment in the emergency setting where peculiar cases and off-label situations may be faced and where decision-making process for the optimal acute treatment may be challenging.

In general, acute treatment of young adult stroke patients is similar to that of older patients. Unfortunately, young patients have been underrepresented in clinical trials on acute treatment. However, it is possible to extrapolate data and draw some conclusions on some aspects of the acute treatment of young stroke, particularly for intravenous thrombolysis (IVT) and decompressive hemicraniectomy.

General acute treatment

Recommendations for general management of blood pressure (BP), body temperature, glucose, and oxygenation are essentially the same as those for older stroke patients (4). BP management in the acute setting is nevertheless controversial. A recent study from the Helsinki Young Stroke Registry focused on the relationship between BP and long-term outcome in 1004 patients with a first-ever acute ischaemic stroke (IS) (mean age of 44 years; 63% males) of whom 39% had previous hypertension and 36% were on antihypertensive treatment. Systolic BP (SBP), diastolic BP (DBP), and mean arterial pressure at baseline and at 24 hours were significantly higher in patients with recurrent stroke compared to those without, during a median follow-up period of 8.9 years. For SBP of 160 mmHg or greater, the hazard ratio (HR) was 3.3 (95% confidence interval (CI), 2.05–4.55), P <0.001); for DBP of 100 mmHg or greater, the HR was 3.2 (95% CI, 2.36–4.09, P <0.001). In multivariate analysis, higher admission SBP, DBP, pulse pressure, and mean arterial pressure were independently associated with the risk of recurrent stroke (after adjustment for age, sex, previous transient ischaemic attack, type 1 and type 2 diabetes mellitus, obesity, hyperlipidaemia, and current smoking), whereas the 24-hour BP levels were not (5). These findings are consistent with what has been observed in older patients, suggesting that, also in young patients a careful lowering of acute BP may have a crucial impact on long-term prognosis.

Similarly to older patients, young patients with stroke benefit from access to stroke centres, preferably to expert comprehensive stroke centres with neuro-critical care units in order to guarantee aggressive management when indicated.

Intravenous thrombolysis

The response to IVT with tissue plasminogen activator (tPA) by age categories has always been an issue to address. The pivotal trials (NINDS, ECASS I, ECASS II, ATLANTIS) (6) showed that age itself is the most significant independent risk factor for stroke-associated mortality, mainly because elderly people are more prone to complications and have more comorbidity than their younger counterparts. In these trials, parenchymal haematoma type 2 correlated not only with treatment but also with age (6).

Age greater than 80 years has therefore been considered a relative exclusion criterion for safety reasons, namely haemorrhagic transformation of the infarct in biologically frail elderly subjects. However, according to randomized controlled trials (RCTs), an upper age limit is no longer justified (7, 8).

For younger patients below 18 years, US Food and Drug Administration and European Medicines Agency labels emphasize that the use of tPA in children and adolescents is not indicated because safety and effectiveness in this age category have not been established. Indeed, only a few case reports and single case series of children and adolescents receiving intravenous (IV) or intra-arterial (IA) thrombolysis for acute IS have been published. Moreover, the Thrombolysis in Pediatric Stroke Study (TIPS), a multi-institutional, multidisciplinary trial aiming to determine safety, best dose, and feasibility of IV tPA in children with acute IS, was interrupted due to problems in recruiting patients (9). Based on data from the US Nationwide Inpatient Sample, despite the absence of clear evidence, thrombolytic therapy is being administered to children (10).

No trial on thrombolytic therapy in young adult stroke patients has been conducted and most published sub-analyses by age have used 80 years of age as a cut-off (11–13). The comparison between 80 years or older and younger than 80 years does not allow any conclusion on young patients aged 18 to 45–55 years. Therefore, data on the young can be derived only from very few published sub-analyses from RCTs or observational studies.

The NINDS trial showed that patients aged 60 years or younger benefit from IV thrombolysis more than older patients, irrespective of the baseline stroke severity. However, no age threshold for benefit was demonstrated (14).

A Finnish single-centre cohort study (48 patients 16–49 years vs 96 older control subjects) (15) and a Canadian multicentre study (CASES, Canadian Alteplase for Stroke Effectiveness Study) (99 patients ≤50 years vs 1021 patients of >50 years) (16), did not find statistically significant differences in terms of functional excellent outcome (modified Rankin Scale (mRS) score 0–1) compared with the older counterparts (40% vs 48%, $P=0.343$ and 50% vs 35.5% with an adjusted risk ratio of 1.24 (95% CI 0.85–1.84), respectively) (15, 16). However, it seems that there is an inverse relationship between age and the probability of achieving an excellent outcome, and for each decade older this probability falls by 6.3%, after taking into account baseline neurological severity, early ischaemic radiological signs, admission blood glucose levels, onset-to-treatment time, and gender (16). In the Canadian CASES, mortality was statistically significantly decreased in young patients treated with IVT, after adjustment for gender, baseline National Institutes of Health Stroke Scale (NIHSS) score, and blood glucose levels (10.2% vs 23.5%; risk ratio 0.40, 95% CI 0.18–0.89) (16). Conversely, the Finnish study found no significant difference in the risk of death between younger and older patients, albeit with a trend towards a statistical significance (0 vs 7%; $P=0.095$) (15). The risk of symptomatic intracerebral haemorrhage (SICH) in the young was consistently comparable to that observed in the older counterparts in both CASES and Finnish studies (3.0% vs 4.7%, $P=0.62$ and 0 vs 3%, $P=0.551$, respectively), although in the latter study no SICH occurred in the young patients (15, 16). Younger patients tend to have a higher rate of protocol violations, a shorter median length of hospitalization after their stroke, and a greater chance to be discharged directly home (16).

Other small studies on acute stroke care and IVT in the young have been published (17, 18). Overall, the few young patients treated in each of these studies make translating their results into daily clinical practice quite difficult.

More reliable evidence comes from a post-hoc analysis of the Safe Implementation of Thrombolysis in Stroke–International Stroke Thrombolysis Register (SITS-ISTR) (19). This analysis included 3246 patients aged 18–50 years (median age 45 years) treated with IVT within 4.5 hours. Compared with the older patients, young patients were more likely to be women, current smokers, and functionally independent prior to the index stroke, whereas classical vascular risk factors such as hypertension, diabetes mellitus, hyperlipidaemia, atrial fibrillation, congestive heart failure, and previous IS, as well as previous antiplatelet treatment, were significantly less prevalent. Furthermore, neurological deficit at baseline measured by the NIHSS was less severe and blood glucose and BP levels at admission were lower in young patients. Young patients tend to have more strokes from other determined aetiology or from undetermined aetiology (including multiple causes) and less large vessel disease and cardioembolic strokes than do patients aged greater than 50 years.

The SITS-ISTR data showed that functional independence, mortality and SICH differ between two age groups in favour of younger patients. Patients aged 50 years or less had a higher functional independence (mRS 0–2) at 3 months as compared to those aged greater than 50 years (72.1% vs 54.5%; adjusted odds ratio (OR) 1.61, 95% CI 1.43–1.80; $P <0.001$). No or minimal disability (mRS 0–1) at 3 months was significantly more frequent in young patients (52% vs 38.6%; adjusted OR 1.26, 95% CI 1.14–1.39, $P <0.001$). A mRS score of 0–1 is likely a more appropriate target in young patients, because it indicates an ability to return to working activities.

Patients aged 50 years or less had lower 3-month mortality (4.9% vs 14.4%, adjusted OR 0.49, 95% CI 0.40–0.60, $P <0.001$). They also had lower SICH rates by any definition, that is, from any ICH (SICH by NINDS definition: 3.8% vs 7.8%, OR 0.77 (95% CI 0.62–0.95), $P=0.01$) to the more severe symptomatic ICH (SICH by ECASS definition: 2.2% vs 5.4%, OR 0.67 (95% CI 0.51–0.89), $P=0.005$; SICH by SITS-MOST definition: 0.6% vs 1.9%, OR 0.53 (95% CI 0.31–0.90), $P=0.02$).

When 10-year age bands were considered (i.e. ranges ≤30, 31–40, 41–50, and >50 years), an increase in functional dependence, mortality, and SICH rates with increasing age was observed, with the steepest change of SICH rates after 50 years. This highlights the higher clinical advantage of IVT in younger patients compared to the older ones, also in terms of safety. Based on the SITS-ISTR data, the risk of SICH should be considered a minor concern in young individuals, whatever definition of SICH is adopted, either the more inclusive but clinically less significant according to NINDS criteria or the less inclusive but clinically more meaningful according to ECASS and SITS-MOST definitions.

When the NIHSS score was trichotomized as 0–7, 8–14, and greater than 14 points, the difference between younger and older patients was highly significant for mortality and functional independence across the NIHSS subgroups ($P <0.0001$), whereas for SICH/SITS-MOST the difference increases over an NIHSS value of 8. Therefore, the worse the initial deficit, the higher the clinical gain for young patients as compared to older ones.

It seems that independent predictive variables for all outcome measures are shared between young and old and are similar to those in the overall population of SITS-ISTR, with the exception of those variables with low prevalence in the young age category, such as elevated baseline DBP, diabetes mellitus, congestive heart failure, and antiplatelet treatment other than aspirin. In young patients, NIHSS score at baseline was an independent predictor of SICH, and SBP was independently associated with larger and more severe SICH (SITS-MOST definition). Baseline NIHSS score and serum glucose levels and signs of current infarction on the pre-treatment imaging scans were related to both independence and mortality at 3 months. SBP, previous stroke, and age were other predictors of independence at 3 months. Increased mortality was also independently associated with male gender, as it has been also observed in other studies, and with atrial fibrillation, stressing the prognostic relevance of this heart arrhythmia even among young patients despite its low prevalence in this age group. Treatment response appeared not to be affected by stroke subtype, which is reassuring concerning safety and efficacy of IVT in stroke with uncommon aetiologies.

How strongly good outcome is due to young age rather than to thrombolytic treatment is difficult to assess. Some variables influencing outcome in young patients, but usually not captured by clinical studies, may be the lower burden of significant medical and vascular comorbidities, better brain plasticity, more aggressive medical care, decreased risk, or higher chance of recovery from in-hospital complications; lower chance to be exposed to potential medical complications of institutionalized long-term care; and more family and social support (16). Moreover, data on outcome measures particularly important for young individuals, such as cognitive function, post-stroke depression, and psychosocial factors, are usually not specifically collected and should be investigated in future studies (16).

Endovascular treatment

Also in this setting, age represents an issue to consider in order to fully evaluate the response to the endovascular approach. But as for IVT, the discussion has mainly focused on the elderly. Reliable results from well-designed trials showing the efficacy and safety of endovascular treatment (i.e. thrombectomy) for acute IS have recently been published (7).

These five RCTs on endovascular treatment (MR CLEAN, ESCAPE, EXTEND-IA, SWIFT-PRIME, and REVASCAT) (20–24) achieved results of both statistical significance and clinical relevance by showing consistent efficacy and safety of mechanical thrombectomy, mainly when given after IV tPA in comparison with tPA alone.

In general, although these trials examined anterior circulation, their results can be extrapolated to posterior circulation strokes as well. Therefore, mechanical thrombectomy is recommended within 6 hours of stroke onset in patients with major intracerebral occlusions as bridging therapy or when they do not respond to or cannot be treated with IVT (7, 8, 25).

Most participants of the five positive endovascular treatment RCTs were in their mid 60s to early 70s. Results on outcome measures were adjusted for prognostic factors including age. Subgroup analyses by age performed in some of these trials, again used 80 (MR CLEAN, ESCAPE, EXTEND-IA) (20–22) or 70 (SWIFT-PRIME, REVASCAT) (23, 24) years as a cut-off for the stratification for age. However, because of the low number of young patients in these trials, results were not separately analysed or reported specifically for young patients. Therefore, the magnitude of benefit of mechanical thrombectomy in the young is currently unknown.

Some single-centre observational studies focused on the safety and benefits of endovascular treatment in young patients. One single-centre study, the RECOST (Prognostic Factors related to Clinical Outcome Following Thrombectomy in Ischaemic Stroke) study (26), evaluated benefit and safety of endovascular treatment in acute IS with an anterior circulation major-vessel occlusion within 6 hours depending on age classes less than 50 years, 50–59, 60–69, 70–79, and greater than 80 years. An Alberta Stroke Program Early CT Score (ASPECTS) of 5 or greater on diffusion-weighted imaging sequences and an NIHSS score of 8 or higher were the only pre-specified inclusion criteria of the study. Overall, 165 patients were enrolled; the mean age was 67.4 years (range 29–90). The mean baseline NIHSS score was 17.2 (range 3–27) and was slightly lower in the younger age groups (16.4 in <50 years and 15.2 in 50–59 years vs 16.5 in 60–69 years, 17.8 in 70–79 years, and 18.8 in >80 years). There was no significant difference in Thrombolysis in Cerebral Infarction (TICI) 2b/3 recanalization rate or in peri/post-procedural complication rate between young and old patients, although patients younger than 50 years tended to have a lower risk of complications than older patients. There was a graded prognosis dependent on age with a cut-off at 70 years, that is, patients younger than 70 years benefited the most from acute mechanical recanalization in anterior circulation stroke. However, no substantial differences between endovascular therapy alone and combined treatment across the age categories was observed. The mean age of patients with good outcome (mRS 0–2) was 61.5 years. In addition, 90% of elderly patients who were considered to have protocol deviations on initial diffusion-weighted imaging–magnetic resonance imaging (high initial necrotic core with ASPECT <5) demonstrated a bad outcome at 3 months. On the contrary, we observed a good outcome for diffusion-weighted imaging–magnetic resonance imaging protocol deviation (ASPECTS <5) in 60% of patients younger than 70 years, suggesting that younger patients may still benefit from acute recanalization despite more extensive initial necrotic cores (26).

Stroke-volume threshold for endovascular treatment eligibility should probably be adjusted to the patient's age, and probably could be even very high in the young patient category.

Other small, retrospective, single-centre studies evaluating patients with IS aged 18–35 years or less than 55 years and admitted within 6–8 hours of symptom onset, suggest that a favourable outcome can be achieved (27–29). In these studies, mean age ranged from 26 to 45 years and mean NIHSS score ranged from 13 to 14. Recanalization in terms of Thrombolysis in Myocardial Infarct (TIMI) score of 2/3 was achieved in most patients (83–93%) independent of the systems used and was related to a better short-term (3 months) outcome. Favourable outcome (mRS 0–2 or 0–3) at 3 months ranged from 62.5% to 77.5% and mortality from 0% to 7.5%. Peri- or post-procedural complications occurred in very few patients, while SICH occurred in 2.2–9.5% of cases. In one of these studies, independence (mRS 0–2) at long-term follow-up (approximately 29 months), was observed regardless of whether recanalization was obtained or not, and there were no deaths (28).

These data support a strategy of aggressive intervention in young patients with acute IS and large vessel occlusion. A more effective collateral blood supply, more vascular reserve, less rapid infarct progression, lower baseline disability, lower rate of comorbidities, and in-hospital complications may be mechanisms underlying better prognosis of young stroke patients (26). Moreover, less tortuous arterial anatomy, relative lack of underlying vessel atherosclerosis and calcification, potentially more robust vascular wall, and a baseline quality of health that allows a better tolerability of procedural stresses, may facilitate endovascular intervention and potentially reduce procedural complications in young patients (29). It is still not clear whether in the long term, the advantages of youth may complement or replace the short-term benefit of recanalization (28).

Further sub-analyses on young patients from the recently published RCTs or larger prospective studies focused on young patients treated with endovascular therapy are indicated.

Reperfusion/recanalization therapy in peculiar cases in young stroke patients

Intravenous thrombolysis in stroke due to craniocervical dissection

Craniocervical arterial dissection (CAD) is one of the causes of stroke in young adult (10–25% of ISs <50 years), occurring spontaneously, but also related to trauma or sudden neck movement such as chiropractic neck manipulation or vigorous exercise (30).

RCTs on thrombolysis did not exclude patients with CAD but did not specifically investigate this particular group. CAD is not an exclusion criterion for IVT according to the product characteristics of alteplase, but may be seen as such by less experienced clinicians, particularly for fear of haemorrhagic transformation and intramural haematoma enlargement (7).

In the SITS-ISTR analysis, although not specifically noted, the subgroup with stroke of other determined aetiology probably includes also arterial dissection. Therefore, outcome by stroke subtype from SITS-ISTR indirectly confirms that withholding of IVT in stroke due to CAD is not justified, although efficacy is not proven due to the observational nature of SITS-ISTR (19).

A meta-analysis pooled individual patient data from available retrospective series (n=14) or case reports (n=22) on CAD-related stroke treated with thrombolysis (31). Overall, 180 patients with CAD (carotid artery n=131, basilar artery n=48, both arteries n=1) treated with IVT (n=121, 67%) or IA (n=59, 33%) were included. Patients were predominantly females, with a mean (SD) age of 46 (11) years, a median NIHSS score of 16, and were treated within a median onset-to-treatment time of 165 minutes (interquartile range, 125–225). The 121 patients with CAD receiving IVT were compared with 170 matched controls with stroke from all causes treated with IVT in SITS-ISTR. No relevant differences were observed (3-month mRS 0–2: 58.2% vs 52.2%; SICH defined as any ICH associated with any clinical deterioration: 3.3% vs 5.9%; mortality: 6.7% vs 8.8%) (31). When all patients treated with both IV and IA thrombolysis were considered, vertebral artery dissection was significantly associated with excellent functional outcome (mRS 0–1) compared with carotid artery dissection after adjustment for stroke severity (OR 3.94, 95% CI 1.40–11.12, P=0.01), but not with favourable outcome (mRS 0–2). However, the small numbers included in this meta-analysis do not allow drawing definite conclusions on possible differences in outcome between these two subgroups of CAD. Larger studies would be needed to better understand whether a different, more aggressive therapeutic approach is required for vertebral and carotid artery dissection-related stroke (31).

In general, placebo-controlled trials on thrombolysis in patients presenting with IS due to cervical artery dissection do not seem to be ethical anymore. The meta-analysis of individual data suggests that IVT is safe and should not be denied to these patients (7, 31).

Thrombolysis in menstruating women

In the setting of acute stroke treatment in young adults, particular situations could be faced, such as that of a menstruating woman potentially eligible for thrombolysis, since active bleeding is a contraindication for thrombolytic treatment. However, the limited data available in literature on 31 patients (six with acute IS and 25 treated with tPA and/or streptokinase for myocardial infarction or deep venous thrombosis), show that tPA may be safely administered in menstruating women (32). Five of the menstruating women with IS, were treated in the NINDS trial. In only one of these cases, persistent vaginal bleeding, tachycardia, and mild hypotension led to tPA discontinuation, blood transfusion, and uterine artery embolization. Transfusion due to increased menstrual flow became necessary also for three (one treated for acute stroke) of the remaining 26 cases reported in literature. Indeed, bleeding may increase after thrombolytic treatment and may require blood transfusion, particularly at the beginning of menstruation or if the woman has a history of dysmenorrhea (7).

Available data suggest that thrombolytic therapy may be administered relatively safely in women who are menstruating and should not be withheld or delayed. The potential benefits of the treatment with IVT may outweigh the risks of serious bleedings in those women with recent or active menorrhagia in the absence of significant anaemia or hypotension (8). In patients with a history of recent or active vaginal bleeding causing a clinically significant anaemia, a consultation by a gynaecologist should be taken into account before a decision on thrombolytic treatment is made (8).

If the decision of treating a menstruating woman with IVT is made, the patient has to be informed adequately about the risks and possible transfusion should be considered (7). The degree of vaginal bleeding should be monitored for 24 hours after tPA administration (8).

Thrombolysis and endovascular treatment in pregnancy/puerperium

Another challenging situation in the management of acute stroke in young adult patients is pregnancy. Stroke in pregnancy is relatively rare, but it has been estimated to have a threefold increase in incidence compared with non-pregnant women. Although strokes during pregnancy/puerperium are mostly secondary to cerebral vein thrombosis, arterial occlusion has also been reported as a cause of cerebral infarctions (33). Stroke due to cerebral vein thrombosis often occurs at the time of delivery or postpartum, whereas arterial occlusion may occur at all times of pregnancy, although particularly in the first and third trimesters, for hypercoagulability state, venous stasis, and patent foramen ovale (33). tPA is a large molecule, does not cross the placenta, and has no teratogenic effects in animal models (33). It can, however, act on the placenta with a potential risk of maternal and fetal complications such as premature labour, placenta detachment, fetal death, or postpartum haemorrhage (33).

There are no specific large or controlled studies regarding the efficacy and safety of thrombolytic therapy in pregnant women (34, 35), since pregnancy and the immediate postpartum period have generally been excluded from clinical trials because of the concern of an increased risk of maternal and fetal haemorrhage. However, case reports on the use of IV or IA thrombolysis during pregnancy, even during the first trimester, for various thromboembolic diseases, mainly pulmonary embolism but also for stroke, have been published; a systematic review of 172 of these cases reported bleeding complications in 8% of cases (7, 8, 33, 36).

The largest stroke study on acute reperfusion therapy in pregnancy/postpartum period is a retrospective analysis of the Get-With-The Guidelines database (37). In this study, 40 women among those receiving some form of acute reperfusion treatment were pregnant or in the postpartum period. Overall, 15 received IV tPA monotherapy only (4.4% (15/338) vs 7.9% (1913/24,303) of non-pregnant women; P=0.03). There was a trend towards increased SICH (i.e. any ICH associated with any clinical deterioration) in pregnant/postpartum versus non-pregnant tPA-treated patients (7.5% vs 2.6%, P=0.06) with only one case among those treated with IV tPA alone (6.7%). Patients with stroke during pregnancy/postpartum treated with any form of acute reperfusion therapy had no cases of major systemic bleeding or in-hospital deaths and had similar rates of discharge to home and disability (i.e. independent ambulation at discharge) as did their non-pregnant counterparts (37).

Literature also reports case series of pregnant women with stroke treated with IV or IA thrombolysis. In a series of 12 patients, 11 in the first or second trimester and one in the third trimester of pregnancy, six were treated with IVT and six received IA treatment (7, 8, 33, 38). Among the six patients treated with IVT, four had a good outcome; one patient had a minor intrauterine haematoma that was successfully evacuated, one had a buttock haematoma that was managed conservatively, and one patient died by a massive cerebral infarction due to arterial dissection during subsequent angioplasty, not clearly related to the use of IV. Fetal outcome was good in four cases and there were two elective abortions (7, 8, 33, 38).

Of the six patients treated with IA thrombolysis, two received IA tPA, one IA urokinase, and three received local urokinase, two of whom had a cerebral sinus thrombosis. Two patients had haemorrhagic complications (haematoma in the basal ganglia, asymptomatic intracerebral haemorrhage) (36). Three women had healthy deliveries at term, one woman had an elective abortion, one pregnancy was terminated for medical reasons, and one patient had a fetal demise (7, 8, 33, 36).

Regarding endovascular treatment with the novel thrombectomy devices during pregnancy, two cases of 24- and 28-year old women were published, both under anticoagulant therapy for mitral valve replacement, one in the third trimester and another at 37 weeks of gestation. Both had M1 occlusion treated with a Penumbra device. No haemorrhagic events occurred and both patients had a favourable outcome at 6-month follow-up (mRS 0–2) (39).

Vascular wall changes that are common in pregnancy could increase the risk of vascular wall injury with devices. In theory, if the angiographic team is available on site and ready for the intervention, endovascular treatment with mechanical thrombectomy devices should limit any systemic bleeding risk, particularly uterine haemorrhage, if only a mechanical device is used and IA tPA avoided (38). However, the risk of SICH associated with reperfusion does not decrease (35). Radiation exposure to the fetus may be a concern, but the risk can be minimized with optimal protection (34).

There are many factors that might also influence the decision of whether IV tPA or endovascular treatment should be considered: timing of stroke-onset during the course of pregnancy, location of clot, availability of endovascular team, imaging findings, and other potential medical conditions (34, 35).

There is no definite evidence on the safety and efficacy of thrombolysis in the early postpartum period (<14 days after delivery). There are only two case reports of acute stroke reperfusion therapy in mothers in the early postpartum period, neither of whom received IV tPA (40, 41).

Overall, in most of these case series thrombolytic therapy in pregnancy resulted in favourable outcomes. Based on the currently available data, it could be concluded that women with acute stroke during pregnancy/puerperium should be referred to stroke centres where advanced technology and expertise for fetal and maternal care should be available (38). A scientific statement by the American Heart Association/American Stroke Association (AHA/ASA) highlights that treatment with IVT may be taken into account, particularly in case of moderate or severe stroke, if the expected benefits outweigh the increased risk of uterine bleeding (8). Rescue endovascular treatment may be considered, if indicated, in situations where no clinical improvement is observed after IVT (38).

In any case, as the experience is limited and fetal effects remain unproven, it is recommended to carefully weigh risks and benefits of the treatment for the patient and fetus on an individual basis, to discuss risks and benefits with the patient, and to consider a consultation by a gynaecologist and obstetrician (7, 8).

An international registry of patients may be particularly useful to obtain and provide information on the expected neurological benefit versus the possible risk of haemorrhage or other complications with thrombolysis during pregnancy (33).

Intravenous thrombolysis in stroke due to illicit drug use

Neither the US Food and Drug Administration or European Medicines Agency label of tPA nor the 2013 AHA/ASA guidelines make specific reference to IS secondary to drug use. Patients pertaining to this category are mostly young patients, although use of cocaine and other drugs is not restricted to the young age. Use of illicit drug, mainly cocaine, is a recognized risk factor for acute IS in young patients occurring in 9% of a young stroke population (8). Illicit drug use was the fifth most common cause of stroke in the Baltimore–Washington Young Stroke study of patients aged 18–44 years (8). In a population-based study conducted in 2005, it was observed that one in five stroke patients aged 18–54 years used illicit drugs, with 6.6% of patients using cocaine (8). This sub-group of stroke patients was, in most instances, excluded from participating in thrombolysis trials.

The largest available published retrospective series on the use of tPA within 3 hours of symptom onset in cocaine-associated IS comprised 29 patients who were compared with 75 tPA-treated patients with IS without drug use (42). Cocaine users were younger (median age 48), more frequently male, had higher initial DBP, but similar baseline NIHSS score. There were no significant differences between the two groups in outcome measures in terms of SICH (1.3% vs 0, P=1.0), favourable mRS score at discharge (mRS 0–2) (52% vs 50%, P=1.0), discharge disposition (inpatient rehabilitation or home) (72% vs 82.8%, P=0.319), or mortality (12% vs 3.4%, P=0.276). When patients with cocaine-associated stroke treated with tPA were compared with patients not treated with tPA (n=58), the first group had more severe strokes but no SICH, and the observed overall functional outcomes and mortality were similar between the two groups (42).

IS in subjects using amphetamine and marijuana has been also reported (8). No published data are available on the use of tPA in these patients.

Overall, limited data on thrombolysis in illicit drug-related IS are available. However, withholding treatment in otherwise eligible IS patients who have no other exclusion criteria seems not to be justified (8).

Decompressive hemicraniectomy

Patients with malignant middle cerebral artery infarction (MMI) are about 10 years younger than the average patients with IS. Only patients up to 60 years of age were included in the first RCTs on decompressive hemicraniectomy (DHC) (DECIMAL, DESTINY, HAMLET) (43). A pooled analysis of the three RCTs included 93 patients aged 18–60 years with space-occupying middle cerebral artery infarction treated within 48 hours after stroke onset, showed that DHC not only lowers mortality (survival: 78% vs 24%, pooled risk reduction 51% (95% CI 34–69)), but also improves long-term functional outcome (mRS ≤4: 75% vs 24%, pooled absolute risk reduction 51% (95% CI 34–69); mRS ≤3: 43% vs 21%, pooled absolute risk reduction 23% (95% CI 5–41)) (43). Surgery was beneficial (P <0.01) in all predefined subgroups including age less than 50 years and 50–60 years or greater. Number needed to treat (NNT) to avoid death (mRS 6) is 2, to avoid death or most severe disability (mRS 5 or 6) is 2, while the NNT to avoid death and most severe and moderately severe disability (mRS 4–6) is 4. The effect of surgery was highly consistent across the three trials and consistency was also observed between the results of the RCTs with comparative data from non-randomized studies. The results also seem to be reproducible in medical centres without previous experience with DHC (44). In younger patients, DHC is associated with more quality-adjusted life years than medical treatment is; as a consequence, utilization of DHC increased steadily in the last years, but the total numbers of procedures remained low (0.15–0.3%) (45).

After the final publication of HAMLET, two meta-analyses including different sets of patients from HAMLET were published (46, 47). Both meta-analyses were post hoc and not stratified by time since stroke onset. Mortality rates in patients treated before and after 48 hours of stroke onset in HAMLET differed significantly (45–47). Conversely, pooled data from DESTINY and DECIMAL show the same significant reduction of mortality, most severe disability, and severe disability at 12 months as the prospective pooled analysis did (43).

There are some uncertainties that need to be resolved. Regarding timing of surgery, early DHC is effective and there is no indication for a wait-and-see strategy (i.e. waiting for midline shift or further clinical deterioration) once the diagnosis of MMI has been made (45). Further uncertainties still remain regarding whether a functional outcome defined as mRS score of 4 may be considered 'favourable', and what degree of disability is still acceptable for the individual survivor of MMI, particularly for young patients (45). The mRS focuses more on disability derived by motor deficit but not on neuropsychological functions and quality of life (45). A systemic review on quality of life and outcome satisfaction of survivors after DHC reported that the majority of survivors and caregivers (76.6%) expressed satisfaction with quality of life despite severe disability (mRS 4–5) in more than 50% of those patients (45, 48). It is crucial that in the context of quality of life, special attention is given to the possible development of post-stroke depression, which unfortunately is still not treated sufficiently in many survivors of MMI (43, 45).

Although DCH is considered a live-saving procedure, still more than 20% of younger patients die despite surgery (43). This underlines the need for improving intensive care treatment of these patients. Implementation of hypothermia in patients who underwent DHC might reduce early mortality due to potential anti-oedematous and neuroprotective effects (45, 49).

In conclusion, young patients with large stroke, especially MMI, need an adequate evaluation, aggressive neurocritical care, monitoring of intracranial pressure, and early assessment for DHC. However, the decision should always be made on an individual basis and based on the willingness to accept survival with moderate or even severe disability. With DHC, the probability of survival increases from 28% to nearly 80% and the probability of survival with a mRS score of 3 or less doubles, but the probability of survival in a condition requiring assistance from others (mRS score of 4) increases more than ten times, although the risk of very severe disability (mRS score of 5) is not increased. Information about quality of life of survivors is essential for guiding treatment decisions (43).

Hopefully, ongoing and future trials will answer questions such as long-term outcome and quality of life, the importance of aphasia or other neuropsychological functions, the best timing of DHC, and the further reduction of early mortality (45).

Future perspectives and conclusions

Strategies directed towards raising awareness of stroke at young ages, teaching about young stroke and its risk factors, and warning signs should be promoted and/or implemented in schools, workplaces, the primary care physician's office, and media. In particular, websites and social media can allow networking for survivors to tell their stories, for supporting information, and for promoting research and educational activities (2).

Finally, due to under-representation of young patients in past trials, new RCTs focusing on this age group are needed to confirm the benefits of available acute stroke treatments. Indeed, more research is needed for reducing the burden of stroke in the young, through setting up multicentre collaborative research groups and national young stroke registries, for the identification of research priorities, facilitation of specific clinical trials on treatments and rehabilitative strategies for stroke in the young, and through development of protocols and guidelines that specifically focus on and optimize acute treatment of stroke in young adults (2).

References

1. **Singhal AB, Biller J, Elkind MS, Fullerton HJ, Jauch EC, Kittner SJ**, et al. Recognition and management of stroke in young adults and adolescents. Neurology. 2013;**81**:1089–97.

2. **Putaala J, Curtze S, Hiltunen S, Tolppanen H, Kaste M, Tatlisumak T.** Causes of death and predictors of 5-year mortality in young adults after first-ever ischemic stroke: the Helsinki young stroke registry. Stroke. 2009;**40**:2698–703.

3. **Ji R, Schwamm LH, Pervez MA, Singhal AB.** Ischemic stroke and transient ischemic attack in young adults: risk factors, diagnostic yield, neuroimaging, and thrombolysis. JAMA Neurol. 2013;**70**:51–57.

4. **Jauch EC, Saver JL, Adams HP.** Guidelines for the early management of patients with acute ischemic stroke. a guideline for healthcare professionals from the American Heart Association/American Stroke Association. Stroke. 2013;**44**:870–947.

5. **Mustanoja S, Putaala J, Gordin D, Tulkki L, Aarnio K, Pirinen J,** et al. Acute-phase blood pressure levels correlate with a high risk of recurrent strokes in young-onset ischemic stroke. Stroke. 2016;**47**:1593–98.

6. **Hacke W, Donnan G, Fieschi C, Kaste M, von Kummer R, Broderick JP,** et al. Association of outcome with early stroke treatment: pooled analysis of ATLANTIS, ECASS, and NINDS rt-PA stroke trials. Lancet. 2004;**363**:768–74.

7. **Toni D, Mangiafico S, Agostoni E, Bergui M, Cerrato P, Ciccone A,** et al. Intravenous thrombolysis and intra-arterial interventions in acute ischemic stroke: Italian Stroke Organisation (ISO)-SPREAD guidelines. Int J Stroke. 2015;1119–29.

8. **Demaerschalk BM, Kleindorfer DO, Adeoye OM, Demchuk AM, Fugate JE, Grotta JC,** et al. Scientific rationale for the inclusion and exclusion criteria for intravenous alteplase in acute ischemic stroke: a statement for healthcare professionals from the American Heart Association/American Stroke Association. Stroke. 2016;**47**:581–641.

9. **Rivkin MJ, deVeber G, Ichord RN, Kirton A, Chan AK, Hovinga CA,** et al. Thrombolysis in pediatric stroke study. Stroke. 2015;**46**:880–85.

10. **Janjua N, Nasar A, Lynch JK, Qureshi AI.** Thrombolysis for ischemic stroke in children: data from the nationwide inpatient sample. Stroke. 2007;**38**:1850–54.

11. **Toni D, Lorenzano S.** Intravenous thrombolysis with rt-PA in acute ischemic stroke patients aged older than 80 years in Italy. Cerebrovasc Dis. 2008;**25**:129–35.

12. **The IST-3 collaborative group.** The benefits and harms of intravenous thrombolysis with recombinant tissue plasminogen activator within 6 h of acute ischaemic stroke (the Third International Stroke Trial (IST-3)): a randomized controlled trial. Lancet. 2012;**379**:2352–63.

13. **Emberson J, Lees KR, Lyden P, Blackwell L, Albers G, Bluhmki E,** et al. Effect of treatment delay, age, and stroke severity on the effects of intravenous thrombolysis with alteplase for acute ischaemic stroke: a meta-analysis of individual patient data from randomised trials. Lancet. 2014;**384**:1929–35.

14. **The NINDS-tPA Stroke Study Group.** Generalized efficacy of tPA for acute stroke: subgroup analysis of the NINDS tPA stroke trial. Stroke. 1997;**28**:2119–25.

15. **Putaala J, Metso TM, Metso AJ, Mäkelä E, Haapaniemi E, Salonen O,** et al. Thrombolysis in young adults with ischemic stroke. Stroke. 2009;**40**:2085–91.

16. **Poppe AY, Buchan AM, Hill MD.** Intravenous thrombolysis for acute ischaemic stroke in young adult patients. Can J Neurol Sci. 2009; **36**:161–67.

17. **Ji R, Schwamm LH, Pervez MA, Singhal AB.** Ischemic stroke and transient ischemic attack in young adults. JAMA Neurol. 2013;**70**:51–57.

18. **Tancredi L, Martinelli Boneschi F, Braga M, Santilli I, Scaccabarozzi C, Lattuada P,** et al. Stroke care in young patients. Stroke Res Treat. 2013;**2013**:715380.

19. Toni D, Ahmed N, Anzini A, Lorenzano S, Brozman M, Kaste M, et al. Intravenous thrombolysis in young stroke patients Results from the SITS-ISTR. Neurology. 2012;**78**:880–87.

20. Berkhemer OA, Fransen PSS, Beumer D, van den Berg LA, Lingsma HF, Yoo AJ, et al. A Randomized trial of intraarterial treatment for acute ischemic stroke. N Engl J Med. 2015;**372**:11–20. [Erratum in N Engl J Med. 2015;**372**:394.]

21. Goyal M, Demchuk AM, Menon BK Eesa M, Rempel JL, Thornton J, et al. Randomized assessment of rapid endovascular treatment of ischemic stroke. N Engl J Med. 2015;**372**:1019–30.

22. Campbell BCV, Mitchell PJ, Kleinig TJ, Dewey HM, Churilov L, Yassi N, et al. Endovascular therapy for ischemic stroke with perfusion-imaging selection. N Engl J Med. 2015;**372**:1009–18.

23. Saver JL, Goyal M, Bonafe A, Diener HC, Levy EI, Pereira VM, et al. Stent-retriever thrombectomy after intravenous t-PA vs. t-PA alone in stroke. N Engl J Med. 2015;**372**:2285–95.

24. Jovin TG, Chamorro A, Cobo E, de Miquel MA, Molina CA, Rovira A, et al. Thrombectomy within 8 hours after symptom onset in ischemic stroke. N Engl J Med. 2015;**372**:2296–306.

25. Touma L, Filion KB, Sterling LH, Atallah R, Windle SB, Eisenberg MJ. Stent retrievers for the treatment of acute ischemic stroke. a systematic review and meta-analysis of randomized clinical trials. JAMA Neurol. 2016;**73**:275–81.

26. Danière F, Lobotesis K, Machi P, Eker O, Mourand I, Riquelme C, et al. Patient selection for stroke endovascular therapy-DWI-ASPECTS thresholds should vary among age groups: insights from the RECOST study. AJNR Am J Neuroradiol. 2015;**36**:32–39.

27. Singhal S, Sidhu N, El-Chalouhi N, Thakkar V, Tjoumakaris S. Acute stroke intervention in young patients. JHN Journal. 2013;**8**:Art. 5.

28. Mocco J, Tawk RG, Jahromi BS, Samuelson RM, Siddiqui AH, Hopkins LN, et al. Endovascular intervention for acute thromboembolic stroke in young patients: an ideal population for aggressive intervention? J Neurosurg. 2009;**110**:30–34.

29. Chalouhi N, Tjoumakaris S, Starke RM, Hasan D, Sidhu N, Singhal S, et al. Endovascular stroke intervention in young patients with large vessel occlusions. Neurosurg Focus. 2014;**6**(1):E6.

30. Putaala J, Metso AJ, Metso TM, Konkola N, Kraemer Y, Haapaniemi E, et al. Analysis of 1008 consecutive patients aged 15 to 49 with first-ever ischemic stroke: the Helsinki young stroke registry. Stroke. 2009;**40**:1195–203.

31. Zinkstok SM, Vergouwen MDI, Engelter ST, Lyrer PA, Bonati LH, Arnold M, et al. Safety and functional outcome of thrombolysis in dissection-related ischemic stroke a meta-analysis of individual patient data. Stroke. 2011;**42**:2515–20.

32. Wein TH, Hickenbottom SL, Morgenstern LB, Demchuk AM, Grotta JC. Safety of tissue plasminogen activator for acute stroke in menstruating women. Stroke. 2002;**33**:2506–508.

33. Tassi R, Acampa M, Marotta G, Cioni S. Systemic thrombolysis for stroke in pregnancy. Am J Emerg Med. 2013;**31**:448.e1–448.e3.

34. Selim MH, Molina CA. The use of tissue plasminogen activator in pregnancy. A taboo treatment or a time to think out of the box. Stroke. 2013;**44**:868–69.

35. **Broderick JP.** Should intravenous thrombolysis be considered the first option in pregnant women? Stroke. 2013;**44**:866–67.

36. **Cronin CA, Weisman CJ, Llinas RH.** Stroke treatment beyond the three-hour window and in the pregnant patient. Ann NY Acad Sci. 2008;**1142**:159–78.

37. **Leffert LR, Clancy CR, Bateman BT, Cox M, Schulte PJ, Smith EE,** et al. Treatment patterns and short-term outcomes in ischemic stroke in pregnancy or postpartum period. Am J Obstet Gynecol. 2016;**214**:723.e1–723.e11.

38. **Demchuk AM.** Yes, intravenous thrombolysis should be administered in pregnancy when other clinical and imaging factors are favorable. Stroke. 2013;**44**:864–65.

39. **Aaron S, Shyamkumar NK, Alexander S, Babu PS, Prabhakar AT, Moses V,** et al. Mechanical thrombectomy for acute ischemic stroke in pregnancy using the penumbra system. Ann Indian Acad Neurol. 2016;**19**:261–63.

40. **Rønning OM, Dahl A, Bakke SJ, Hussain AI, Deilkås E.** Stroke in the puerperium treated with intra-arterial rt-PA. J Neurol Neurosurg Psychiatry. 2010;**81**:585–86.

41. **Méndez JC, Masjuán J, García N, de Leciñana M.** Successful intra-arterial thrombolysis for acute ischemic stroke in the immediate postpartum period: case report. Cardiovasc Intervent Radiol. 2008;**31**:193–95.

42. **Martin-Schild S, Albright KC, Misra V, Philip M, Barreto AD, Hallevi H,** et al. Intravenous tissue plasminogen activator in patients with cocaine-associated acute ischemic stroke. Stroke. 2009;**40**:3635–37.

43. **Vahedi K, Hofmeijer J, Juettler E, Vicaut E, George B, Algra A,** et al. Early decompressive surgery in malignant infarction of the middle cerebral artery: a pooled analysis of three randomised controlled trials. Lancet Neurol. 2007;**6**:215–22.

44. **Lucas C, Thines L, Dumont F, Leclerc X, Riegel B, Cordonnier C,** et al. Decompressive surgery for malignant middle cerebral artery infarcts: the results of randomized trials can be reproduced in daily practice. Eur Neurol. 2012;**68**:145–49.

45. **Neugebauer H, Jüttler E.** Hemicraniectomy for malignant middle cerebral artery infarction: current status and future directions. Int J Stroke. 2014;**9**:460–67.

46. **Hofmeijer J, Kapelle LJ, Algra A, Amelink GJ, van Gijn J, van der Worp HB,** et al. Surgical decompression for space-occupying cerebral infarction (the Hemicraniectomy After Middle Cerebral Artery infarction with Life-threatening Edema Trial (HAMLET)): a multicentre, open, randomised trial. Lancet Neurol. 2009;**8**:326–33.

47. **Mitchell P, Gregson BA, Crossman J, Gerber C, Jenkins A, Nicholson C,** et al. Reassessment of the HAMLET study. Lancet Neurol. 2009;**8**:602–603.

48. **Rahme R, Zuccarello M, Kleindorfer D, Adeoye OM, Ringer AJ.** Decompressive hemicraniectomy for malignant middle cerebral artery territory infarction: is life worth living? J Neurosurg. 2012;**117**:749–54.

49. **Els T, Oehm E, Voigt S, Klisch J, Hetzel A, Kassubek J.** Safety and therapeutical benefit of hemicraniectomy combined with mild hypothermia in comparison with hemicraniectomy alone in patients with malignant ischemic stroke. Cerebrovasc Dis. 2006;**21**:79–85.

Chapter 15

Secondary prevention

José M. Ferro and Ana Catarina Fonseca

Stroke in the young adult has some epidemiological features which influence the management of secondary stroke prevention. There is a lower prevalence of classical stroke risk factors, such as hypertension, diabetes mellitus, hyperlipidaemia, and atrial fibrillation, than in older adults although their prevalence is higher than that expected in the general population of the same age (1–3). On the other hand, young adults have specific risk factors including pregnancy and puerperium, hormonal contraception, infections, trauma, and illicit drug use (4). Concerning ischaemic stroke subtypes, stroke due to atherosclerosis, small vessel disease, and atrial fibrillation is less common than in older adults while other determined causes (e. g. dissection) are more frequent (5).

There are only a few studies specifically analysing secondary stroke prevention in young adults (6–8). Young adults are under-represented in secondary stroke prevention clinical trials with antiplatelet drugs, anticoagulants, statins, and antihypertensive drugs. As a consequence, there are no specific guidelines regarding risk factors control in young patients. Recommendations for secondary prevention of ischaemic stroke in young adults are mainly extrapolated from data obtained from older individuals (9, 10).

There are two main points to address regarding secondary stroke prevention: (a) screening and control of vascular risk factors, and (b) identification and treatment of specific causes of ischaemic stroke.

Screening and control of vascular risk factors

Vascular risk factors can be divided into traditional and non-traditional risk factors. Young adults have a lower prevalence of traditional vascular risk factors such as hypertension, diabetes mellitus, or dyslipidaemia, but have particular risk factors such as pregnancy, hormonal contraception, or illicit drug use. Over the past years, traditional risk factors have been increasing and this is reflected in the increasing incidence of young stroke in developed countries (2).

Strategies to control modifiable vascular risk factors can be divided into pharmacological and non-pharmacological. Non-pharmacological treatments are important but are difficult to implement as they require a change in lifestyle. In this setting, multimodal strategies tend to be more effective than unimodal strategies.

Hypertension

Hypertension is one of the most prevalent risk factors for stroke in all age groups. A retrospective study of the outcome of young patients with ischaemic stroke found that high acute-phase blood pressure was independently associated with a high risk of recurrent stroke (11). There are no specific data regarding what target values of blood pressure should be achieved or which specific antihypertensive drug should be used for secondary ischaemic stroke prevention in young patients. Although many clinical trials included young patients, these patients were a minority. The recommendations therefore usually refer to patients in general. The Perindopril Protection Against Recurrent Stroke Study (PROGRESS) trial included young individuals, but the mean age was 64 years, and concluded that the combination of an angiotensin-converting enzyme inhibitor (perindopril) and a thiazide diuretic (indapamide) reduced recurrent stroke in patients with or without hypertension, defined as blood pressure higher than 160/90 mmHg, compared to double placebo (12). Treatment with perindopril (2–4 mg) and indapamide (2–2.5 mg) was associated with a reduction in mean blood pressure of 9 to 4 mmHg and a 4% absolute risk reduction in recurrent stroke. Patients treated with perindopril alone showed blood pressure reduction but had a risk of stroke similar to patients treated with placebo (12). The MOSES trial showed that an angiotensin receptor antagonist (eprosartan) could be more effective than a calcium channel blocker (nitrendipine) in reducing total mortality and all cardiovascular and cerebrovascular events, including all recurrent events (13). No clinical trials evaluated the effect of non-pharmacological interventions that reduce blood pressure for secondary prevention of ischaemic stroke. However, several lifestyle modifications have been shown to be associated with blood pressure reduction and should be considered. Examples of these lifestyle modifications include salt restriction, consumption of fruit and vegetables, regular physical activity, and weight reduction. The American Heart Association (AHA) guidelines (10), recommend that, after the first days of a transient ischaemic attack (TIA) or ischaemic stroke, hypertension should be treated if systolic blood pressure (SBP) is higher than 140 mmHg or diastolic blood pressure (DBP) is higher than 90 mmHg with a class of recommendation I and level of evidence B (I, B). There is uncertain benefit regarding treatment of lower blood pressure levels (IIb, C). It is recommended to reinitiate blood pressure treatment in all patients who were previously medicated with an antihypertensive drugs (I, A), aiming to achieve a blood pressure target of SBP lower than 140 mmHg or DBP lower than 90 mmHg (IIa, B). In lacunar stroke, it is considered reasonable to achieve a SBP of less than 130 mmHg (IIb, B) taking into accounts the results of the Secondary Prevention of Small Subcortical Strokes (SPS3) trial (14). The SPS3 trial excluded patients aged under 30 years.

Disorders of glucose metabolism and diabetes

In a study conducted with patients from the Helsinki Young Stroke Registry, diabetes mellitus previous to stroke was a risk factor for ischaemic stroke recurrence and other vascular events (15). The 'Follow-up of transient ischaemic attack and stroke patients and unelucidated risk factor evaluation' (FUTURE) study, which included young patients from the Netherlands, also showed that diabetes or impaired fasting glucose diagnosed after stroke is associated with recurrent vascular events (16). These data suggest that screening for diabetes or impaired fasting glucose in young patients is important for secondary prevention, namely in patients with higher age, other vascular risk factors, or with a family history of diabetes (16). It is recommended to screen for diabetes after stroke (IIa, C) (10). Determinations of HbA1c are probably more accurate as acute illness can cause temporary increases in fasting plasma glucose or in glucose oral tolerance tests. Diabetes should be managed with lifestyle modification and individualized pharmacological therapy according to the European Stroke Organization (ESO) guidelines (IV, good clinical practice (GCP)) (9). In a sub-analysis of the Prospective Pioglitazone Clinical Trial in Macrovascular Events (PROactive), pioglitazone was associated with a 47% relative risk reduction in recurrent stroke (hazard ratio (HR) 0.53; 95% confidence interval (CI) 0.34–0.85) (17). The Insulin Resistance Intervention After Stroke (IRIS) trial included patients above 40 years with insulin resistance but without diabetes, and evaluated the effectiveness of pioglitazone titrated to 45 mg for secondary stroke prevention. The risk of stroke was lower among patients who received pioglitazone than among those who received placebo. Pioglitazone was also associated with a lower risk of diabetes but with a higher risk of weight gain, oedema, and fracture than placebo (18).

Dyslipidaemia

The Stroke Prevention by Aggressive Reduction in Cholesterol Levels (SPARCL) trial included adults above 18 years with recent ischaemic stroke or intracranial haemorrhage and showed that 80 mg of atorvastatin reduced stroke recurrence compared with placebo (19). Patients with cardioembolic stroke were excluded from the SPARCL trial. In the Heart Protection Study that included patients aged 40–80 years old, simvastatin 40 mg/day reduced vascular events in patients with prior stroke compared to placebo (20). In a retrospective, observational study of 312 young patients with a first-ever ischaemic stroke of undetermined aetiology, those who used statin post stroke had lower rates of new vascular events (stroke, myocardial infarction, other arterial thrombosis, revascularization, or vascular death) in a long-term follow-up (21). There is currently no evidence supporting the use of statins in patients with cervical arterial dissections. The ESO recommends treatment with statins in subjects with non-cardioembolic stroke. The AHA guidelines (10) state that statin therapy is recommended to reduce the risk of stroke in patients with stroke of atherosclerotic origin and low-density lipoprotein cholesterol (LDL-C) level of 100 mg/dL or greater (I, B). A statin is also recommended if LDL-C level is less than 100 mg/dL (I, C). An important part of the recommendations include lifestyle modifications and diet changes (I, A) (10).

Obesity

Although obesity is an established risk factor for a first stroke, it has not been established as a risk factor for recurrent stroke. There are no clinical trials directly evaluating the association between weight reduction and risk of recurrent stroke. In a post hoc analysis of the Telemedical Project for Integrative Stroke Care (TEMPiS), obese patients had a lower risk of death and recurrent stroke (odds ratio 0.56, 95% CI 0.37–0.86) (22) than leaner patients. This study reproduced the results of another post hoc analysis of 20246 patients with a previous ischaemic stroke. The researchers found that obesity was not related to recurrent stroke risk, but obese patients with stroke were at lower overall vascular risk than their leaner counterparts (23). This association of obesity with improved prognosis after stroke has been termed the *obesity paradox*. Some authors suggest that the reduced risk of vascular events in obese patients may be due to high levels of treatment with antihypertensive drugs.

Patients admitted due to stroke should have an evaluation of their body mass index. Despite the uncertainty regarding the role of weight reduction in prevention of stroke recurrence, the AHA guidelines suggest that a weight loss programme may be beneficial for improvement of cardiovascular risk factors and useful for recent TIA or stroke (IIb, C) (10).

Nutrition

A nutritional assessment should be performed in patients with stroke (IIa, C) (10). Patients who have signs of undernutrition should be referred to individual nutritional counselling (I, B). Currently, there is no evidence for prescribing supplemental vitamins routinely to all patients (III, A). Dietary recommendations include reduction of sodium intake to less than 2.4 g/day or

1.5 g/day (IIa, C) and adoption of a Mediterranean type of diet (high in fruit, vegetables, and whole grains, with low-fat dairy products, and limitation of red meat intake).

Physical activity

Physical activity improves stroke risk factors, but no randomized clinical trials have directly evaluated the effectiveness of physical activity for secondary stroke prevention. Regular physical activity is recommended (IV, GCP). If the patient is capable of engaging in physical activity, three or four sessions per week with 40 minutes of moderate–vigorous intensity aerobic exercise are recommended (IIa, C). Also advised is a comprehensive behavioural-oriented programme (IIa, C) and supervision by a health care professional on at least the initiation of an exercise regimen (IIB, C) (10).

Sleep apnoea

Sleep apnoea is associated with an increased risk of hypertension, heart arrhythmias, and stroke in the young (24). It has also been shown that young patients with sleep apnoea have reduced cerebrovascular reactivity (25). There may be clues in the clinical history indicating sleep apnoea, such as snoring, day-time somnolence, obesity, and short neck. Lifestyle measures can be adopted to reduce sleep apnoea, such as losing weight, side sleeping instead of back sleeping, and stopping nightly alcohol or sedative intake, but the most effective treatment is continuous positive airway pressure (CPAP) (IIb, B) (10). CPAP therapy initiated on the first night after stroke seems to be feasible and not associated with neurological deterioration (26). However, in a clinical trial that compared the regular use of CPAP with usual care versus usual care alone (advice on healthful sleep habits and lifestyle changes to minimize sleep apnoea) in patients with moderate to severe sleep apnoea and established cardiovascular disease, the use of CPAP did not reduce the risk of recurrent vascular events, including stroke, as compared to usual care (27). This clinical trial included patients aged between 45 and 75 years.

Smoking

Smoking cessation should be recommended. Measures to support smoking cessation include counselling, nicotine replacement, and oral smoking cessation treatments. Studies in general show that although a high number of patients with a stroke attempt to stop smoking, only a few are successful in the long term (28). In one cohort of young stroke patients with ischaemic stroke, only 22% of patients gave up smoking in the long term (29). This suggests that interventions should be targeted at multiple points.

Illicit drug use

Cessation of intake of drugs including marijuana should be recommended.

Migraine

In patients with migraine who have an ischaemic stroke, treatment with triptans and ergots is contraindicated due to their vasoconstrictive effects.

Hormonal contraception

Hormonal contraception should be discontinued after stroke.

Identification and treatment of specific causes of ischaemic stroke

Cardioembolic stroke

Common causes of cardioembolic stroke found in the young include cardiomy-opathy, atrial myxomas, patent foramen ovale, ventricular wall hypokinesia and atrial fibrillation. Rheumatic heart disease has been progressively decreasing in developed countries due to timely treatment with antibiotics, but is still a leading disease in low- and middle-income countries (30). Infective endocar-ditis may be caused by intravenous drug use. Treatment recommendations for young patients are similar to those for older individuals (9, 10).

Atrial fibrillation

The European Atrial Fibrillation trial showed that anticoagulation with vita-min k antagonists (VKAs) (international normalized ratio (INR) 2.0–3.0) in patients with atrial fibrillation reduced the risk of stroke when compared with aspirin (31). Young patients over 25 years old were included in this trial. More recently, patients aged 18 years or older were included in the clinical trials which evaluated the new oral anticoagulants (NOACs) dabigatran (RELY) (32), rivar-oxaban (ROCKET-AF) (33), and apixaban (ARISTOTLE) (34) versus warfarin for prevention of stroke or systemic embolism in patients with non-valvular atrial fibrillation. The clinical trial that evaluated edoxaban in this clinical set-ting (ENGAGE–AF TIMI) (35) included patients aged 21 years or older. These trials showed that the NOACs were at least non-inferior to warfarin, therefore young patients with an ischaemic stroke or a TIA may be anticoagulated with VKAs (INR 2–3) or NOACs (9, 10). When compared to VKAs, the NOACs have the advantage of being administered in a fixed dose as the cytochrome P450 enzymes metabolize them less. VKAs have the disadvantage of needing fre-quent monitoring and dose adjustments and having a higher number of inter-actions with food and other drugs. The NOACs have a faster onset and offset of action than VKAs requiring a strict adherence to dose schedule. Currently, the NOACs do not have widely available monitoring tests. As young patients tend to have a more active lifestyle than older patients (e.g. frequently working, having children to care for), NOACs may have the advantage of freeing their time. An antidote for dabigatran (36) is already used in clinical practice. An antidote for anti-Xa anticoagulants has been shown to be effective in clinical trials, but is not yet available for general use (37).

Rheumatic heart disease

Rheumatic heart disease can lead to cardiac changes associated with an increased risk of stroke. The major cause of stroke in patients with rheumatic heart disease is atrial fibrillation, but mitral stenosis and infective and mechanical prosthetic valves can also cause ischaemic strokes. The effectiveness of antithrombotic therapy in mitral stenosis has not been examined in clinical trials. Nevertheless, there is general agreement that anticoagulation is indicated in mitral stenosis complicated by atrial fibrillation, prior embolism, or left atrial thrombus (10). Patients with valvular atrial fibrillation should be treated with VKAs aiming for an INR of 2.0–3.0 or of 2.5–3.5 when the patient has a mechanical prosthetic valve. In patients with ischaemic stroke who have rheumatic heart disease without atrial fibrillation, anticoagulation may be considered instead of treatment with antiplatelet drugs (IIb, C). In patients with rheumatic mitral valve disease who have an ischaemic stroke while being treated with adequate VKA therapy, aspirin might be added (IIb, C). A phase II clinical trial with dabigatran showed that this anticoagulant was not as effective as warfarin for the prevention of thromboembolic complication and was associated with an increased risk of bleeding in patients with mechanical heart valves (38). There is currently no indication for the use of NOACs in patient with valvular atrial fibrillation.

Dilated cardiomyopathy

In patients with ischaemic stroke in sinus rhythm with dilated cardiomyopathy (left ventricular ejection fraction $\leq35\%$) without evidence of intracardiac thrombus, the effectiveness of anticoagulation compared with antiplatelet therapy is uncertain, and the choice should be individualized (IIb, B). Patients with an intracardiac thrombus should be anticoagulated with a VKA for 3 months or more (I, C). Regarding anticoagulation, effectiveness of treatment with dabigatran, rivaroxaban, or apixaban is uncertain compared with VKA therapy for prevention of recurrent stroke.

Atrial myxomas

Cardiac myxoma is the most common primary cardiac tumour. It is usually located in the left atrium and tends to occur during the third to sixth decades of life. Long-term prognosis after total surgical resection is usually very good with sporadic reports of tumour recurrence (39).

Patent foramen ovale

Three randomized controlled trials (RCTs) compared patent foramen ovale (PFO) percutaneous closure versus medical therapy in patients with cryptogenic stroke or TIA. None of the trials proved that closure was superior to conservative treatment. It was also evident in all trials that the risk of recurrent stroke in PFO was very low (6–8). A Cochrane systematic review and meta-analysis (40) which included those three RCTs found that there was a high risk of bias in all the trials and that there was no risk reduction, neither for the primary outcome (recurrent stroke or TIA) nor stroke recurrence. A pooled analysis of individual participant data from 2303 patients (41) included in these three RCTs of PFO closure versus medical therapy in patients with cryptogenic stroke confirmed that closure was not significantly associated with the primary composite outcome (stroke, TIA, or death). There was no heterogeneity for subgroups namely patients with large shunts or associated atrial septal aneurysm. However, the difference between closure and conservative treatment became significant after covariate adjustment (HR 0.68; P=0.049). For the outcome recurrent stroke, all comparisons were significant, unadjusted and adjusted HRs being respectively 0.58 (P=0.043) and 0.58 (P=0.044). Atrial fibrillation was more common among closure patients in both the Cochrane and the individual participant data meta-analysis. Two RCTs of PFO closure (REDUCE and the CLOSE) are still ongoing. The REDUCE trial evaluates if PFO closure with the Septal Occluder/GORE® plus antiplatelet medication is safe and more effective than antiplatelet medication alone. The CLOSE trial is a three-arm trial comparing chronic anticoagulation, transcatheter closure, and antiplatelet therapy in preventing stroke recurrence.

Considering (a) that PFO is a condition with a very low risk of stroke recurrence, (b) the evidence from three negative trials, albeit with methodological limitations and insufficient sample size, and (c) two partially contradictory meta-analyses, what can be recommended? Our recommendation is that PFO closure should only be used in selected patients considering patient option, younger age, presence of deep venous thrombosis at stroke onset or of a large atrial septal aneurysm, and the risk of paradoxical embolism score (RoPE score) (42), which enables the calculation of the risk of recurrent stroke in individual patients and of the pathogenic role of PFO on the incident stroke, which is probable if the RoPE score is greater than 6 points.

If a patient with cryptogenic stroke and PFO under antiplatelet treatment suffers a recurrent stroke it is recommended to shift to oral anticoagulants or to close the PFO.

Stroke due to large artery atheroma

Secondary prevention of atherothrombotic stroke includes lifestyle modification, risk factors control, antihypertensive medication if the SBP is 140 mmHg or higher, or DBP is 90 mmHg or higher (IIb, C), statins even if LDL-cholesterol levels are below 100 mg/dL (IC), antiplatelet therapy, and surgery or endovascular treatment for severe symptomatic carotid stenosis.

Most of the large RCTs which demonstrated the efficacy of statins and antiplatelet drugs to prevent recurrent stroke and other vascular events excluded patients younger than 40–50 years. The mean age of included patients was above 55 years. So the recommendations concerning these treatments for younger stroke patients are extrapolations with limited external validity.

Dual antiplatelet treatment is only recommended for a short period, from day 1 to 21 after ischaemic stroke (IIb, B). Concerning the selection of antiplatelet drugs, the ESO (9) recommends as first line clopidogrel or the combination of low-dose aspirin with dipyridamole, and for second line low-dose aspirin alone or triflusal, where available. Cilostazol is commonly prescribed in Asian countries. Selection of the most appropriate antiplatelet drug for the individual patient must also consider contraindications, side effects, tolerability, interactions with other drugs, and costs.

Extracranial atheroma

Severe symptomatic stenosis of the internal carotid artery is associated with a high risk of recurrent stroke in particular during the days and weeks (up to 6 months) after the index stroke and also of myocardial infarction and vascular death. Severe carotid stenosis is a stenosis of greater than 70% measured by the NASCET method (43) on an angiography. If the stenosis is detected by ultrasound it is advisable to corroborate its severity by a repeated echo-Doppler performed by a different operator or by angiography (computed tomography, magnetic resonance or intra-arterial). Age is a risk factor for recurrent stroke in patients with recent symptomatic carotid stenosis of greater than 50%. Patients aged 30–40 are at lower risk than those aged 40–50, and the latter have a lower risk than older patients. Other risk factors which increase the risk of recurrence are the severity of the stenosis (up to near occlusion—99% with post-stenosis collapse of the arterial wall), irregular or ulcerated plaque, male sex, time since event, cerebral event (vs ocular), multiple events, major stroke, diabetes, hypertension, and previous myocardial infarction (44, 45).

Severe symptomatic carotid stenosis should be treated by endarterectomy (I, A) as soon as the patient is neurologically and systemically stable, preferably within 15 days of the index event (IIa, B). Women and patients with contralateral carotid occlusion benefit less from surgery. Carotid angioplasty and stenting (CAS) is an alternative for surgical endarterectomy (IIa, B). Angioplasty and stenting have a lower risk of myocardial infarction and of lower cranial nerve injury than endarterectomy, but have a higher periprocedural risk. Angioplasty/stenting is indicated when endarterectomy is not technically feasible (e.g. to high carotid bifurcation) or is contraindicated (e.g. severe cardiac, coronary, or pulmonary disease) and also in severe carotid stenosis due to radiation and in the rare event of symptomatic carotid restenosis after endarterectomy (IIa, B). Individual patient data meta-analysis from four RCTs comparing CAS with carotid surgery in patients with symptomatic stenosis showed that CAS had a higher risk for periprocedural HR for stroke and death higher but only in patients aged over 65 years (patients aged 65–69 years vs <60 years: HR 2.16; patients aged ≥70 years: 4.0). For carotid endarterectomy (CAE), there was no increased periprocedural risk by age group. The comparison of the two interventions (CAS vs CEA periprocedural risk) favoured CAE for patients aged 65–69 years (HR 1.61) and patients aged 70–74 years (HR 2.09), but the risk was similar for those patients younger than 65 years. For all ages the periprocedural event rate should be below 6% (I, B). Age is not associated with the postprocedural stroke risk for either procedure (46). Therefore, for younger patients the two procedures are equivalent (IIa, B).

Intracranial atheroma

Dual antiplatelet treatment may be used for a more extended period (up to 90 days) if there is severe intracranial stenosis (IIb, B). Otherwise, preventive treatment follows the above-enumerated secondary prevention recommendations for atheroma-related stroke. There is no advantage of using oral anticoagulants, because they are not superior to antiplatelet drugs, as demonstrated in the WASID trial (47). In this trial, age below 40 was an exclusion criterion. Angioplasty/stenting of severely stenosed intracranial arteries is not recommended (III, B), because this intervention is not superior to best medical treatment, as shown in the SAMMPRIS trial (48), whose exclusion criteria listed age less than 30 years

Stroke due to small vessel disease

The secondary prevention of stroke after a lacunar stroke due to small cerebral vessel disease follows the general rules of secondary prevention with a few remarks concerning management of hypertension and dual antiplatelet therapy, based on evidence from the SPS3 trial (14). The recommended target value for treated hypertension is to keep DBP below 130 mmHg (IIa, B). Long- or short-term dual antiplatelet therapy is not recommended, because of lack of efficacy and safety concerns.

Stroke of other determined cause

Cervical artery dissection

The risk of early recurrence after cervical artery dissection is low (<1%). The risk is higher in patients presenting as stroke/TIA than with local signs. Most of the recurrent strokes occur during the first 2 months after the initial event. Long-term risk of recurrent dissection (0.3–1.4%), stroke (0.3–3.4%/year), and vascular death are low (49, 50). Antithrombotic treatment (antiplatelet or anticoagulant) is reasonably safe after carotid or vertebral artery dissection. In a serial cervical magnetic resonance imaging study, asymptomatic limited growth of the mural haematoma was detected in one-third of treated patients, with no differences between antiplatelet and anticoagulant treatments (51).

Two meta-analysis of observational studies comparing antiplatelet versus anticoagulation after cervical dissection on several outcomes (recurrent stroke, death, intracranial bleeding) reported very low risk of these outcomes and no significant differences between the two preventive regimens.

One recent RCT (CADISS) compared antiplatelet versus anticoagulation after carotid dissection (52). The study included patients up to 7 days after symptoms onset. The trial failed to reach the planned sample size. The results from the non-randomized arm (88 patients unsuitable for randomization, 59 treated with antiplatelets and 28 with anticoagulation) showed very low number of recurrent events: one stroke (1.7%) and three TIAs (5.1%) in patients on antiplatelets and one stroke (3.6%) in those on anticoagulants (53). The randomized study succeeded to include only 250 patients, with a mean onset-to-inclusion of 3.7 days (52). No patients died, only four strokes (2%; three on antiplatelet and one on anticoagulants) and one serious bleeding (on anticoagulants) occurred, with no significant difference between the two preventive regimens. This trial has several limitations and should be considered a phase II feasibility trial, underpowered to detect small differences. In 52 patients, the diagnosis of dissection was not confirmed by central adjudication, but again no difference between antiplatelet and oral anticoagulant was found, if these patients were excluded. Other limitations were the onset-to-inclusion up to 7 days, missing early recurrences, the open-label, non-blind treatment allocation, and variable antiplatelet regimen, which surprisingly included dual antiplatelet therapy in 28% of the patients.

A few single-centre series reported the use of direct anticoagulants after cervical dissection (54, 55). NOACs appear to be safe for this indication, but numbers were too small and comparisons were neither randomized nor blindly assessed, and robust conclusions regarding the use of NOACs after cervical artery dissection are therefore not possible.

In conclusion, after cervical artery dissection there is a very low rate of recurrent events. The available evidence for recommendations is of low quality. Antiplatelets and anticoagulants are safe and have probably a similar efficacy. Antiplatelet drugs or oral anticoagulants (VKAs) can be used for 3–6 months (IIa, B). In the unusual instance of recurrence of ischaemic events despite antiplatelet drugs or oral anticoagulants, stenting (IIb, C) or surgery (IIb, C) are alternatives.

Antiphospholipid syndrome

Stroke in the young adult and antiphospholipid syndrome (APS) can be associated in three scenarios: (a) a patient with known APS suffers a stroke, (b) stroke is the first manifestation of APS confirmed by repeated laboratory tests 12 weeks apart, or (c) laboratory tests for APS are positive once but not confirmed in repeated testing. A systematic review and meta-analysis on anticoagulation in patients with antiphospholipid antibodies, showed that patients with stroke and a single positive testing had no increased risk of recurrence, and that risk was successively higher in those fulfilling the criteria for APS and past venous thrombosis, an arterial thrombosis, and recurrent thrombotic events (56, 57). A few clinical trials compared anticoagulation aiming at different INR levels and anticoagulation with heparin to prevent thrombotic events in patients with APS (57–60). In two studies (58, 60) which included patients with APS and with previous thrombosis, high-intensity (INR 3–4) was not superior to moderate-intensity (INR 2–3) oral anticoagulation. In the APPS study, which included stroke patients with positive lupus anticoagulant or cardiolipin antibodies (on at least one occasion), no difference was found between oral anticoagulation and antiplatelet therapy. Currently, AHA/American Stroke Association guidelines state that (a) for patients with ischaemic stroke or TIA who meet the criteria for the APS, anticoagulant therapy might be considered (I, B); (b) for patients with ischaemic stroke or TIA who have an antiphospholipid antibody but who do not fulfil the criteria for antiphospholipid antibody syndrome, antiplatelet therapy is recommended (I, B); and (c) for patients with ischaemic stroke or TIA who meet the criteria for the antiphospholipid antibody syndrome but in whom anticoagulation is not begun, antiplatelet therapy is indicated (I, A).

Sickle cell disease

Sickle cell disease is an important cause of stroke in children and young adults of African descent. The main treatment to prevent ischaemic crisis is repeated blood transfusions, with the target of decreasing the levels of Hg S to less than 30%. Based on the results of the STOP trial (61), which showed a risk reduction from 10% to less than 1%, repeated blood transfusions are recommended both in the primary prevention (I, A) and secondary prevention (I, B) of thrombotic events. The STOP II trial (62) showed an increased risk of stroke if repeated transfusions were stopped after 30 months. This treatment policy should continue for at least 5 years or until the patient is 8 years old. The SIT trial (63) demonstrated a reduction from 14% to 6% of new silent infarcts with repeated blood transfusions.

Other preventive measures include detection and treatment of hypertension and other risk vascular risk factors (IIa), prevention of iron overload and antiplatelets (IIa, B). The DOVE trial (64) failed to demonstrate the efficacy of prasugrel in sickle cell disease. Hydroxyurea and phlebotomy were evaluated in patients on transfusion/chelation therapy at risk of iron overload in the SWiTCH trial (65), which was closed for futility. More strokes occurred in the hydroxyurea/phlebotomy arm (10% vs 0%). Hydroxyurea and phlebotomy should only be used if transfusion is not available/practical. Bone marrow transplantation (IIb, C) is a promising intervention, which in the future may become the first option for secondary prevention of stroke and other ischaemic events in patients with sickle cell disease.

Moyamoya syndrome and disease

The goals of preventive treatments in moyamoya syndrome are to prevent stroke and cognitive decline, the latter being secondary both to stroke and chronic cerebral hypoperfusion (66). Patients are at risk of both ischaemic (early in the course of the disease) and haemorrhagic stroke (later in life). The preventive treatments used in moyamoya by consensus are surgical revascularization procedures (IIb, C). Revascularization can be direct (superficial temporal artery—middle cerebral artery anastomosis) but is more commonly indirect (encephaloduroarteriosynangiosis and encephalomyoarteriosynangiosis). There are no RCTs evaluating these procedures, but they are routinely used worldwide with an acceptable safety profile. The 30-day risk of stroke is 4% and the probability of no stroke within 5 years is very high (96%). Current indications for revascularization surgery are recurrent or progressive ischaemic symptoms, cognitive deterioration, or evidence of inadequate cerebral blood flow or cerebral perfusion reserve. Antiplatelet drugs (IIb, C) are used after surgery or if surgery is not anticipated.

Fabry disease

The aetiological treatment of Fabry disease is enzyme replacement therapy with agalsidase 1 mg/kg or 0.2 mg/kg every other week. Trials showed a reduction in death and an improvement on several surrogate (plasma levels of GL-3a, accumulation in skin, kidney, and heart) and renal, cardiac, and peripheral nervous system clinical outcomes and quality of life. However, agalsidase does not change the risk of stroke/TIA or prevent the occurrence of white matter lesions and is of doubtful benefit in advanced disease (67–72).

CADASIL

In patients with cerebral autosomal dominant arteriopathy with subcortical infarcts and leucoencephalopathy (CADASIL), it is not known if blood pressure control and aspirin prevent further strokes or the progression of white matter lesions. The safety (risk of intracerebral bleeding) of antiplatelet drugs in these patients is also questionable (73).

MELAS

MELAS is a mitochondrial disease featuring myopathy, encephalopathy, lactic acidosis, and stroke-like episodes. Several drugs have been tried to prevent recurrent stroke-like episodes and new infarcts, including coenzyme Q10, L-carnitine, L-arginine, idebenone, vitamins (C, E, and B) and dichloroacetate, all with inconclusive results (74). Allogenic stem cell transplant and mitochondrial replacement (75, 76) are promising new therapeutic techniques.

Stroke of undetermined cause

In more than one-third of the cases, the cause of stroke in the young adult remains elusive despite extensive investigation. The cause of the stroke may be missed by incomplete or by delayed investigation (e.g. in cervical artery dissection) or because stroke is the first manifestation of atrial fibrillation or of a systemic disease (e.g. cancer, essential thrombocythaemia). An antiplatelet drug is currently recommended for secondary prevention after a stroke of undetermined cause. Statins are also recommended. Putaala et al. (12) followed 215 ischaemic strokes of unknown aetiology in patients with a mean age of 39 years. Some of them were prescribed statins. Patients on a statin at any time during follow-up were less likely to experience outcome events (HR 0.23). Of 143 patients never on a statin, 29 (20%) suffered recurrent events (stroke, myocardial infarction, other arterial thrombosis, revascularization, or vascular death). None of the 36 patients on continuous statin treatment experienced a recurrent event, while among 36 with discontinuous statin use, 11% had recurrent events.

A subgroup of strokes of undetermined cause with complete investigation has clinical and imaging features suggesting embolism. They are now labelled embolic strokes of unknown source (77). Two RCTs are currently evaluating if NOACs are superior to antiplatelet treatment to prevent recurrent strokes in patients with embolic stroke of undetermined source. The RESPECT-ESUS trial compares dabigatran versus aspirin and includes young adult stroke patients (78). The NAVIGATE-ESUS study evaluates rivaroxaban versus aspirin, but only includes patients older than 50 years (79).

Conclusion

Young adults who suffer an ischaemic stroke and survive have a shorter-life span than age-matched controls (80). Nevertheless, because of their young age they will have a longer exposure to risk factors and survival time than older stroke patients. Added to the exposure to risk factors and aetiologies at inception, we have to consider the additional effect of incident risk factors, which may be detected during follow-up. There is then an opportunity for lifelong prevention of vascular events. On the other hand, young adults will also have a longer exposure to the potential side effects of drugs used in secondary prevention. Very few therapeutic trials have been performed in young adult stroke patients and there has been a low inclusion rate of young adults in secondary prevention RCTs, because young age (<40 or <50 years) was an exclusion criteria. Most of the recommendations we presented in this chapter are therefore extrapolated from older age groups.

References

1. Viana-Baptista M, Melo T, Carvalho M, Cruz V, Fernandes C, Silva F, et al. Long-term prognosis of stroke in young adults: the PORTYSTROKE study. Cerebrovasc Dis. 2013;35:325.

2. Singhal AB, Biller J, Elkind MS, Fullerton HJ, Jauch EC, Kittner SJ, et al. Recognition and management of stroke in young adults and adolescents. Neurology. 2013;81(12):1089–97.

3. von Sarnowski B, Putaala J, Grittner U, Gaertner B, Schminke U, Curtze S, et al. Lifestyle risk factors for ischemic stroke and transient ischemic attack in young adults in the Stroke in Young Fabry Patients study. Stroke. 2013;44(1):119–25.

4. Ferro JM, Massaro AR, Mas JL. Aetiological diagnosis of ischaemic stroke in young adults. Lancet Neurol. 2010;9(11):1085–96.

5. Putaala J, Metso AJ, Metso TM, Konkola N, Kraemer Y, Haapaniemi E, et al. Analysis of 1008 consecutive patients aged 15 to 49 with first-ever ischemic stroke: the Helsinki young stroke registry. Stroke. 2009;**40**(4):1195–203.

6. Furlan AJ, Reisman M, Massaro J, Mauri L, Adams H, Albers GW, et al. Closure or medical therapy for cryptogenic stroke with patent foramen ovale. N Engl J Med. 2012;**366**(11):991–99.

7. Meier B, Kalesan B, Mattle HP, Khattab AA, Hildick-Smith D, Dudek D, et al. Percutaneous closure of patent foramen ovale in cryptogenic embolism. N Engl J Med. 2013;**368**(12):1083–91.

8. Carroll JD, Saver JL, Thaler DE, Smalling RW, Berry S, MacDonald LA, et al. Closure of patent foramen ovale versus medical therapy after cryptogenic stroke. N Engl J Med. 2013;**368**(12):1092–100.

9. European Stroke Organisation (ESO) Executive Committee; ESO Writing Committee. Guidelines for management of ischaemic stroke and transient ischaemic attack 2008. Cerebrovasc Dis. 2008;**25**(5):457–507.

10. Kernan WN, Ovbiagele B, Black HR, Bravata DM, Chimowitz MI, Ezekowitz MD, et al. Guidelines for the prevention of stroke in patients with stroke and transient ischemic attack: a guideline for healthcare professionals from the American Heart Association/American Stroke Association. Stroke. 2014;**45**(7):2160–236.

11. Mustanoja S, Putaala J, Gordin D, Tulkki L, Aarnio K, Pirinen J, et al. Acute-phase blood pressure levels correlate with a high risk of recurrent strokes in young-onset ischemic stroke. Stroke. 2016;**47**(6):1593–98.

12. Arima H, Anderson C, Omae T, Woodward M, Hata J, Murakami Y, et al. Effects of blood pressure lowering on major vascular events among patients with isolated diastolic hypertension: the perindopril protection against recurrent stroke study (PROGRESS) trial. Stroke. 2011;**42**(8):2339–41.

13. Schrader J, Luders S, Kulschewski A, Hammersen F, Plate K, Berger J, et al. Morbidity and mortality after stroke, eprosartan compared with nitrendipine for secondary prevention: principal results of a prospective randomized controlled study (MOSES). Stroke. 2005;**36**(6):1218–26.

14. Benavente OR, Coffey CS, Conwit R, Hart RG, McClure LA, Pearce LA, et al. Blood-pressure targets in patients with recent lacunar stroke: the SPS3 randomised trial. Lancet. 2013;**382**(9891):507–15.

15. Putaala J, Liebkind R, Gordin D, Thorn LM, Haapaniemi E, Forsblom C, et al. Diabetes mellitus and ischemic stroke in the young: clinical features and long-term prognosis. Neurology. 2011;**76**(21):1831–37.

16. Rutten-Jacobs LC, Keurlings PA, Arntz RM, Maaijwee NA, Schoonderwaldt HC, Dorresteijn LD, et al. High incidence of diabetes after stroke in young adults and risk of recurrent vascular events: the FUTURE study. PLoS One. 2014;**9**(1):e87171.

17. Wilcox R, Bousser MG, Betteridge DJ, Schernthaner G, Pirags V, Kupfer S, et al. Effects of pioglitazone in patients with type 2 diabetes with or without previous stroke: results from PROactive (PROspective pioglitAzone Clinical Trial In macroVascular Events 04). Stroke. 2007;**38**(3):865–73.

18. Kernan WN, Viscoli CM, Furie KL, Young LH, Inzucchi SE, Gorman M, et al. Pioglitazone after ischemic stroke or transient ischemic attack. N Engl J Med. 2016;**374**(14):1321–31.

19. **Amarenco P, Bogousslavsky J, Callahan A, 3rd, Goldstein LB, Hennerici M, Rudolph AE,** et al. High-dose atorvastatin after stroke or transient ischemic attack. N Engl J Med. 2006;**355**(6):549–59.

20. MRC/BHF Heart Protection Study of cholesterol lowering with simvastatin in 20,536 high-risk individuals: a randomised placebo-controlled trial. Lancet. 2002;**360**(9326):7–22.

21. **Putaala J, Haapaniemi E, Kaste M, Tatlisumak T.** Statins after ischemic stroke of undetermined etiology in young adults. Neurology. 2011;**77**(5):426–30.

22. **Doehner W, Schenkel J, Anker SD, Springer J, Audebert HJ.** Overweight and obesity are associated with improved survival, functional outcome, and stroke recurrence after acute stroke or transient ischaemic attack: observations from the TEMPiS trial. Eur Heart J. 2013;**34**:268–77.

23. **Ovbiagele B, Bath PM, Cotton D, Vinisko R, Diener HC.** Obesity and recurrent vascular risk after a recent ischemic stroke. Stroke. 2011;**42**(12):3397–402.

24. **Chang CC, Chuang HC, Lin CL, Sung FC, Chang YJ, Hsu CY,** et al. High incidence of stroke in young women with sleep apnea syndrome. Sleep Med. 2014;**15**(4):410–14.

25. **Buterbaugh J, Wynstra C, Provencio N, Combs D, Gilbert M, Parthasarathy S.** Cerebrovascular reactivity in young subjects with sleep apnea. Sleep. 2015;**38**(2):241–50.

26. **Minnerup J, Ritter MA, Wersching H, Kemmling A, Okegwo A, Schmidt A,** et al. Continuous positive airway pressure ventilation for acute ischemic stroke: a randomized feasibility study. Stroke. 2012;**43**(4):1137–39.

27. **McEvoy RD, Antic NA, Heeley E, Luo Y, Ou Q, Zhang X,** et al. CPAP for Prevention of cardiovascular events in obstructive sleep apnea. N Engl J Med. 2016;**375**(10):919–31.

28. **Ives SP, Heuschmann PU, Wolfe CD, Redfern J.** Patterns of smoking cessation in the first 3 years after stroke: the South London Stroke Register. Eur J Cardiovasc Prev Rehabil. 2008;**15**(3):329–35.

29. **Leys D, Bandu L, Henon H, Lucas C, Mounier-Vehier F, Rondepierre P,** et al. Clinical outcome in 287 consecutive young adults (15 to 45 years) with ischemic stroke. Neurology. 2002;**59**(1):26–33.

30. **Wang D, Liu M, Lin S, Hao Z, Tao W, Chen X,** et al. Stroke and rheumatic heart disease: a systematic review of observational studies. Clin Neurol Neurosurg. 2013;**115**(9):1575–82.

31. **Secondary prevention in non-rheumatic atrial fibrillation after transient ischaemic attack or minor stroke.** EAFT (European Atrial Fibrillation Trial) Study Group. Lancet. 1993;**342**(8882):1255–62.

32. **Connolly SJ, Ezekowitz MD, Yusuf S, Eikelboom J, Oldgren J, Parekh A,** et al. Dabigatran versus warfarin in patients with atrial fibrillation. N Engl J Med. 2009;**361**(12):1139–51.

33. **Patel MR, Mahaffey KW, Garg J, Pan G, Singer DE, Hacke W,** et al. Rivaroxaban versus warfarin in nonvalvular atrial fibrillation. N Engl J Med. 2011;**365**(10):883–91.

34. **Granger CB, Alexander JH, McMurray JJ, Lopes RD, Hylek EM, Hanna M,** et al. Apixaban versus warfarin in patients with atrial fibrillation. N Engl J Med. 2011;**365**(11):981–92.

35. **Giugliano RP, Ruff CT, Braunwald E, Murphy SA, Wiviott SD, Halperin JL,** et al. Edoxaban versus warfarin in patients with atrial fibrillation. N Engl J Med. 2013;**369**(22):2093–104.

36. **Pollack CV, Jr., Reilly PA, Eikelboom J, Glund S, Verhamme P, Bernstein RA**, et al. Idarucizumab for dabigatran reversal. N Engl J Med. 2015;**373**(6):511–20.

37. **Connolly SJ, Milling TJ, Jr., Eikelboom JW, Gibson CM, Curnutte JT, Gold A**, et al. Andexanet alfa for acute major bleeding associated with factor Xa inhibitors. N Engl J Med. 2016;**375**(12):1131–41.

38. **Eikelboom JW, Connolly SJ, Brueckmann M, Granger CB, Kappetein AP, Mack MJ**, et al. Dabigatran versus warfarin in patients with mechanical heart valves. N Engl J Med. 2013;**369**(13):1206–14.

39. **Vistarini N, Alloni A, Aiello M, Vigano M.** Minimally invasive video-assisted approach for left atrial myxoma resection. Interact Cardiovasc Thorac Surg. 2010;**10**(1):9–11.

40. **Li J, Liu J, Liu M, Zhang S, Hao Z, Zhang J**, et al. Closure versus medical therapy for preventing recurrent stroke in patients with patent foramen ovale and a history of cryptogenic stroke or transient ischemic attack. Cochrane Database Syst Rev. 2015(9):CD009938.

41. **Kent DM, Dahabreh IJ, Ruthazer R, Furlan AJ, Reisman M, Carroll JD**, et al. Device closure of patent foramen ovale after stroke: pooled analysis of completed randomized trials. J Am Coll Cardiol. 2016;**67**(8):907–17.

42. **Thaler DE, Ruthazer R, Weimar C, Mas JL, Serena J, Di Angelantonio E**, et al. Recurrent stroke predictors differ in medically treated patients with pathogenic vs. other PFOs. Neurology. 2014;**83**(3):221–6.

43. Beneficial effect of carotid endarterectomy in symptomatic patients with high-grade carotid stenosis. N Engl J Med. 1991;**325**(7):445–53.

44. **Rothwell PM, Eliasziw M, Gutnikov SA, Fox AJ, Taylor DW, Mayberg MR**, et al. Analysis of pooled data from the randomised controlled trials of endarterectomy for symptomatic carotid stenosis. Lancet. 2003;**361**(9352):107–16.

45. **Rothwell PM, Eliasziw M, Gutnikov SA, Warlow CP, Barnett HJ.** Endarterectomy for symptomatic carotid stenosis in relation to clinical subgroups and timing of surgery. Lancet. 2004;**363**(9413):915–24.

46. **Howard G, Roubin GS, Jansen O, Hendrikse J, Halliday A, Fraedrich G**, et al. Association between age and risk of stroke or death from carotid endarterectomy and carotid stenting: a meta-analysis of pooled patient data from four randomised trials. Lancet. 2016;**387**(10025):1305–11.

47. **Chimowitz MI, Lynn MJ, Howlett-Smith H, Stern BJ, Hertzberg VS, Frankel MR**, et al. Comparison of warfarin and aspirin for symptomatic intracranial arterial stenosis. N Engl J Med. 2005;**352**(13):1305–16.

48. **Derdeyn CP, Chimowitz MI, Lynn MJ, Fiorella D, Turan TN, Janis LS**, et al. Aggressive medical treatment with or without stenting in high-risk patients with intracranial artery stenosis (SAMMPRIS): the final results of a randomised trial. Lancet. 2014;**383**(9914):333–41.

49. **Debette S, Leys D.** Cervical-artery dissections: predisposing factors, diagnosis, and outcome. Lancet Neurol. 2009;**8**(7):668–78.

50. **Dittrich R, Nassenstein I, Bachmann R, Maintz D, Nabavi DG, Heindel W**, et al. Polyarterial clustered recurrence of cervical artery dissection seems to be the rule. Neurology. 2007;**69**(2):180–86.

51. **Machet A, Fonseca AC, Oppenheim C, Touze E, Meder JF, Mas JL**, et al. Does anticoagulation promote mural hematoma growth or delayed occlusion in spontaneous cervical artery dissections? Cerebrovasc Dis. 2013;**35**(2):175–81.

52. **Markus HS, Hayter E, Levi C, Feldman A, Venables G, Norris J.** Antiplatelet treatment compared with anticoagulation treatment for cervical artery dissection (CADISS): a randomised trial. Lancet Neurol. 2015;**14**(4):361–67.

53. **Kennedy F, Lanfranconi S, Hicks C, Reid J, Gompertz P, Price C,** et al. Antiplatelets vs anticoagulation for dissection: CADISS nonrandomized arm and meta-analysis. Neurology. 2012;**79**(7):686–89.

54. **Caprio FZ, Bernstein RA, Alberts MJ, Curran Y, Bergman D, Korutz AW,** et al. Efficacy and safety of novel oral anticoagulants in patients with cervical artery dissections. Cerebrovasc Dis. 2014;**38**(4):247–53.

55. **Mustanoja S, Metso TM, Putaala J, Heikkinen N, Haapaniemi E, Salonen O,** et al. Helsinki experience on nonvitamin K oral anticoagulants for treating cervical artery dissection. Brain Behav. 2015;**5**(8):e00349.

56. **Ruiz-Irastorza G, Hunt BJ, Khamashta MA.** A systematic review of secondary thromboprophylaxis in patients with antiphospholipid antibodies. Arthritis Rheum. 2007;**57**(8):1487–95.

57. **Arachchillage DR, Machin SJ, Cohen H.** Antithrombotic treatment for stroke associated with antiphospholipid antibodies. Expert Rev Hematol. 2014;**7**(2):169–72.

58. **Crowther MA, Ginsberg JS, Julian J, Denburg J, Hirsh J, Douketis J,** et al. A comparison of two intensities of warfarin for the prevention of recurrent thrombosis in patients with the antiphospholipid antibody syndrome. N Engl J Med. 2003;**349**(12):1133–38.

59. **Levine SR, Brey RL, Tilley BC, Thompson JL, Sacco RL, Sciacca RR,** et al. Antiphospholipid antibodies and subsequent thrombo-occlusive events in patients with ischemic stroke. JAMA. 2004;**291**(5):576–84.

60. **Finazzi G, Marchioli R, Brancaccio V, Schinco P, Wisloff F, Musial J,** et al. A randomized clinical trial of high-intensity warfarin vs. conventional antithrombotic therapy for the prevention of recurrent thrombosis in patients with the antiphospholipid syndrome (WAPS). J Thromb Haemost. 2005;**3**(5):848–53.

61. **Lee MT, Piomelli S, Granger S, Miller ST, Harkness S, Brambilla DJ,** et al. Stroke Prevention Trial in Sickle Cell Anemia (STOP): extended follow-up and final results. Blood. 2006;**108**(3):847–52.

62. **Adams RJ, Brambilla D.** Discontinuing prophylactic transfusions used to prevent stroke in sickle cell disease. N Engl J Med. 2005;**353**(26):2769–78.

63. **DeBaun MR, Gordon M, McKinstry RC, Noetzel MJ, White DA, Sarnaik SA,** et al. Controlled trial of transfusions for silent cerebral infarcts in sickle cell anemia. N Engl J Med. 2014;**371**(8):699–710.

64. **Heeney MM, Hoppe CC, Abboud MR, Inusa B, Kanter J, Ogutu B,** et al. A Multinational trial of prasugrel for sickle cell vaso-occlusive events. N Engl J Med. 2016;**374**(7):625–35.

65. **Ware RE, Schultz WH, Yovetich N, Mortier NA, Alvarez O, Hilliard L,** et al. Stroke With Transfusions Changing to Hydroxyurea (SWiTCH): a phase III randomized clinical trial for treatment of children with sickle cell anemia, stroke, and iron overload. Pediatr Blood Cancer. 2011;**57**(6):1011–17.

66. **Kim JS.** Moyamoya disease: epidemiology, clinical features, and diagnosis. J Stroke. 2016;**18**(1):2–11.

67. **Rolfs A, Fazekas F, Grittner U, Dichgans M, Martus P, Holzhausen M**, et al. Acute cerebrovascular disease in the young: the Stroke in Young Fabry Patients study. Stroke. 2013;**44**(2):340–49.

68. **Rombach SM, Smid BE, Bouwman MG, Linthorst GE, Dijkgraaf MG, Hollak CE.** Long term enzyme replacement therapy for Fabry disease: effectiveness on kidney, heart and brain. Orphanet J Rare Dis. 2013;**8**:47.

69. **Wyatt K, Henley W, Anderson L, Anderson R, Nikolaou V, Stein K**, et al. The effectiveness and cost-effectiveness of enzyme and substrate replacement therapies: a longitudinal cohort study of people with lysosomal storage disorders. Health Technol Assess. 2012;**16**(39):1–543.

70. **Viana-Baptista M.** Stroke and Fabry disease. J Neurol. 2012;**259**(6):1019–28.

71. **Schaefer RM, Tylki-Szymanska A, Hilz MJ.** Enzyme replacement therapy for Fabry disease: a systematic review of available evidence. Drugs. 2009;**69**(16):2179–205.

72. **Eng CM, Guffon N, Wilcox WR, Germain DP, Lee P, Waldek S**, et al. Safety and efficacy of recombinant human alpha-galactosidase A—replacement therapy in Fabry's disease. N Engl J Med. 2001;**345**(1):9–16.

73. **Oh JH, Lee JS, Kang SY, Kang JH, Choi JC.** Aspirin-associated intracerebral hemorrhage in a patient with CADASIL. Clin Neurol Neurosurg. 2008;**110**(4):384–86.

74. **Muqtadar H, Testai FD.** Single gene disorders associated with stroke: a review and update on treatment options. Curr Treat Options Cardiovasc Med. 2012;**14**(3):288–97.

75. **Halter JP, Michael W, Schupbach M, Mandel H, Casali C, Orchard K**, et al. Allogeneic haematopoietic stem cell transplantation for mitochondrial neurogastrointestinal encephalomyopathy. Brain. 2015;**138**(Pt 10):2847–58.

76. **Falk MJ, Decherney A, Kahn JP.** Mitochondrial replacement techniques—implications for the clinical community. N Engl J Med. 2016;**374**(12):1103–106.

77. **Hart RG, Diener HC, Coutts SB, Easton JD, Granger CB, O'Donnell MJ**, et al. Embolic strokes of undetermined source: the case for a new clinical construct. Lancet Neurol. 2014;**13**(4):429–38.

78. **ClinicalTrials.gov.** Dabigatran Etexilate for Secondary Stroke Prevention in Patients With Embolic Stroke of Undetermined Source (RE-SPECT ESUS). https://clinicaltrials.gov/ct2/show/NCT02239120 (accessed 14 October 2016).

79. **ClinicalTrials.gov.** Rivaroxaban Versus Aspirin in Secondary Prevention of Stroke and Prevention of Systemic Embolism in Patients With Recent Embolic Stroke of Undetermined Source (ESUS) (NAVIGATE ESUS). https://clinicaltrials.gov/ct2/show/NCT02313909 (accessed 14 October 2016).

80. **Waje-Andreassen U, Naess H, Thomassen L, Eide GE, Vedeler CA.** Long-term mortality among young ischemic stroke patients in western Norway. Acta Neurol Scand. 2007;**116**(3):150–56.

Chapter 16

Long-term prognosis

Halvor Naess

Introduction

Because of longer expected survival, prognosis is an important issue among young adults. Causes of cerebral infarction and risk factor profile often differ between young and older patients. It is important to identify young patients with cerebral infarction at risk of premature death, recurrent cerebral infarction, or other vascular events in order to adapt secondary preventive treatment. Knowledge of prognosis is important for patients in the prime of their life in order to make informed decisions about choice of education and profession.

Search strategy and selection criteria

References for this review were identified through searches of PubMed from 1966 until March 2016 with the terms 'cerebral infarction', 'ischemic stroke', 'ischaemic stroke', 'young adults', 'prognosis', 'follow-up', 'recurrence', 'mortality', and 'long-term'. Only studies including more than 100 patients were included. Studies with mean follow-up of less than 2 years were excluded. Articles were also identified through searches of the author's own files. Only papers published in English were reviewed.

Mortality

Mortality rate

Compared to matched controls, young patients with stroke have much higher long-term mortality than old patients with stroke (1).

  A number of mostly hospital-based, long-term follow-up studies including exclusively young patients with cerebral infarction have been published, showing varying mortality rates. Table 16.1 summarizes the main findings from these studies. The mortality rates range from 3.9% after a mean follow-up time

Table 16.1 Long-term mortality after cerebral infarction or TIA among young adults

Population, *N*, study type	Age (years)	Mean follow-up (years)	Mortality (%)	First year mortality rate (%)	Annual mortality rate[a] (%)	Reference
Population based						
Hordaland, *N*=232, R	15–49	5.7	9.9	–	–	8
Hordaland,[b] *N*=232, R	15–49	11	19.4	5.2	1.8	9
Hospital based						
Taiwan,[c] *N*=231, P	25–49	2.4	3.9	–	–	4
Lille, *N*=287, P	15–45	3	7.7	4.5	1.6	2
Iowa, *N*=296, P	14–45	6	21	–	–	3
Helsinki, *N*=731, P	15–49	5	10.7	4.7	1.5	5
Nijmegen, *N*=606, P	18–50	11.1	–	2.4	1.5[d]	6
Athens, *N*=253, P	15–45	4.4	7.1	1.2	1.7	7
Portugal, *N*=215, P[e]	≤45	2.8	2.8	–	–	13
Italy, *N*=155, P[e]	16–45	6	5.8	–	–	11
Italy, *N*=330, P[e]	15–44	8	7.9	3.9	0.6	12
Spain, *N*=272, R[e]	15–45	11.7	16	4.9	0.9	14
Italy, *N*=1,867, P[e]	18–45	3.5[f]	4.6	3.2	1.9	27

P, prospective study; R, retrospective study.

[a] From the second year after cerebral infarction.
[b] Second follow-up.
[c] Cerebral infarction of non-cardiac origin.
[d] Excluding the first 30 days.
[e] Both cerebral infarction and TIA.
[f] Median.

of 2.4 years to 21% after a mean follow-up time of 6 years (2–8). After about 10 years of mean follow-up time, about 17–19% have died (9, 10). Some studies have included patients with either transient ischaemic attack (TIA) or cerebral infarction. In these studies, mortality rates range from 2.8% after a mean follow-up of 2.8 years to 7.9% after a mean follow-up of 8 years (11–13).

While 19.4% of the patients had died after a mean follow-up of 11 years in a population-based study (9), in the age- and sex-matched control group only 2.0% had died, showing that the mortality rate was ten times higher among the patients (9) which accords with an Italian study that also found the mortality rate to be about ten times higher than among the general population of the same age (12).

The mortality is higher during the first year after cerebral infarction than in subsequent years. The first-year mortality frequency in most studies ranges from around 4% to 5% (median 3.9% for cerebral infarction) (2, 9, 12, 14). However, one study reported 1-year mortality to be only 1.2% (7). After TIA, the first-year mortality is lower: 0.7% according to one study (12).

The annual average mortality rates following the first year of first ever cerebral infarction is rather consistently reported to be about 1.5–1.9% (median 1.7%) (2, 9, 12, 14). Studies including patients with TIA show lower annual mortalities.

The annual average mortality rate among age- and sex-matched controls was 0.15% in a population-based study (9). Long-term annual average mortality is lower among patients with TIA than among patients with cerebral infarction: 0.4% according to one study (12). However, long-term mortality was similar among patients with cerebral infarction and TIA in a recent large study (6).

A recent study reported on change in long-term mortality among 17,149 patients hospitalized because of cerebral infarction surviving the first 28 days in Sweden during 1987–2006. Overall there was about a tenfold higher risk of death among patients aged 18–44 years, and among patients aged 45–54 there was a sixfold increased risk of death compared to the general population (15). From the first to the last 4-year period the mortality decreased by 32% in males and 45% in females.

Predictors for mortality

A number of predictors for mortality have been detected in different studies. After cerebral infarction, long-term mortality was significantly associated with large-vessel atherosclerosis according to a prospective hospital-based study (3). On univariate analyses, a prospective, multicentre, hospital-based study including patients with either TIA or cerebral infarction showed that long-term mortality was significantly associated with male gender (hazard ratio (HR) 2.6), age over 35 years (HR 3.7), cerebral infarction (HR 4.2), cardiac diseases (HR 4.5), and hypertension (HR 2.3). On multivariate analysis, long-term mortality was associated with cerebral infarction (HR 3.3) and cardiac diseases (HR 3.7) (12). Long-term mortality after cerebral infarction was significantly associated with male gender (relative risk (RR) 1.9), age over 35 years (RR 2.0), and severe handicap at discharge (RR 5.1) in a retrospective, hospital-based study. No patient with cerebral infarction due to dissection of extracranial vessels died during follow-up (*P* <0.01) (14).

Neither aetiology, hypertension, diabetes mellitus, smoking, age, sex, nor sex were significantly associated with time to death after a mean follow-up of 6 years in a population-based study in Norway (8). A second follow-up was performed on average 11 years after stroke onset. Another 9.5% had died between the first and second follow-up. Multivariate analysis showed that mortality between the first and second follow-up was independently associated with malignant tumour, alcoholism, coronary atherosclerosis, living alone, and seizures. Between the first and second follow-up, 60% of alcoholics, 54% of patients with malignant tumours, 47% of patients with peripheral artery disease, 28% of patients with epilepsy, 27% of patients with coronary disease, 24% of heavy smokers, and 22% of patients living alone had died (all P ≤0.001) (9). No patients with dissection of neck vessels died. A third follow-up was performed on average 18 years after the index stroke. Mortality between the first and the third follow-up was significantly associated with fatigue, depression, low health-related quality of life, and elevated C-reactive protein present at the first follow-up on average 6 years after the index stroke (16–18).

A study from Athens in 2010 found 10-year mortality after cerebral infarction to be associated with heart failure and stroke severity on multivariate Cox regression analyses (7). Among 30-day survivors in Finland, death within 5 years of cerebral infarction was associated with increasing age, heart failure, diabetes mellitus type 1, heavy drinking, malignancy, and large artery atherosclerosis based on multivariate Cox regression analyses (5). A study from the Netherlands showed that death among 30-day survivors after cerebral infarction was associated with increasing age and cardioembolic stroke (6).

Two studies have reported an association between the number of traditional risk factors known at the time of the index stroke and subsequent long-term mortality. A study from Finland showed long-term mortality to be significantly associated with the number of well-documented risk factors known at the time of the index stroke (19). A population-based study in Norway showed that after a mean follow-up time of 18 years, 12.5% with no risk factor had died while the corresponding frequencies in patients with one to three or more risk factors known at the time of the index stroke were 18.5%, 25.4%, and 53.1%, respectively (20). Table 16.2 summarizes predictors for mortality.

Causes of death among patients discharged alive

Causes of death were cardiac disease (29%), malignancy (20%), infections (16%), recurrent cerebral infarction (15%), and others (20%) in a study from the

Table 16.2 Risk factors associated with mortality, recurrence of cerebral infarction, and other vascular events in young adults with first-ever cerebral infarction or TIA

	Mortality	Recurrence	Composite events
Male	+		+[a]
Age	+	+	+[a]
Cerebral infarction	+		
Cardiac disease	+		+[a]
Hypertension	+		+[a]
Severe handicap at discharge	+		
Alcoholism	+		
Coronary disease	+		
Post-infarction epilepsy	+		
Peripheral artery disease	+		
Heart failure	+		
Malignancy	+		
Cardiac embolism	+		
Discontinuation of antiplatelets		+	
Discontinuation of antihypertensive drugs		+	
Partial anterior circulation syndrome		+	
Haematological abnormalities		+	
Antiphospholipid antibodies		+	
Diabetes mellitus	+	+	+[b,c]
Anterior circulation infarction		+	
Atherosclerosis	+	+	+[c]
TIA prior to cerebral infarction		+	+[c]
Small vessel disease		+	
Carotid abnormalities			+[a]
Myocardial infarction prior to index stroke			+[b]
Angina pectoris			+[b]
Intermittent claudication			+[b]
Smoking			+[b,c]
Family history of coronary heart disease			+[c]
Family history of stroke		+	

[a] Mortality, recurrence of stroke, or myocardial infarction.

[b] Recurrent cerebral infarction or myocardial infarction.

[c] Recurrent cerebral infarction, symptomatic coronary heart disease, or symptomatic peripheral artery disease.

Netherlands with a mean follow-up time of 11.1 years among 30-day survivors with cerebral infarction (6). Causes of death were cardioaortic disease (31%), recurrent cerebral infarction (16%), malignancy (12%), infections (9%), and others (32%) in a study from Finland among 30-day survivors after the index stroke (5). A population-based study from Norway reported causes of death after a mean follow-up time of 6 years to be cardiac disease (20%), sudden death (20%), intoxication (13%), recurrent cerebral infarction (7%), and others (40%) (8). A study comprising all (17,149) patients with cerebral infarction surviving the first 28 days aged 18–55 years hospitalized in Sweden during 1987–2006 reported the following causes of long-term mortality: cardiovascular disease (46%), malignancies (19%), recurrent cerebral infarction (7%), haemorrhagic stroke (5%), and others (22%). Malignancies were more frequent among females (28% vs 15%) and cardiovascular disease was more frequent among males (50% vs 36%) (15).

Recurrence of cerebral infarction and other vascular events

Recurrence rate of cerebral infarction

Among patients with first-ever cerebral infarction irrespective of age, more than 30% suffered from recurrence of cerebral infarction during a prospective 5-year follow-up study in Perth, Australia (1). Among old patients with cerebral infarction, the recurrence rate is about 10% in the first year and subsequently 5% per year (21, 22). Among young patients with cerebral infarction the recurrence rate is lower.

Table 16.3 summarizes the main findings from studies reporting recurrence of cerebral infarction. The recurrence rates of cerebral infarction range from 3.5% during a 3-year mean follow-up to 12.1% during a 10-year mean follow-up period (2, 3, 7, 8, 23–25). Studies including both patients with cerebral infarction and TIA report recurrence rates of cerebral infarction ranging from 4.1% during a mean follow-up of 3.5 years to 3.2% during a mean follow-up of 8 years (11–13). In a prospective, multicentre, hospital-based study including 140 patients with TIA there were no recurrent cerebral infarction during the first year (12).

Studies with follow-up periods of longer than 10 years have shown recurrence rates of cerebral infarction ranging from 25% after a mean follow-up of 12 years in two studies. One was population based and included only patients with cerebral infarction whereas the other study included both patients with cerebral infarction and TIA (14, 26).

The recurrence rates of cerebral infarction during the first year after first-ever cerebral infarction or TIA in hospital-based studies range from 1.4% to 3.6%

Table 16.3 Recurrence of cerebral infarction or TIA among young adults with cerebral infarction

Population, N, study type	Age (years)	Mean follow-up (years)	Recurrence (%)	First year recurrence rate (%)	Annual recurrence rate[a] (%)	Reference
Population based						
Hordaland, N=232, R	15–49	6	9.9	2	1.5	8
Hordaland, N=144,[b] R	15–49	12	26			26
Hospital based						
Switzerland, N=203, P	16–45	2.2	7.4	–	3.0[c]	24
Italy, N=135, P	16–45	2.3	11.1	–	2.3[c]	
Taiwan,[d] N=231, P	25–49	2.4	12.1	–	–	4
Lille, N=287, P	15–45	3	3.5	1.4	1.0	2
Iowa, N=296, P	15–45	6	9	–	–	3
Helsinki, N=807	15–49	5	8.9	3	1.5	25
Athens, N=253, P	15–45	4.4	8.7	–	–	7
Portugal, N=184, P[e]	≤45	3.6	4.4	–	–	13
Italy, N=155, P[e]	16–45	5.8	3	–	–	11
Italy, N=330, P[e]	15–44	8	3.2	1.6	0.3	12
Spain, N=272, R[e]	15–45	12	25	3.6	1.7	14

P, prospective study; R, retrospective study.

[a] From the second year after cerebral infarction.

[b] Including only surviving patients on second follow-up.

[c] Including the first year after cerebral infarction.

[d] Cerebral infarction of non-cardiac origin.

[e] Both cerebral infarction and TIA.

(2, 12–14). In a population-based study, the recurrence rate during the first year after first-ever cerebral infarction was 2.0% (8). The median recurrence rate of recurrent cerebral infarction during the first year is 2% including both population- and hospital-based studies.

Hospital-based studies have reported the average annual incidence rate of recurrent ischaemic stroke including the first year to range from 1.2% to 3.0% (23, 24).

The average annual recurrence rate of cerebral infarction following the first year after cerebral infarction or TIA ranges from 0.3% to 1.7% in hospital-based studies (2, 12, 14) and 0.18% following the first year after TIA (12). The average annual rate of recurrent cerebral infarction was 1.5% for surviving patients following the first year after cerebral infarction in a population-based study including patients with first-ever cerebral infarction (8, 26). Among sex- and age-matched controls, the average annual frequency of first-ever stroke was 0.42% per year (26). The median recurrence rate of cerebral infarction after the first year is 1.5% including both population- and hospital-based studies.

A large multicentre study in Italy including 1867 30-day survivors after cerebral infarction aged 18–45 years reported cumulative risk of recurrent cerebral infarction or TIA to be 3.2% at 1 year, 10.9% at 5 years, and 14.0% at 10 years (27).

A study comprising all (17,149) patients with cerebral infarction surviving the first 28 days, aged 18–55 years, and hospitalized in Sweden during 1987–2006 reported a reduction of 55% in males and 59% in females in long-term recurrence of stroke (28).

Predictors for recurrent cerebral infarction or composite vascular outcome events

As for mortality, predictors for recurrent cerebral infarction vary much from one study to another. The recurrence of cerebral infarction was significantly associated with partial anterior circulation syndrome (PACS) and haematological abnormalities including antiphospholipid antibodies, protein S, and protein C deficiency in a prospective, hospital-based study (23). The frequency of recurrent cerebral infarction was significantly higher among patients with cardiovascular risk factors (RR 1.6), diabetes mellitus (RR 2.3), cerebral infarction in the carotid territory (RR 1.7), and atherosclerosis (RR 1.9) in a retrospective, hospital-based study (14). Dissection of neck vessels (RR 0.4) and cerebral infarction associated with classical migraine (RR 0.4) were significantly associated with lower recurrence rate of cerebral infarction (14). The recurrence of cerebral infarction was significantly associated with TIA prior to the index stroke in a prospective, hospital-based study (24). Another prospective, hospital-based study showed that a composite outcome event comprising stroke, myocardial infarction, and death was significantly associated with male gender, age over 35 years, cardiac diseases, carotid abnormalities, and hypertension (12).

Diabetes mellitus was the only variable significantly associated with recurrence of cerebral infarction after a mean follow-up of 6 years in a population-based study (8). After a mean time of 12 years after the index stroke, a second follow-up was performed (26). Multivariate analysis showed that arterial events (recurrent cerebral infarction, symptomatic coronary heart disease, or symptomatic peripheral artery disease) were independently associated with age (odds ratio (OR) 1.1), family history of coronary heart disease (OR 3.7), current smoking on follow-up (OR 7.5), ex-smoking (OR 4.8), and diabetes mellitus (OR 5.5). There were no significant differences as to smoking, hypertension, diabetes mellitus, body mass index, or family history of coronary heart disease between patients without arterial events during follow-up and age- and sex-matched controls (26).

A study from Finland found that recurrent cerebral infarction after a follow-up period of 5 years was significantly associated with increasing age, a history of TIA, diabetes mellitus type 1, and large artery atherosclerosis on multivariate Cox regression analyses (25).

A composite outcome event (cerebral infarction or myocardial infarction) was significantly associated with the following variables present before the index stroke: diabetes mellitus, myocardial infarction, angina pectoris, intermittent claudication, and smoking after a mean follow-up of 6 years in a population-based study in Norway (29). The composite outcome event was significantly associated with small vessel disease, but no other aetiology. The proportion of patients with composite outcome event and none to five traditional risk factors present before stroke onset (hypertension, smoking, hypercholesterolaemia, diabetes mellitus, myocardial infarction, angina pectoris, and peripheral artery disease) was 2.1%, 6%, 19%, 26%, 30%, and 67% (*P* <0.001) (29). The average annual frequency of the composite outcome event among patients with no traditional risk factor was only 0.35% per year which was similar to the annual incidence of first-ever stroke among age- and sex-matched controls.

A study from Finland showed that after a follow-up period of 5 years, recurrent cerebral infarction was significantly associated with the number of risk factors. Likewise, myocardial infarction subsequent to the index stroke was also significantly associated with the number of risk factors (19).

A large multicentre study from Italy identified the following predictors for recurrent cerebral infarction or TIA using Cox regression analyses: family history of stroke, discontinuation of antiplatelets, discontinuation of antihypertensive drugs, and antiphospholipid antibodies (27).

Table 16.2 summarizes predictors for recurrent cerebral infarction and composite end points.

Other vascular events

The rate of myocardial infarction is lower than the rate of recurrent cerebral infarction in all studies.

A prospective hospital-based study including 190 patients with cerebral infarction showed that none had myocardial infarction during the first year after the index stroke. After the first year of the index stroke, the average annual frequency of myocardial infarction was 0.7% per year (12). A retrospective, hospital-based study including 272 patients with cerebral infarction showed that 10% had non-cerebral cardiovascular events (angina pectoris, myocardial infarction, cardiac failure, and arrhythmia) during a mean follow-up time of 12 years (14). Non-cerebral cardiovascular events were significantly associated with male gender, age over 35 years, diabetes mellitus, and atherosclerosis. Migraine, dissection, and non-atherosclerotic vasculopathy were significantly associated with a low frequency of non-cerebral vascular events (14).

Other studies have also reported low frequencies of later myocardial infarction in patients with cerebral infarction or TIA. Three studies totalling 653 patients with cerebral infarction or TIA reported the annual rate of later myocardial infarction to be less than 0.5% (2, 4, 11). A hospital-based study from Finland including 807 patients reported that 10 (1.2%) patients had myocardial infarction during the 5-year observation period. The annual rate was about 0.5% (25).

A population-based study in Norway had a first follow-up at a mean time of 6 years after the index stroke (8). In total, 4.3% had suffered from myocardial infarction after the index stroke, and the annual rate was about 0.6%. At a second follow-up on average 12 years after the index stroke with new clinical examinations, 13.2% had coronary heart disease and 11.8% peripheral artery disease among 144 surviving patients (26).

Long-term functional outcome, cognitive function, and employment

A follow-up was performed on average 6 years after cerebral infarction in a population-based study in Norway. Among 194 survivors, 87% had good functional outcome (modified Rankin Scale score ≤2) (8). Poor functional outcome was significantly associated with large index stroke and diabetes mellitus, but not time to follow-up. A hospital-based study from France also reported 87% of patients to have good functional outcome after a mean follow-up period of 3 years (2). A recent study reported that 55% had good functional outcome after a mean follow-up period of 13.9 years. Poor functional outcome was associated with age, female sex, large index stroke, and cardiovascular disease (including peripheral artery disease) (30).

Prior to cerebral infarction, the employment (including studying) rate was 85% in a population-based study in Norway. On a follow-up on average 6 years later, the rate had fallen to 58% with 33% being granted disability pension. More patients were part-time on follow-up than prior to the index stroke (18% vs 11%) (8). Hospital-based studies have reported that 42–91% have resumed work on long-term follow-up (2, 3, 11, 13).

There is one study evaluating cognitive function on long-term follow-up on average 11 years after the index stroke compared to a matched reference group. The patients had worse cognitive performance compared to the reference group on six cognitive domains (processing speed, working memory, immediate memory, delayed memory, attention, and executive functioning). Cognitive impairment was associated with long follow-up duration (partly due to recurrent stroke). Worst cognitive impairment was found among patients with left supratentorial territory infarction (31).

The Mini Mental State Examination was performed among 193 surviving patients on average 6 years after the index stroke in a population-based study in Norway. A top score (30/30 points) was obtained by 31% whereas 73% had scores of 28 or higher. A low score (≤24) was disclosed among 8%. Among patients employed before the stroke, 24% with scores of 28 or higher and 45% with scores of 25–27 had lost employment (32). A second follow-up was performed on average 12 years after stroke onset. A questionnaire was sent to patients and matched controls. Self-assessed memory problems were reported by 41% of the patients compared to 5% of the controls (33).

Depression, fatigue, and health-related quality of life

Depression was evaluated in a population-based study in Norway on average 6 years after the index stroke. Montgomery-Åsberg Depression Rate Scale score was 7 or higher in 29% of the patients. Most had mild depression (88%) and none had severe depression. Multivariate analyses showed depression to be associated with depression prior to the index stroke and severe stroke (32). A second follow-up was performed on average 12 years after the index stroke. A questionnaire was sent to the patients and matched controls. Self-assessed depression was reported by 29% of the patients and by 13% of the controls. Anxiety (19% vs 9%) and sleeping problems (36% vs 19%) were also reported more frequently among patients compared to controls (33).

Many patients complain of fatigue after stroke. Long-term follow-up in a hospital-based study in Norway on average 6 years after the index stroke showed that fatigue (Fatigue Severity Scale score ≥4) was detected among 37% of the patients and among 23% of matched controls (34). Patients reporting depressive symptoms were excluded from this analysis. Multivariate analyses including all patients showed fatigue to be associated with depression, poor functional outcome, and basilar artery infarction through interaction with the functional outcome (34). Another study reported similar findings 9.8 years after the stroke. Fatigue was reported by 41% of young ischaemic stroke patients compared to 18% among matched controls. Fatigue was associated with poor functional outcome and impaired speed of information processing (35). Fatigue is probably an unspecific symptom related to a large number of factors as reported in a study including stroke patients irrespective of age where multivariate analyses showed post-stroke fatigue to be independently associated with prior depression, present depression, poor functional outcome, leucoaraiosis, prior myocardial infarction, diabetes mellitus, present pain, and present sleeping disturbances (36).

A population-based study in Norway compared health-related quality of life on average 6 years after the index stroke with a matched control group. Compared with the controls, a low level of health-related quality of life was most pronounced in regard to physical functioning among the patients. Low health-related quality of life was mostly found among patients who were depressed, unemployed, or suffered from fatigue (37). Similar findings were reported in a study from the Netherlands. Among young patients with mild ischaemic stroke, quality of life was affected by fatigue, depression, and anxiety (38).

Post-stroke epilepsy

A hospital-based study in Norway reported that on average 6 years after the index stroke 10.5% had developed post-stroke seizures (1.8% with early and 8.8% with late onset seizures). Most patients developed seizures within 2 years and none beyond 4 years of the stroke, and most (92%) were considered seizure free on follow-up (8). One-third of the patients with severe stroke developed post-stroke seizures. Reported cumulative risk of post-stroke epilepsy 10 years after the index stroke was 16% in a large hospital-based study in the Netherlands (39). Severe stroke was associated with post-stroke epilepsy. Cumulative risk of post-stroke epilepsy 10 years after the index stroke was 12% in a large hospital-based study from Finland. A large majority had the first seizure within 3 years of the index stroke. Multivariate analyses showed late-onset epilepsy to be associated with males, total or partial anterior circulation infarct (vs posterior circulation infarct), haemorrhagic infarction, and use of antidepressants at the time of the seizure (40).

Conclusion

Median first-year mortality after first-ever cerebral infarction among young adults is about 4% while median annual average mortality after the first year is about 1.7% (2, 5–7, 9, 12, 14, 27). High long-term mortality is associated with cardiac diseases, large vessel atherosclerosis, hypertension, smoking, and alcoholism (9). In contrast, long-term mortality seems to be low among patients with dissection of neck vessels.

The median frequency of recurrent cerebral infarction during the first year after first-ever cerebral infarction is about 2% (2, 26). The median annual frequency of recurrent cerebral infarction after the first year is about 1.5% (2, 5, 7, 9, 12, 14, 27). Recurrence of cerebral infarction is highly associated with modifiable risk factors such as hypertension, diabetes mellitus, symptomatic atherosclerosis, and smoking (8, 14). The risk of recurrent vascular events (including cerebral infarction and myocardial infarction) is strongly linked to the number of traditional risk factors (19, 29). Discontinuation of antiplatelets or discontinuation of antihypertensive drugs is associated with recurrent stroke (27).

There are several shortcomings in the studies included in this review. Most are hospital based and therefore suffering from possible bias in patient selection. Some studies are retrospective as to patient inclusion which may affect case finding and case ascertainment. Only one study was population based, but a limitation of that study was retrospective case finding. There are also differences as to the upper age limit which ranges from 30 to 49 years. Most studies include patients younger than 45 years. Furthermore, the study periods range from the 1970s up until the present and both investigation and treatment of stroke have changed substantially during these decades. It seems likely that the prognosis both as to mortality and recurrence of stroke or other vascular events has improved as indicated by studies from Sweden (15, 28). This should be taken into account when interpreting the study results.

References

1. **Hardie K, Jamrozik K, Hankey GJ, Broadhurst RJ, Anderson C.** Trends in five-year survival and risk of recurrent stroke after first-ever stroke in the Perth Community Stroke Study. Cerebrovasc Dis. 2005;**19**(3):179–85.

2. **Leys D, Bandu L, Hénon H, Lucas C, Mounier-Vehier F, Rondepierre P**, et al. Clinical outcome in 287 consecutive young adults (15 to 45 years) with ischemic stroke. Neurology. 2002;**59**(1):26–33.

3. **Kappelle LJ, Adams HP Jr, Heffner ML, Torner JC, Gomez F, Biller J.** Prognosis of young adults with ischemic stroke. A long-term follow-up study assessing recurrent vascular events and functional outcome in the Iowa Registry of Stroke in Young Adults. Stroke. 1994;**25**(7):1360–65.

4. **Yeh PS, Lin HJ, Li YH, Lin KC, Cheng TJ, Chang CY**, et al. Prognosis of young ischemic stroke in Taiwan: impact of prothrombotic genetic polymorphisms. Thromb Haemost. 2004;**92**(3):583–89.

5. Putaala J, Curtze S, Hiltunen S, Tolppanen H, Kaste M, Tatlisumak T. Causes of death and predictors of 5-year mortality in young adults after first-ever ischemic stroke: the Helsinki Young Stroke Registry. Stroke. 2009;**40**(8):2698–703.

6. Rutten-Jacobs LC, Arntz RM, Maaijwee NA, Schoonderwaldt HC, Dorresteijn LD, van Dijk EJ, et al. Long-term mortality after stroke among adults aged 18 to 50 years. JAMA. 2013;**309**(11):1136–44.

7. Spengos K, Vemmos K. Risk factors, etiology, and outcome of first-ever ischemic stroke in young adults aged 15 to 45—the Athens young stroke registry. Eur J Neurol. 2010;**17**(11):1358–64.

8. Naess H, Nyland HI, Thomassen L, Aarseth J, Myhr KM. Long-term outcome of cerebral infarction in young adults. Acta Neurol Scand. 2004;**110**(2):107–12.

9. Waje-Andreassen U, Naess H, Thomassen L, Eide GE, Vedeler CA. Long-term mortality among young ischemic stroke patients in western Norway. Acta Neurol Scand. 2007;**116**(3):150–56.

10. Aarnio K, Haapaniemi E, Melkas S, Kaste M, Tatlisumak T, Putaala J. Long-term mortality after first-ever and recurrent stroke in young adults. Stroke. 2014;**45**(9):2670–76.

11. Lanzino G, Andreoli A, Di Pasquale G, Urbinati S, Limoni P, Serracchioli A, et al. Etiopathogenesis and prognosis of cerebral ischemia in young adults. A survey of 155 treated patients. Acta Neurol Scand. 1991;**84**(4):321–25.

12. Marini C, Totaro R, Carolei A. Long-term prognosis of cerebral ischemia in young adults. National Research Council Study Group on Stroke in the Young. Stroke. 1999;**30**(11):2320–25.

13. Ferro JM, Crespo M. Prognosis after transient ischemic attack and ischemic stroke in young adults. Stroke. 1994;**25**(8):1611–16.

14. Varona JF, Bermejo F, Guerra JM, Molina JA. Long-term prognosis of ischemic stroke in young adults. Study of 272 cases. J Neurol. 2004;**251**(12):1507–14.

15. Giang KW, Björck L, Nielsen S, Novak M, Sandström TZ, Jern C, et al. Twenty-year trends in long-term mortality risk in 17,149 survivors of ischemic stroke less than 55 years of age. Stroke. 2013;**44**(12):3338–43.

16. Naess H, Nyland H. Poststroke fatigue and depression are related to mortality in young adults: a cohort study. BMJ Open. 2013;**3**(3).

17. Naess H, Nyland H, Idicula T, Waje-Andreassen U. C-reactive protein and homocysteine predict long-term mortality in young ischemic stroke patients. J Stroke Cerebrovasc Dis. 2013;**22**(8):e435–40.

18. Naess H, Nyland H. Poor health-related quality of life is associated with long-term mortality in young adults with cerebral infarction. J Stroke Cerebrovasc Dis. 2013;**22**(7):e79–83.

19. Putaala J, Haapaniemi E, Kaste M, Tatlisumak T. How does number of risk factors affect prognosis in young patients with ischemic stroke? Stroke. 2012;**43**(2):356–61.

20. Naess H, Waje-Andreassen U, Nyland H. Risk factor burden predicts long-term mortality in young patients with arterial cerebral infarction. Acta Neurol Scand. 2013;**127**(2):92–6.

21. Burn J, Dennis M, Bamford J, Sandercock P, Wade D, Warlow C. Long-term risk of recurrent stroke after a first-ever stroke. The Oxfordshire Community Stroke Project. Stroke. 1994;**25**(2):333–37.

22. **Eriksson SE, Olsson JE.** Survival and recurrent strokes in patients with different subtypes of stroke: a fourteen-year follow-up study. Cerebrovasc Dis. 2001;**12**(3):171–80.

23. **Camerlingo M, Casto L, Censori B, Ferraro B, Caverni L, Manara O,** et al., Recurrence after first cerebral infarction in young adults. Acta Neurol Scand. 2000;**102**(2):87–93.

24. **Nedeltchev K, der Maur TA, Georgiadis D, Arnold M, Caso V, Mattle HP,** et al. Ischaemic stroke in young adults: predictors of outcome and recurrence. J Neurol Neurosurg Psychiatry. 2005;**76**(2):191–95.

25. **Putaala J, Haapaniemi E, Metso AJ, Metso TM, Artto V, Kaste M,** et al. Recurrent ischemic events in young adults after first-ever ischemic stroke. Ann Neurol. 2010;**68**(5):661–71.

26. **Waje-Andreassen U, Naess H, Thomassen L, Eide GE, Vedeler CA.** Arterial events after ischemic stroke at a young age: a cross-sectional long-term follow-up of patients and controls in western Norway. Cerebrovasc Dis. 2007;**24**(2–3):277–82.

27. **Pezzini A, Grassi M, Lodigiani C, Patella R, Gandolfo C, Zini A,** et al. Predictors of long-term recurrent vascular events after ischemic stroke at young age: the Italian Project on Stroke in Young Adults. Circulation. 2014;**129**(16):1668–76.

28. **Giang KW, Björck L, Ståhl CH, Nielsen S, Sandström TZ, Jern C,** et al. Trends in risk of recurrence after the first ischemic stroke in adults younger than 55 years of age in Sweden. Int J Stroke. 2016;**11**(1):52–61.

29. **Naess H, Waje-Andreassen U, Thomassen L, Nyland H, Myhr KM.** Do all young ischemic stroke patients need long-term secondary preventive medication? Neurology. 2005;**65**(4):609–11.

30. **Synhaeve NE, Arntz RM, van Alebeek ME, van Pamelen J, Maaijwee NA, Rutten-Jacobs LC,** et al. Women have a poorer very long-term functional outcome after stroke among adults aged 18-50 years: the FUTURE study. J Neurol. 2016;**263**(6):1099–105.

31. **Schaapsmeerders P, Maaijwee NA, van Dijk EJ, Rutten-Jacobs LC, Arntz RM, Schoonderwaldt HC,** et al. Long-term cognitive impairment after first-ever ischemic stroke in young adults. Stroke. 2013;**44**(6):1621–28.

32. **Naess H, Nyland HI, Thomassen L, Aarseth J, Myhr KM.** Mild depression in young adults with cerebral infarction at long-term follow-up: a population-based study. Eur J Neurol. 2005;**12**(3):194–98.

33. **Waje-Andreassen U, Thomassen L, Jusufovic M, Power KN, Eide GE, Vedeler CA,** et al. Ischaemic stroke at a young age is a serious event--final results of a population-based long-term follow-up in Western Norway. Eur J Neurol. 2013;**20**(5):818–23.

34. **Naess H, Nyland HI, Thomassen L, Aarseth J, Myhr KM.** Fatigue at long-term follow-up in young adults with cerebral infarction. Cerebrovasc Dis. 2005;**20**(4):245–50.

35. **Maaijwee NA, Arntz RM, Rutten-Jacobs LC, Schaapsmeerders P, Schoonderwaldt HC, van Dijk EJ,** et al. Post-stroke fatigue and its association with poor functional outcome after stroke in young adults. J Neurol Neurosurg Psychiatry. 2015;**86**(10):1120–26.

36. **Naess H, Lunde L, Brogger J, Waje-Andreassen U.** Fatigue among stroke patients on long-term follow-up. The Bergen Stroke Study. J Neurol Sci. 2012;**312**(1–2):138–41.

37. **Naess H, Waje-Andreassen U, Thomassen L, Nyland H, Myhr KM.** Health-related quality of life among young adults with ischemic stroke on long-term follow-up. Stroke. 2006;**37**(5):1232–36.

38. **de Bruijn MA, Synhaeve NE, van Rijsbergen MW, de Leeuw FE, Mark RE, Jansen BP,** et al. Quality of life after young ischemic stroke of mild severity is mainly influenced by psychological factors. J Stroke Cerebrovasc Dis. 2015;**24**(10):2183–88.

39. **Arntz R, Rutten-Jacobs L, Maaijwee N, Schoonderwaldt H, Dorresteijn L, van Dijk E,** et al. Post-stroke epilepsy in young adults: a long-term follow-up study. PLoS One. 2013;**8**(2):e55498.

40. **Roivainen R, Haapaniemi E, Putaala J, Kaste M, Tatlisumak T.** Young adult ischaemic stroke related acute symptomatic and late seizures: risk factors. Eur J Neurol. 2013;**20**(9):1247–55.

Index